PN Nursing Care of Children
REVIEW MODULE EDITION 10.0

P9-DFM-893

Contributors

Norma Jean E. Henry, MSN/Ed, RN

Honey C. Holman, MSN, RN

Brenda S. Ball, MEd, BSN, RN

Debborah Williams, MSN, RN

Kellie Wilford, MSN, RN

Marsha S. Barlow, MSN RN

Mendy G. McMichael, DNP, MSN, RN

Consultants

Susan Adcock, MS, RN

Christi Blair, MSN, RN

Donna B. Sheaffer, BSN, RN

Judy Drumm, DNS, RN, CPN

LaKeisha Wheless, MSN, RN

Director of content review: Kristen Lawler

Director of development: Derek Prater

Project management: Nicole Burke

Coordination of content review: Norma Jean E. Henry, Honey C. Holman

Copy editing: Kelly Von Lunen, Bethany Phillips

Layout: Spring Lenox, Randi Hardy, Charves Hervey, Rachel Cohen

Illustrations: Randi Hardy

Online media: Morgan Smith, Ron Hanson, Nicole Lobdell, Brant Stacy

Cover design: Jason Buck

Interior book design: Spring Lenox

IMPORTANT NOTICE TO THE READER

User's Guide

Welcome to the Assessment Technologies Institute® PN Nursing Care of Children Review Module Edition 10.0. The mission of ATI's Content Mastery Series® Review Modules is to provide user-friendly compendiums of nursing knowledge that will:

- Help you locate important information quickly.
- Assist in your learning efforts.
- Provide exercises for applying your nursing knowledge.
- Facilitate your entry into the nursing profession as a newly licensed nurse.

This newest edition of the Review Modules has been redesigned to optimize your learning experience. We've fit more content into less space and have done so in a way that will make it even easier for you to find and understand the information you need.

ORGANIZATION

This Review Module is organized into units covering the foundations of nursing care of children, nursing care of children who have systems disorders, and nursing care of children who have other specific needs. Chapters within these units conform to one of four organizing principles for presenting the content.

- Nursing concepts
- Growth and development
- Procedures
- System disorders

Nursing concepts chapters begin with an overview describing the central concept and its relevance to nursing. Subordinate themes are covered in outline form to demonstrate relationships and present the information in a clear, succinct manner.

Growth and development chapters cover expected growth and development, including physical and psychosocial development, age-appropriate activities, and health promotion, including immunizations, health screenings, nutrition, and injury prevention.

Procedures chapters include an overview describing the procedure(s) covered in the chapter. These chapters provide nursing knowledge relevant to each procedure, including indications, nursing considerations, interpretation of findings, and complications.

System disorders chapters include an overview describing the disorder(s) and/or disease process. These chapters address assessments, including risk factors, expected findings, laboratory tests, and diagnostic procedures. Next, you will focus on patient-centered care, including nursing care, medications, therapeutic procedures, interprofessional care, and client education. Finally, you will find complications related to the disorder, along with nursing actions in response to those complications.

ACTIVE LEARNING SCENARIOS AND APPLICATION EXERCISES

Each chapter includes opportunities for you to test your knowledge and to practice applying that knowledge. Active Learning Scenario exercises pose a nursing scenario and then direct you to use an ATI Active Learning Template (included at the back of this book) to record the important knowledge a nurse should apply to the scenario. An example is then provided to which you can compare your completed Active Learning Template. The Application Exercises include NCLEX-style questions, such as multiple-choice and multiple-select items, providing you with opportunities to practice answering the kinds of questions you might expect to see on ATI assessments or the NCLEX. After the Application Exercises, an answer key is provided, along with rationales.

NCLEX® CONNECTIONS

To prepare for the NCLEX-PN, it is important to understand how the content in this Review Module is connected to the NCLEX-PN test plan. You can find information on the detailed test plan at the National Council of State Boards of Nursing's website, www.ncsbn.org. When reviewing content in this Review Module, regularly ask yourself, "How does this content fit into the test plan, and what types of questions related to this content should I expect?"

To help you in this process, we've included NCLEX Connections at the beginning of each unit and with each question in the Application Exercises Answer Keys. The NCLEX Connections at the beginning of each unit point out areas of the detailed test plan that relate to the content within that unit. The NCLEX Connections attached to the Application Exercises Answer Keys demonstrate how each exercise fits within the detailed content outline. These NCLEX Connections will help you understand how the detailed content outline is organized, starting with major client needs categories and subcategories and followed by related content areas and tasks. The major client needs categories are:

- Safe and Effective Care Environment
  - Management of Care
  - Safety and Infection Control
- Health Promotion and Maintenance
- Psychosocial Integrity
- Physiological Integrity
  - Basic Care and Comfort
  - Pharmacological and Parenteral Therapies
  - Reduction of Risk Potential
  - Physiological Adaptation

An NCLEX Connection might, for example, alert you that content within a unit is related to:

- Physiological Adaptation
  - Alterations in Body Systems
    - Identify clinical manifestations and incubation periods of infectious diseases.

QSEN COMPETENCIES

As you use the Review Modules, you will note the integration of the Quality and Safety Education for Nurses (QSEN) competencies throughout the chapters. These competencies are integral components of the curriculum of many nursing programs in the United States and prepare you to provide safe, high-quality care as a newly licensed nurse. Icons appear to draw your attention to the six QSEN competencies.

Safety: The minimization of risk factors that could cause injury or harm while promoting quality care and maintaining a secure environment for clients, self, and others.

Patient-Centered Care: The provision of caring and compassionate, culturally sensitive care that addresses clients' physiological, psychological, sociological, spiritual, and cultural needs, preferences, and values.

Evidence-Based Practice: The use of current knowledge from research and other credible sources, on which to base clinical judgment and client care.

Informatics: The use of information technology as a communication and information-gathering tool that supports clinical decision-making and scientifically based nursing practice.

Quality Improvement: Care related and organizational processes that involve the development and implementation of a plan to improve health care services and better meet clients' needs.

Teamwork and Collaboration: The delivery of client care in partnership with multidisciplinary members of the health care team to achieve continuity of care and positive client outcomes.

ICONS

Icons are used throughout the Review Module to draw your attention to particular areas. Keep an eye out for these icons.

ⓃN This icon is used for NCLEX Connections.

ⒼG This icon indicates gerontological considerations, or knowledge specific to the care of older adult clients.

Q𝗌 This icon is used for content related to safety and is a QSEN competency. When you see this icon, take note of safety concerns or steps that nurses can take to ensure client safety and a safe environment.

Q𝗉𝖼𝖼 This icon is a QSEN competency that indicates the importance of a holistic approach to providing care.

Q𝖾𝖻𝗉 This icon, a QSEN competency, points out the integration of research into clinical practice.

Q𝗂 This icon is a QSEN competency and highlights the use of information technology to support nursing practice.

Q𝗊𝗂 This icon is used to focus on the QSEN competency of integrating planning processes to meet clients' needs.

Q𝗍𝖼 This icon highlights the QSEN competency of care delivery using an interprofessional approach.

M◇ This icon appears at the top-right of pages and indicates availability of an online media supplement, such as a graphic, animation, or video. If you have an electronic copy of the Review Module, this icon will appear alongside clickable links to media supplements. If you have a hard copy version of the Review Module, visit www.atitesting.com for details on how to access these features.

FEEDBACK

ATI welcomes feedback regarding this Review Module. Please provide comments to comments@atitesting.com.

Table of Contents

NCLEX® Connections

When reviewing the following chapters, keep in mind the relevant topics and tasks of the NCLEX outline, in particular:

Safety and Infection Control

ACCIDENT/ERROR/INJURY PREVENTION: Assist in and/or reinforce education to the client about safety precautions.

HOME SAFETY: Reinforce client education on home safety precautions (home disposal of syringes, lighting, handrails, kitchen safety).

Health Promotion and Maintenance

AGING PROCESS
Provide care that meets the needs of the newborn less than 1 month old through the infant or toddler client through 2 years.

Provide care that meets the needs of the preschool, school-age, and adolescent client ages 3 through 17 years.

DATA COLLECTION TECHNIQUES
Collect data for health history (client medical history, family medical history).

Collect baseline physical data (skin integrity, height and weight).

Report the client's physical examination results to the health care provider.

DEVELOPMENTAL STAGES AND TRANSITIONS
Identify occurrence of expected body image changes.

Compare client development to norms.

Modify approaches to care in accordance with the client's development stage.

HEALTH PROMOTION/DISEASE PREVENTION
Identify clients in need of immunizations (required and voluntary).

Identify precautions and contraindications to immunizations.

Provide assistance for screening examinations (scoliosis, breast and testicular self-examinations, blood pressure check).

Monitor incorporation of healthy behaviors into lifestyle by the client (screening examinations, immunizations, limiting risk-taking behaviors).

Basic Care and Comfort

NUTRITION AND ORAL HYDRATION: Monitor and provide for nutritional needs of the client.

REST AND SLEEP: Provide measures to promote sleep/rest.

CHAPTER 1 *Family-Centered Nursing Care*

Families are groups that should remain constant in children's lives. Family is defined as what an individual considers it to be.

Families often include individuals with a biological, marital, or adoptive relationship. In the absence of these characteristics, families also consist of individuals who have a strong emotional bond and commitment to one another. Due to the expanding concepts of family, the term household is sometimes used.

Positive family relationships are characterized by parent-child interactions that show mutual warmth and respect.

COMPONENTS OF CARE

Family-centered nursing care includes the following. **Q**PCC
- Agreed-upon partnerships between families of children, nurses, and providers, in which the families and children benefit
- Respecting cultural diversity, and incorporating cultural views when contributing to the plan of care
- Understanding growth and developmental needs of children and their families
- Treating children and their families as clients
- Working with all types of families
- Collaborating with families regarding hospitalization, home, and community resources
- Allowing families to serve as experts regarding their children's health conditions, usual behaviors in different situations, and routine needs

PROMOTING FAMILY-CENTERED CARE

Assist with comprehensive family data collection to identify strengths and weaknesses.

Characteristics of healthy families
- Members communicate well and listen to each other.
- There is affirmation and support for all members.
- There is a clear set of family rules, beliefs, and values.
- Members teach respect for others.
- There is a sense of trust.
- Members play and share humor together.
- Members interact with one another.
- There is a shared sense of responsibility.
- There are traditions and rituals.
- There is adaptability and flexibility in roles.
- Members seek help for their problems.

NURSING ACTIONS
- Pay close attention when family members state that a child "isn't acting right" or have other concerns.
- Consider the children's opinions when providing care.

FAMILY THEORIES

FAMILY SYSTEMS

The family is viewed as a whole system, instead of the individual members.
- A change to one member affects the entire system.
- The system can both initiate and react to change.
- Too much and too little change can lead to dysfunction.
- Interaction between family members affects the family as a whole.

FAMILY STRESS

Stress is inevitable.
- Stressors can be expected or unexpected.
- Explains the reaction of a family to stressful events.
- Offers guidance for adapting to stress.

DEVELOPMENTAL

Views families as small groups that interact with the larger social system
- Emphasizes similarities and consistencies in how families develop and change
- Uses Duvall's family life cycle stages to describe the changes a family goes through over time
- How the family functions in one stage has a direct effect on how the family will function in the next stage.

FAMILY COMPOSITION

Traditional nuclear family: Married couple and their biologic children (only full siblings)

Nuclear family: Two parents and their children (biologic, adoptive, step, foster)

Single-parent family: One parent and one or more children

Blended family (also called reconstituted): At least one stepparent, stepsibling, or half-sibling

Extended family: At least one parent, one or more children, and other individuals (might not be related)

Foster family: One or more children who are placed in an approved living environment away from the family of origin, usually with one or two parents

Binuclear family: Parents who have terminated spousal roles but continue their parenting roles

Communal family: Individuals who share common ownership of property and goods, and exchange services without monetary consideration

Alternative families: Include extended family members caring for children in the absence of biological parents.

Changes that occur with the birth (or adoption) of the first child
- Parents' sense of self as they transition to the new parental role
- Division of labor and roles within the relationships of couples
- Relationships with grandparents
- Work relationships
- Increased financial responsibilities and possible loss of income
- Necessary sleep habit changes

PARENTING STYLES

TYPES OF PARENTING

Authoritarian

Parents try to control the child's behaviors and attitudes through unquestioned rules and expectations.

> The child is never allowed to watch television on school nights.

Permissive

Parents exert little or no control over the child's behaviors, and consult the child when making decisions.

> The child assists with deciding whether he will watch television.

Authoritative

Parents direct the child's behavior by setting rules and explaining the reason for each rule setting.

> The child can watch television for 1 hr on school nights after completing all of his homework and chores.

Parents negatively reinforce deviations from the rules.

> The privilege is taken away but later reinstated based on new guidelines.

GUIDELINES FOR PROMOTING ACCEPTABLE BEHAVIOR IN CHILDREN

- Set clear and realistic limits and expectations based on the developmental level of the child.
- Validate the child's feelings, and offer sympathetic explanations.
- Provide role modeling and reinforcement for appropriate behavior.
- Focus on the child's behavior when disciplining the child.

FAMILY DATA COLLECTION

History: Medical history for parents, siblings, and grandparents

Structure: Family members (mother, father, son)

Developmental tasks: Tasks a family works on as the child grows (parents with a school-age child helping her to develop peer relations)

Family characteristics: Cultural, religious, and economic influences on behavior, attitudes, and actions

Family stressors: Expected (birth of a child) and unexpected (illness, divorce, disability, death of a family member) events that cause stress

Environment: Availability of and family interactions with community resources

Family support system: Availability of extended family, work and peer relationships, social systems, and community resources to assist the family in meeting needs or adapting to a stressor Q℠

Application Exercises

1. A nurse on a pediatric acute care unit is assisting with an education program on working with families for a group of newly hired nurses. Which of the following should the nurse recommend to include when discussing the developmental theory?

   A. Describes that stress is inevitable

   B. Emphasizes that change with one member affects the entire family

   C. Provides guidance to assist families adapting to stress

   D. Defines consistencies in how families change

2. A nurse is assisting a group of parents of adolescents to develop skills that will improve communication within the family. The nurse identifies the use of an authoritative style of parenting when she hears a parent make which of the following statements?

   A. "My son knows he better do what I say."

   B. "My daughter is mature enough to determine her own curfew."

   C. "My son understands that a part of learning responsibility is helping with household chores."

   D. "I only allow my daughter to date boys that attend our church."

3. A nurse is collecting data about a family. Which of the following should the nurse include? (Select all that apply.)

   A. Medical history

   B. Parents' education level

   C. Child's physical growth

   D. Support systems

   E. Stressors

PRACTICE Active Learning Scenario

A nurse is reinforcing teaching with the mother of a toddler. The nurse learns that the household includes the mother, toddler, an older brother, and a grandmother. Use the ATI Active Learning Template: Basic Concept to complete this item.

RELATED CONTENT: Describe the composition of this family.

UNDERLYING PRINCIPLES
- Describe two methods the parent can use to positively influence the child.
- Describe two ways the parent can promote acceptable behavior in the child.

NURSING INTERVENTIONS: Include two additional family data collections the nurse should perform.

Application Exercises Key

1. A. The family stress theory describes that stress is inevitable.

   B. The family systems theory emphasizes that change with one member affects the entire family.

   C. The family stress theory provides guidance to assist families adapting to stress.

   D. **CORRECT:** The nurse should include that the developmental theory defines consistencies in how families change.

   Ⓝ *NCLEX® Connection: Psychosocial Integrity, Support Systems*

2. A. This statement is reflective of an authoritarian parenting style. The parent controls the adolescent's behaviors and attitudes through unquestioned rules and expectations.

   B. This statement is reflective of a permissive parenting style. The parent exerts little or no control over the adolescent's behaviors, and consults the adolescent when making decisions.

   C. **CORRECT:** This statement is reflective of an authoritative parenting style. The parent directs the adolescent's behavior by setting rules and explaining the reason for each rule setting.

   D. This statement is reflective of an authoritarian parenting style. The parent controls the adolescent's behaviors and attitudes through unquestioned rules and expectations.

   Ⓝ *NCLEX® Connection: Health Promotion and Maintenance, Developmental Stages and Transitions*

3. A. **CORRECT:** The nurse should include a medical history on the parents, siblings, and grandparents when collecting data about a family.

   B. **CORRECT:** The nurse should include the family structure, which includes family members, family size, roles/position within the family, and occupation and education of family members, when collecting data about a family.

   C. The nurse should include the child's physical growth when performing an individual data collection on the child.

   D. **CORRECT:** The nurse should include support systems to determine the availability of extended family, work and peer relationships, and social systems and community resources to assist the family in meeting needs when collecting data about a family.

   E. **CORRECT:** The nurse should include stressors, both expected and unexpected, when collecting data about a family.

   Ⓝ *NCLEX® Connection: Health Promotion and Maintenance, Data Collection Techniques*

PRACTICE Answer

Using the ATI Active Learning Template: Basic Concept

RELATED CONTENT: This is an extended family, which includes at least one parent, one or more children, and other individuals who are either related or not related.

UNDERLYING PRINCIPLES

- Positive parental influences
  - Practice positive self-coping techniques.
  - Maintain structure and routine in the household.
  - Engage in activities with the child.
  - Validate the child's feelings when communicating.
  - Monitor for safety concerns with special consideration for the child's developmental needs.
- Promoting acceptable behavior
  - Validate the child's feelings, and offer sympathetic explanations.
  - Provide role modeling and reinforcement for acceptable behavior.
  - Set clear and realistic limits and expectations based on the child's developmental level.
  - Focus on the behavior when implementing discipline.

NURSING INTERVENTIONS: The nurse should collect the following family data.

- Medical history on parents, siblings, and grandparents
- Family structure for roles/position within the family, as well as occupation and education of family members
- Developmental tasks a family works on as the child grows
- Family characteristics, such as cultural, religious, and economic influences on behavior, attitudes, and actions
- Family stressors, such as expected (birth of a child) and unexpected (illness of a child, divorce, disability, death of a family member) events that cause stress
- Availability of and family interactions with community resources
- Family support systems, such as availability of extended family; work and peer relationships; social systems; and community resources to assist the family in meeting needs or adapting to a stressor

Ⓝ *NCLEX® Connection: Health Promotion and Maintenance, Aging Process*

CHAPTER 2 *Physical Assessment Findings*

Alter exams to accommodate chronological age and developmental needs. Involve children and family members in examinations. Praise children for cooperation during exams. Q℗cc

Observe for behaviors to determine the child's readiness to cooperate (interacting with the nurse, making eye contact, permitting physical touch, willingly sitting on the examination table).

Language, cognition, and fine and gross motor development can be screened using a standardized tool such as the Denver Developmental Screening Test II (Denver II). A combination of data collected from psychosocial and medical histories and a physical examination is used to determine need and make a referral for further evaluation.

NURSING CONSIDERATIONS

- Keep the room warm and well lit.
- Perform examinations in nonthreatening environments.
- Keep medical equipment out of sight.
- Provide privacy. Determine whether older school-age children and adolescents prefer a caregiver to remain during examination.
- Take time to play and develop rapport prior to beginning an examination.
- Observe for behaviors that demonstrate child's readiness to cooperate (interacting with nurse, making eye contact, permitting physical touch, willingly sitting on the examination table).
- Explain each step of the examination to the child.
  ○ Use age-applicable language.
  ○ Demonstrate what will happen using dolls, puppets, or paper drawings.
  ○ Allow the child to manipulate and handle equipment.
  ○ Encourage the child to use equipment on others.
- Examine the child in a secure, comfortable position. For example, a toddler may sit on a parent's lap.

- Proceed to examine the child in an organized sequence when possible.
- If the child is uncooperative, determine reasons, be firm and direct about expected behavior, complete the examination quickly, and use a calm voice.
- Encourage the child and family to ask questions during physical exams. Discuss findings with family after the examination.

PHYSIOLOGIC AND GROWTH MEASUREMENTS

TEMPERATURE

- At 2 hr of age, temperature is approximately 99° F (37.2° C). The temperature stabilizes at 98.6° F (37° C) by 4 hr of age.
- Expected temperature values in children are the same as in an adult.
  ○ Axillary: 97.6° F (36.5° C)
  ○ Oral: 98.6° F (37° C)
  ○ Tympanic: 98.6° F (37° C)
  ○ Rectal: 99.6° F (37.6° C)
- Temperature should be obtained from a newborn or infant less than 1 month old using the axillary route.
- Rectal temperatures are contraindicated in newborns less than 1 month old because the rectal mucosa is fragile, and there is an increased risk of rectal perforation from the thermometer.
- Oral temperatures are contraindicated in children younger than 5 years old.
- Oral temperatures are also contraindicated in children who are receiving oxygen, have had recent trauma to the oral mucosa, or have an altered level of consciousness.

HEART RATE

Values are a range from 2nd to 98th percentile, are recorded as beats/min, and vary depending on activity.

Birth to 2 days: 93 to 159/min

3 days to 3 weeks: 91 to 182/min

1 month to 2 months: 128 to 179/min

3 months to 5 months: 106 to 186/min

6 months to 11 months: 109 to 169/min

1 year to 2 years: 89 to 151/min

3 years to 4 years: 73 to 137/min

5 to 7 years: 65 to 133/min

8 years to 11 years: 62 to 130/min

12 years to 15 years: 60 to 119/min

RESPIRATIONS

Values range from 2nd to 98th percentile, are recorded as breaths/min, and vary depending on activity.

2 to 6 hr: 20 to 80/min (average 50/min)

6 hr to 12 months: 20 to 60/min (average 30 to 40/min)

1 to 2 years: 25 to 30/min

3 to 9 years: 20 to 25/min

10 to 18 years: 16 to 20/min

BLOOD PRESSURE

- Readings should be compared with standard measurements (National High Blood Pressure Education Program Working Group on High Blood Pressure in Children and Adolescents). Q**EBP**
- Age, height, and sex influence blood pressure readings. **(2.1)**

GROWTH

Growth can be evaluated using weight, length/height, body mass index (BMI), and head circumference. Growth charts are tools that can be used to determine the overall health of a child.

- It is recommended to use the World Health Organizations (WHO) growth standards for infants and children ages 0 to 2 in the United States and CDC growth charts for children 2 years and older.
- To see growth charts by age and sex, visit the website for the Centers for Disease Control and Prevention (http://www.cdc.gov/growthcharts) Q**EBP**

EXPECTED FINDINGS

GENERAL APPEARANCE

- Appears content, clean, well-kept, and without body odors.
- Muscle tone: Erect head posture is expected in infants after 4 months of age.
- Makes eye contact when addressed (except infants).
- Follows simple, age-acceptable commands.
- Uses speech, language, and motor skills spontaneously.

SKIN

- Variations in skin color are expected based on race and ethnicity.
- Temperature should be warm or slightly cool to the touch.
- Skin texture should be smooth and slightly dry, not oily.
- Skin turgor exhibits brisk elasticity with adequate hydration.
- Lesions are not expected findings.
- Skin folds should be symmetric.

HAIR AND SCALP

- Hair should be evenly distributed, smooth, and strong.
  - Manifestations of nutritional deficiencies include hair that is stringy, dull, brittle, and dry.
  - Hair loss or balding spots on infants can indicate the child is spending too much time in the same position.
- Scalp should be clean and absent from any flaking, infestations, and trauma.
- Examine children approaching adolescence for secondary hair growth.

NAILS

- Pink over the nail bed and white at the tips
- Smooth and firm (but slightly flexible in infants)

LYMPH NODES

Lymph nodes should be nonpalpable. Lymph nodes that are small, palpable, nontender, and mobile can be an expected finding in children.

HEAD

- The shape of the head should be symmetric.
- Fontanels should be flat. The posterior fontanel usually closes by 6 and 8 weeks of age, and the anterior fontanel usually closes between 12 and 18 months of age.

FACE

- Symmetric appearance and movement
- Proportional features

NECK

- Short in infants
- No palpable masses
- Midline trachea
- Full range of motion present whether checked actively or passively

2.1 Expected blood pressure ranges by age and sex

	Females		Males	
	SYSTOLIC (mm Hg)	DIASTOLIC (mm Hg)	SYSTOLIC (mm Hg)	DIASTOLIC (mm Hg)
INFANTS	76 to 105	64 to 67	87 to 105	63 to 69
1 YEAR	97 to 102	52 to 55	94 to 102	49 to 53
3 YEARS	100 to 106	61 to 64	100 to 108	59 to 63
6 YEARS	104 to 110	68 to 71	105 to 113	68 to 72
10 YEARS	112 to 118	73 to 76	111 to 119	73 to 77
16 YEARS	121 to 127	78 to 81	125 to 133	78 to 82

EYES

Eyebrows should be symmetric and evenly distributed from the inner to the outer canthus.

Eyelids should close completely and open to allow the lower border and most of the upper portion of the iris to be seen.

Eyelashes should curve outward and be evenly distributed with no inflammation around any of the hair follicles.

Conjunctiva
- Palpebral is pink.
- Bulbar is transparent.

Lacrimal apparatus is without excessive tearing, redness, or discharge.

Sclera should be white.

Corneas should be clear.

Pupils should be
- Round
- Equal in size
- Reactive to light
- Accommodating

Irises should be round. The permanent color manifests around 6 to 12 months of age.

Visual acuity
- Can be difficult to determine in children younger than 3 years old.
- Visual acuity in infants can be determined by holding an object in front of the eyes and checking to see whether the infant is able to fixate on the object and follow it.
- Use the tumbling E or HOTV test to check visual acuity of children who are unable to read letters and numbers.
- Older children should be tested using a Snellen chart or symbol chart.

Peripheral visual fields should be
- Upward 50°
- Downward 70°
- Nasally 60°
- Temporally 90°

Extraocular movements
- Might not be symmetric in newborns.
- Corneal light reflex should be symmetric.
- Cover/uncover test should demonstrate equal movement of the eyes.
- Six cardinal fields of gaze should demonstrate no nystagmus.

Internal exam
- Red reflex should be present in infants.
- Arteries, veins, optic discs, and maculae can be visualized in older children and adolescents.

EARS

Alignment: The top of the auricles should meet in an imaginary horizontal line that extends from the outer canthus of the eye.

External ear
- The external ear should be free of lesions and nontender.
- The ear canal should be free of foreign bodies or discharge.
- Cerumen is an expected finding.

Internal ear
- In infants and toddlers, pull the pinna down and back to visualize the tympanic membrane.
- In children older than 3 years, pull the pinna up and back to visualize.
- The ear canal should be pink with fine hairs.
- The tympanic membrane should be pearly pink or gray.
- The light reflex should be visible.
- Umbo (tip of the malleolus) and manubrium (long process or handle) are the bony landmarks that should be visible.

Hearing
- Behavioral audiometry is a test used to observe the behavior of infants in response to sounds projected through speakers or earphones.
- Play audiometry is a test used to observe the behavior of toddlers as an audiometer transmits sounds at different pitches and volumes.
- Tympanometry is a test used to determine how well the middle ear is functioning for children and adolescents. This test can also identify pressure changes in the middle ear.

NOSE

- The position should be midline.
- Patency should be present for each nostril without excessive flaring.
- Smell can be checked in older children.

Internal structures
- Septum is midline and intact.
- Mucosa is deep pink and moist with no discharge.

MOUTH AND THROAT

Lips
- Darker pigmented than facial skin
- Smooth, soft, moist, and symmetric

Gums
- Coral pink
- Tight against the teeth

Mucous membranes
- Without lesions
- Moist, pink, smooth, glistening

Tongue
- Infants can have white coatings on their tongues from milk that can be easily removed. Oral candidiasis coating is not easily removed.
- Children and adolescents should have pink, symmetric tongues that they are able to move beyond their lips.

Teeth
- Infants should have six to eight teeth by 1 year of age.
- Children and adolescents should have teeth that are white and smooth, and begin replacing the 20 deciduous teeth with 32 permanent teeth.

Hard and soft palates: Intact, firm, and concave

Uvula: Intact and moves with vocalization

Tonsils
- Infants: Might not be able to visualize
- Children: Barely visible to prominent, same color as surrounding mucosa

Speech
- Infants: Strong cry
- Children and adolescents: Clear and articulate

THORAX AND LUNGS

Chest shape
- Infants: Shape is almost circular with anteroposterior diameter equaling the transverse or lateral diameter.
- Children and adolescents: The chest typically increases in the transverse direction, causing the anteroposterior diameter to be less than the lateral diameter.

Ribs and sternum: More soft and flexible in infants; symmetric and smooth, with no protrusions or bulges

Movement
- Symmetric, no retractions
- Infants: Irregular rhythms are common.
- Children younger than 7: More abdominal movement is seen during respirations.

Breath sounds
- Inspiration is longer and louder than expiration
- Vesicular (soft, swishing) sounds are heard over most of the lungs
- Bronchovesicular (loud, high pitched inspiration) sounds are heard over intrascapular region
- Bronchial (short inspiratory, long expiratory phase) sounds are heard near the suprasternal notch of the trachea

Breasts
- Newborns: Breasts can be enlarged during the first few days.
- Children and adolescents: Nipples and areolas are darker pigmented and symmetric.
  - Females: Breasts typically develop between 10 and 14 years old. The breasts should appear asymmetric, have no masses, and be palpable.
  - Males can develop gynecomastia, which is unilateral or bilateral breast enlargement that occurs during puberty.

CIRCULATORY SYSTEM

A comprehensive examination of the circulatory system includes data collection of pulses, capillary refill time, neck veins, clubbing of fingers, peripheral cyanosis, edema, blood pressure, and respiratory status.

Heart sounds
- Auscultation should be done in both a sitting and reclining position.
- S_1 and S_2 heart sounds should be clear and crisp. S_1 is louder at the apex of the heart. S_2 is louder near the base of the heart. Physiologic splitting of S_2 and S_3 heart sounds are expected findings in some children. Sinus arrhythmias that are associated with respirations are common.

Pulses
- Infants: Brachial, temporal, and femoral pulses should be palpable, full, and localized.
- Children and adolescents: Pulse locations and expected findings are the same as those in adults.

Abdomen
- Without tenderness, no guarding. Peristaltic waves can be visible in thinner children.
- Shape: Symmetric and without protrusions around the umbilicus
  - Infants and toddlers have rounded abdomens.
  - Children and adolescents should have flat abdomens.
- Bowel sounds should be heard, report absence of bowel sounds or hyperperistalsis.

GENITALIA

Anus: Surrounding skin should be intact with sphincter tightening if the anus is touched. Routine rectal exams are not done with the pediatric population.

MALE: Hair distribution is diamond shaped after puberty in adolescent males. No pubic hair is noted in infants and small children.
- **Penis**
  - Penis should appear straight.
  - Urethral meatus should be at the tip of the penis.
  - Foreskin might not be retractable in uncircumcised infants and small children. Therefore, do not attempt to forcibly retract.
  - Enlargement of the penis occurs during adolescence.
  - The penis can look asymmetrically small in males who are obese because of skin folds partially covering the base.
- **Scrotum**
  - The scrotum hangs separately from the penis.
  - The skin on the scrotum has a wrinkled (rugose) appearance and is loose.
  - The left testicle hangs slighter lower than the right.
  - The inguinal canal should be absent of swelling.
  - During puberty, the testes and scrotum enlarge with darker scrotal skin.

FEMALE: Hair distribution over the mons pubis should be documented in terms of amount and location during puberty. Hair should appear in an inverted triangle. No pubic hair should be noted in infants or small children.
- **Labia:** Symmetric, without lesions, moist on the inner aspects
- **Clitoris:** Small, without bruising or edema
- **Urethral meatus:** Slit-like in appearance with no discharge
- **Vaginal orifice:** The hymen can be absent, or it can completely or partially cover the vaginal opening prior to sexual intercourse.

MUSCULOSKELETAL SYSTEM

Length, position, and size of extremities are symmetric.

Joints

Stable and symmetric with full range of motion and no crepitus or redness

Spine

Infants: Spines should be without dimples or tufts of hair. They should be midline with an overall C-shaped lateral curve.

Toddlers appear squat with short legs and protuberant abdomens.

Preschoolers appear more erect than toddlers.

Children should develop the cervical, thoracic, and lumbar curvatures like that of adults.

Adolescents should remain midline (no scoliosis).

Gait

Toddlers and young children: A bowlegged or knock-kneed appearance is a common finding. Feet should face forward while walking.

Older children and adolescents: A steady gait that appears graceful and balanced is expected.

NEUROLOGIC SYSTEM

Infant reflexes (2.2)

Cranial nerves (2.3)

Deep tendon reflexes

Deep tendon reflexes should demonstrate the following.
- Partial flexion of the lower arm at the biceps tendon
- Partial extension of the lower arm at the triceps tendon
- Partial extension of the lower leg at the patellar tendon
- Plantar flexion of the foot at the Achilles tendon

Cerebellar function (children and adolescents)

Finger to nose test: Rapid coordinated movements

Heel to shin test: Able to run the heel of one foot down the shin of the other leg while standing

Romberg test: Able to stand with slight swaying while eyes are closed

2.2 Infant reflexes

	EXPECTED FINDING	EXPECTED AGE
SUCKING AND ROOTING REFLEXES	Elicited by stroking an infant's cheek or the edge of an infant's mouth. The infant turns her head toward the side that is touched and starts to suck.	Birth to 4 months
PALMAR GRASP	Elicited by touching an infant's palm, near the fingers. The infant's hand flexes into a grasp motion.	Birth to 3 months
PLANTAR GRASP	Elicited by touching the sole of an infant's foot, near the toes. The infant's toes curl/flex downward.	Birth to 8 months
MORO REFLEX	Elicited by allowing the head and trunk of an infant in a semi-sitting position to fall backward to an angle of at least 30°. The infant's arms and legs symmetrically extend, then abduct while fingers spread to form C shape, followed by flexion and adduction of extremities.	Birth to 4 months
STARTLE REFLEX	Elicited by clapping hands or by a loud noise. The newborn abducts arms with flexion at the elbows, and the hands remain clenched.	Birth to 4 months
ASYMMETRIC TONIC NECK REFLEX	Elicited by turning an infant's head to one side. The infant extends the arm and leg on that side and flexes the arm and leg on the opposite side.	Birth to 3 to 4 months
BABINSKI REFLEX	Elicited by stroking the outer edge of the sole, across the ball of an infant's foot up toward the toes. The infant's toes fan upward and out.	Birth to 1 year
DANCING AND STEPPING REFLEXES	Elicited by holding an infant upright with his feet touching a hard, flat surface. The infant makes stepping movements.	Birth to 4 weeks

2.3 Cranial nerves: expected findings

	INFANTS	CHILDREN AND ADOLESCENTS
I OLFACTORY	Difficult to test	Identifies smells through each nostril individually
II OPTIC	Looks at face and tracks with eyes	Has intact visual acuity, peripheral vision, and color vision
III OCULOMOTOR	Blinks in response to light Has pupils that are reactive to light	PERRLA is intact
IV TROCHLEAR	Looks at face and tracks with eyes	Has the ability to look down and in with eyes
V TRIGEMINAL	Has rooting and sucking reflexes	Is able to clench teeth together Detects touch on face with eyes closed
VI ABDUCENS	Looks at face and tracks with eyes	Is able to see laterally with eyes
VII FACIAL	Has symmetric facial movements	Has the ability to differentiate between salty and sweet on tongue Has symmetric facial movements
VIII ACOUSTIC	Tracks a sound Blinks in response to a loud noise	Does not experience vertigo Has intact hearing
IX GLOSSOPHARYNGEAL	Has an intact gag reflex	Has an intact gag reflex Is able to taste sour sensations on back of tongue
X VAGUS	Has no difficulties swallowing	Speech clear, no difficulties swallowing Uvula is midline
XI SPINAL ACCESSORY	Moves shoulders symmetrically	Has equal strength of shoulder shrug against examiner's hands
XII HYPOGLOSSAL	Has no difficulties swallowing Opens mouth when nares are occluded	Has a tongue that is midline Is able to move tongue in all directions with equal strength against tongue blade resistance

Application Exercises

1. A nurse is preparing to examine a preschool-age child. Which of the following actions should the nurse take to prepare the child?

    A. Allow the child to role-play using miniature equipment.

    B. Use medical terminology to describe what will happen.

    C. Separate the child and the parent during the examination.

    D. Keep the medical equipment visible to the child.

2. A nurse is checking the vital signs of a 3-year-old child during a well-child visit. Which of the following findings should the nurse report to the provider?

    A. Temperature 37.2° C (99° F)

    B. Heart rate 106/min

    C. Respirations 30/min

    D. Blood pressure 88/54 mm Hg

3. A nurse is inspecting the ears of a 3-year-old child during a well-child visit. Which of the following findings should the nurse expect?

    A. Light reflex is located at the 2 to 3 o'clock position.

    B. Tympanic membrane is nontransparent gray in color.

    C. Ear canal curves upward and forward.

    D. External auditory canal walls are pink.

4. A nurse is checking the reflexes of a 6-month-old infant. Which of the following reflexes should the nurse expect the infant to exhibit?

    A. Moro

    B. Plantar grasp

    C. Stepping

    D. Tonic neck

5. A school nurse is examining the cranial nerves of an adolescent following a fall during football practice. Which of the following reactions should the nurse expect when checking the trigeminal nerve? (Select all that apply.)

    A. Clenching the teeth together tightly

    B. Recognizing sour tastes on the back of the tongue

    C. Identifying smells through each nostril

    D. Detecting facial touches with eyes closed

    E. Looking down and inward toward the nose with the eyes

PRACTICE Active Learning Scenario

A nurse is preparing to examine a preschooler. Use the ATI Active Learning Template: Basic Concept to complete this item.

UNDERLYING PRINCIPLES: Describe two behaviors that indicate the child is ready to cooperate.

NURSING INTERVENTIONS

- Describe two actions to take if the child is uncooperative.
- Include three actions to promote the child's comfort during the examination.

Application Exercises Key

1. A. **CORRECT:** The nurse should allow the child to role-play or manipulate actual or miniature equipment to reduce anxiety and fear related to the examination.

    B. The nurse should use neutral words and avoid overestimating what the child understands when describing what will happen.

    C. The nurse should encourage parental presence during the examination because this helps the child to feel safe.

    D. The nurse should keep medical equipment out of sight unless showing or using it on the child because this could increase the child's anxiety level.

    Ⓝ *NCLEX® Connection: Health Promotion and Maintenance, Data Collection Techniques*

2. A. A temperature of 37.2° C (99° F) is within the expected reference range for a 3-year-old child and should not be reported to the provider.

    B. A heart rate of 106/min is within the expected reference range for a 3-year-old child and should not be reported to the provider.

    C. **CORRECT:** Respirations of 30/min is above the expected reference range for a 3-year-old child and should be reported to the provider.

    D. A blood pressure of 90/52 mm Hg is within the expected reference range for a 3-year-old child and should not be reported to the provider.

    Ⓝ *NCLEX® Connection: Reduction of Risk Potential, Changes/Abnormalities in Vital Signs*

3. A. The child's light reflex should be located around the 5 or 7 o'clock position, rather than the 2 or 3 o'clock position. Therefore, this is an atypical finding and should be reported to the provider.

    B. The child's tympanic membrane should be translucent gray or light pearly pink, rather than nontransparent gray in color. Therefore, this is an atypical finding and should be reported to the provider.

    C. The child's ear canal should curve downward and forward, rather than upward and forward. Therefore, this is an atypical finding and should be reported to the provider.

    D. **CORRECT:** The walls of the child's external auditory should be pink. Therefore, this is an expected finding by the nurse.

    Ⓝ *NCLEX® Connection: Health Promotion and Maintenance, Data Collection Techniques*

4. A. The Moro reflex is exhibited by infants from birth to the age of 4 months.

    B. **CORRECT:** The plantar grasp is exhibited by infants from birth to the age of 8 months.

    C. The stepping reflex is exhibited by infants from birth to the age of 4 weeks.

    D. The tonic neck reflex is exhibited by infants from birth to the age of 3 to 4 months.

    Ⓝ *NCLEX® Connection: Health Promotion and Maintenance, Data Collection Techniques*

5. A. **CORRECT:** Clenching the teeth together tightly is an expected reaction by the adolescent when the nurse is checking the trigeminal cranial nerve.

    B. Recognizing sour tastes on the back of the tongue is an expected reaction by the adolescent when the nurse is checking the glossopharyngeal nerve.

    C. Identifying smells through each nostril is an expected reaction by the adolescent when the nurse is checking the olfactory nerve.

    D. **CORRECT:** Detecting facial touches with both eyes closed is an expected reaction by the adolescent when the nurse is checking the trigeminal nerve.

    E. Looking down and inward toward the nose with the eyes is an expected reaction by the adolescent when the nurse is checking the trochlear cranial nerve.

    Ⓝ *NCLEX® Connection: Reduction of Risk Potential, Potential for Alterations in Body Systems*

PRACTICE Answer

Using the ATI Active Learning Template: Basic Concept

UNDERLYING PRINCIPLES
- Child is ready to cooperate.
- Interacting with nurse.
- Making eye contact.
- Permitting physical touch.
- Willingly sitting on examination table.
- Accepting and handling equipment.

NURSING INTERVENTIONS
- Actions to take if child is uncooperative
  - Engage both the child and parent.
  - Be firm and direct about expected behavior.
  - Complete the examination as quickly as possible.
  - Use a calm voice.
  - Reduce environmental stimuli.
  - Limit the people in the room.

- Actions to enhance child's comfort
  - Perform examination in nonthreatening environment.
  - Take time to play and develop rapport prior to beginning the examination.
  - Keep the room warm and well lit.
  - Keep medical equipment out of sight until needed.
  - Provide privacy.
  - Explain each step of the examination to the child.
  - Examine the child in a secure, comfortable position.
  - Examine the child in an organized sequence when possible.
  - Encourage the child and family to ask questions during the examination.

Ⓝ *NCLEX® Connection: Health Promotion and Maintenance, Data Collection Techniques*

Health Promotion of Infants (2 Days to 1 Year)

PHYSICAL DEVELOPMENT

Fontanel
- Posterior fontanel closes by 6 to 8 weeks of age.
- Anterior fontanel closes by 12 to 18 months of age.

Infant size is tracked using weight, height, and head circumference measurements.
- **Weight**: Infants gain approximately 680 g (1.5 lb) per month during the first 5 months of life. The average weight of a 6-month-old infant is 7.26 kg (16 lb). Birth weight is at least doubled by the age of 5 months, and tripled by the age of 12 months to an average of 9.75 kg (21.5 lb).
- **Height**: Infants grow approximately 2.5 cm (1 in) per month the first 6 months of life. Growth occurs in spurts after the age of 6 months, and the birth length increases by 50% by the age of 12 months.
- **Head circumference**: The circumference of infants' heads increases approximately 2 cm (0.75 in) per month during the first 3 months, 1 cm (0.4 in) per month from 4 to 6 months, and then approximately 0.5 cm (0.2 in) per month during the second 6 months.

EXPECTED GROWTH AND DEVELOPMENT

GENERAL MEASUREMENTS OF FULL-TERM NEWBORN

Head circumference averages 33 to 35 cm (13 to 14 in).

Crown to rump length is 31 to 35 cm (12.2 to 14 in), approximately equal to head circumference.

Head to heel length averages 48 to 53 cm (19 to 21 in).

Weight averages 2,700 to 4,000 g (6 to 9 lb).

> Newborns lose up to 10% of their birth weight by 3 to 4 days of age. This is due to fluid shifts, loss of meconium, and limited intake, especially in infants who are breastfed. The birth weight is usually regained by the tenth to fourteenth day of life, depending on the feeding method used. Q EBP

3.1 Motor skill development by age

	GROSS MOTOR SKILLS	FINE MOTOR SKILLS
1 MONTH	Demonstrates head lag	Has a strong grasp reflex
2 MONTHS	Lifts head off mattress when prone	Holds hands in an open position Grasp reflex fading
3 MONTHS	Raises head and shoulders off mattress when prone Only slight head lag	No longer has a grasp reflex Keeps hands loosely open
4 MONTHS	Rolls from back to side	Grasps objects with both hands
5 MONTHS	Rolls from abdomen to back	Uses palmar grasp
6 MONTHS	Rolls from back to abdomen	Holds bottle
7 MONTHS	Bears full weight on feet Sits, leaning forward on both hands	Moves objects from hand to hand
8 MONTHS	Sits unsupported	Begins using pincer grasp
9 MONTHS	Pulls to a standing position Creeps on hands and knees instead of crawling	Has a crude pincer grasp Dominant hand preference evident
10 MONTHS	Changes from a prone to a sitting position	Grasps rattle by its handle
11 MONTHS	Cruises or walks while holding onto something Walks with both hands held	Places objects into a container Neat pincer grasp
12 MONTHS	Sits down from a standing position without assistance Walks with one hand held	Tries to build a two-block tower without success Can turn pages in a book

Dentition

- Six to eight teeth should erupt in infants' mouths by the end of the first year. The first teeth typically erupt between 6 and 10 months (average age 8 months).
- Some children show minimal indications of teething (sucking or biting on their fingers or hard objects, drooling). Others are irritable, have difficulty sleeping, have a mild fever, rub their ears, and have decreased appetite for solid foods.
- Teething pain can be eased using frozen teething rings or an ice cube wrapped in a wash cloth and over-the-counter teething gels. With topical anesthetic ointments, absorption rates vary in infants; therefore, parents should be advised to apply them correctly. Acetaminophen and ibuprofen can be used if irritability interferes with sleeping and feeding, but should not be used for more than 3 days. Ibuprofen should be used only if age-appropriate. Qs
- Clean infants' teeth using cool, wet washcloths.
- Bottles should not be given to infants when they are falling asleep, because prolonged exposure to milk or juice can cause early childhood dental caries.

COGNITIVE DEVELOPMENT

Piaget: Sensorimotor stage (birth to 24 months) QEBP
- Infants progress from reflexive to simple repetitive to imitative activities.
- Separation, object permanence, and mental representation are the three important tasks accomplished in this stage.
  - **Separation**: Infants learn to separate themselves from other objects in the environment.
  - **Object permanence**: The process by which infants learn that an object still exists when it is out of view. This occurs at approximately 9 to 10 months of age.
  - **Mental representation**: The ability to recognize and use symbols.

Language development

- Crying is the first form of verbal communication.
- Infants cry for 1 to 1.5 hr each day up to 3 weeks of age and build up to 2 to 4 hr by 6 weeks.
- Crying decreases by 12 weeks of age.
- Vocalizes with cooing noises by 3 to 4 months.
- Shows considerable interest in the environment by 3 months.
- Turns head to the sound of a rattle by 3 months.
- Laughs and squeals by 4 months.
- Makes single vowel sounds by 2 months.
- By 3 to 4 months, the consonants are added.
- Begins speaking two-word phrases and progresses to speaking three-word phrases.
- Says three to five words by the age of 1 year.
- Comprehends the word "no" by 9 to 10 months and obeys single commands accompanied by gestures.

PSYCHOSOCIAL DEVELOPMENT

Erikson: Trust vs. mistrust (birth to 1 year) QEBP
- Achieving this task is based on the quality of the caregiver-infant relationship and the care received by the infant.
- The infant begins to learn delayed gratification. Failure to learn delayed gratification leads to mistrust.
- Trust is developed by meeting comfort, feeding, stimulation, and caring needs.
- Mistrust develops if needs are inadequately or inconsistently met, or if needs are continuously met before being vocalized by the infant.

Social development

- Social development is initially influenced by infants' reflexive behaviors and includes attachment, separation, recognition/anxiety, and stranger fear.
- Attachment is seen when infants begin to bond with their parents. This development is seen within the first month, but it actually begins before birth. The process is enhanced when infants and parents are in good health, have positive feeding experiences, and receive adequate rest.
- Separation-individuation occurs during the first year of life as infants first distinguish themselves and their primary caregiver as separate individuals at the same time that object permanence is developing.
- Separation anxiety begins around 4 to 8 months of age. Infants protest when separated from parents, which can cause considerable anxiety for parents. By 11 to 12 months, infants are able to anticipate the mother's imminent departure by watching her behaviors.
- Stranger fear becomes evident between 6 and 8 months of age, when infants have the ability to discriminate between familiar and unfamiliar people.
- Reactive attachment disorder results from maladaptive or absent attachment between the infant and primary caregiver and continues through childhood and adulthood.

Body-image changes

- Infants discover that mouths are pleasure producers.
- Hands and feet are seen as objects of play.
- Infants discover that smiling causes others to react.

AGE-APPROPRIATE ACTIVITIES

- Play should provide interpersonal contact and educational stimulation.
- Infants have short attention spans and will not interact with other children during play (solitary play). Appropriate toys and activities stimulate the senses and encourage development. QPCC
  - Rattles
  - Soft stuffed toys
  - Teething toys
  - Nesting toys
  - Playing pat-a-cake
  - Playing with balls
  - Reading books
  - Mirrors
  - Brightly colored toys
  - Playing with blocks

HEALTH PROMOTION

CARE OF THE NEWBORN AFTER DISCHARGE

- Newborn infants should be placed in a federally approved car seat at a 45° angle to prevent slumping and airway obstruction. The car seat is placed rear-facing in the rear seat of the vehicle and secured using the safety belt. The shoulder harnesses are placed in the slots at or below the level of the infant's shoulders. The harness should be snug and the retainer clip placed at the level of the infant's armpits.
- Assist parents to schedule follow-up appointments with the provider according to the infant's needs and the age of the infant at the time of discharge. The American Academy of Pediatrics recommends infants who are less than 48 hr old at the time of discharge receive a physical assessment by a provider within 48 hr of discharge. QPCC

IMMUNIZATIONS

The Centers for Disease Control and Prevention (CDC) immunization recommendations for healthy infants less than 12 months of age include the following. QEBP
- Birth: hepatitis B (Hep B)
- 2 months: diphtheria and tetanus toxoids and pertussis (DTaP), rotavirus vaccine (RV), inactivated poliovirus (IPV), Haemophilus influenzae type B (Hib), pneumococcal vaccine (PCV), and Hep B
- 4 months: DTaP, RV, IPV, Hib, PCV
- 6 months: DTaP, IPV (6 to 18 months), PCV, and Hep B (6 to 18 months); RV; Hib
- 6 to 12 months: seasonal influenza vaccination yearly (the trivalent inactivated influenza vaccine is available as an IM injection)

CDC immunization recommendations change periodically. Check the CDC's website (www.cdc.gov) for its latest recommendations.

NUTRITION

- Feeding options
  - Breastfeeding provides a complete diet for infants during the first 6 months.
  - Iron-fortified formula is an acceptable alternative to breast milk. Cow's milk is not recommended.
  - It is recommended to begin vitamin D supplements within the first few days of life to prevent rickets and vitamin D deficiency. QEBP
  - Iron supplements are recommended for infants who are being exclusively breastfed after the age of 4 months.
  - Alternative sources of fluids (juice, water) are not needed during the first 4 months of life. Excessive intake of water could result in hyponatremia and water intoxication.
  - After the age of 6 months, 100% fruit juice should be limited to 4 to 6 oz per day.
- Solids are introduced around 4 to 6 months of age.
  - Indicators for readiness include interest in solid foods, voluntary control of the head and trunk, and disappearance of the extrusion reflex.
  - Iron-fortified cereal is typically introduced first due to its high iron content.
  - New foods should be introduced one at a time, over a 5- to 7-day period, to observe for indications of allergy or intolerance, which can include fussiness, rash, vomiting, diarrhea, and constipation.
  - Vegetables or fruits are started around 6 months of age depending on provider recommendations and family history of food allergies. After both have been introduced, meats can be added.
  - Breast milk/formula should be decreased as intake of solid foods increases, but should remain the primary source of nutrition through the first year.
  - Table foods that are well-cooked, chopped, and unseasoned are appropriate by 1 year of age.
  - Suggested finger foods include ripe bananas, toast strips, graham crackers, cheese cubes, noodles, firmly-cooked vegetables, and raw pieces of fruit (except grapes).
- Weaning can be accomplished when infants show indications of readiness and are able to drink from a cup (sometime in the second 6 months).
  - Gradually replace one bottle or breastfeeding at a time with breast milk or formula in a cup with handles.
  - Bedtime feedings are the last to be stopped.

SLEEP AND REST

- Nocturnal sleep pattern is established by 3 to 4 months of age.
- Infants sleep 14 to 15 hr daily (of those, 9 to 11 hr at nighttime) around the age of 4 months.
- Infants sleep through the night and take one to two naps during the day by the age of 12 months.

INJURY PREVENTION Qs

Aspiration of foreign objects
- Hold the infant for feedings; do not prop bottles.
- Avoid small objects that can become lodged in the throat (grapes, coins, candy).
- Provide age-appropriate toys.
- Check clothing for safety hazards (loose buttons).

Bodily harm
- Keep sharp objects out of reach.
- Anchor heavy objects and furniture so they cannot be overturned on top of the infant.
- Infants should not be left unattended with any animals present.

Burns
- Avoid warming formula in a microwave; check temperature of liquid before feeding.
- Check the temperature of bath water.
- Set hot water thermostats at or less than 49° C (120° F).
- Keep working smoke detectors in the home.
- Turn handles of pots and pans to the back of stoves.
- Use sunscreen infants are exposed to the sun.
- Cover electrical outlets.

Drowning
- Infants should not be left unattended in bathtubs or around water sources (toilets, cleaning buckets, drainage areas).
- Secure fencing around swimming pools.
- Close bathroom doors.

Falls
- Keep crib mattresses in the lowest position possible with the rails all the way up.
- Use restraints in infant seats.
- Infant seats should be placed on the ground or floor if used outside of the car, and they should not be left unattended or on elevated surfaces.
- Place safety gates at the top and bottom of stairs.

Poisoning
- Avoid exposure to lead paint.
- Keep toxins and plants out of reach.
- Keep safety locks on cabinets that contain cleaners and other household chemicals.
- Keep the phone number for a poison control center near the phone.
- Keep medications in childproof containers, away from the reach of infants.
- Keep a working carbon monoxide detector in the home.

Motor-vehicle injuries
- Infant-only and convertible infant-toddler car seats are available.
- Infants and toddlers remain in a rear-facing car seat until the age of 2 years or the height recommended by the manufacturer.
- The safest area for infants and children is the backseat of the car.
- Do not place rear-facing car seats in the front seat of vehicles with passenger airbags.
- Do not leave infants in parked cars.

Suffocation
- Avoid plastic bags.
- Keep balloons away from infants.
- Crib mattresses should fit snugly.
- Crib slats should be no farther apart than 6 cm (2.375 in).
- Remove crib mobiles and/or crib gyms by 4 to 5 months of age.
- Keep pillows out of the crib.
- Place infants on their backs for sleep.
- Keep toys with small parts out of reach.
- Remove drawstrings from jackets and other clothing.

Application Exercises

1. A nurse is collecting data from a 12-month-old infant during a well-child visit. Which of the following findings should the nurse report to the provider?

    A. Closed anterior fontanel

    B. Eruption of six teeth

    C. Birth weight doubled

    D. Birth length increased by 50%

2. A nurse is assisting with data collection for a developmental screening on a 10-month-old infant. Which of the following fine motor skills should the nurse expect the infant to perform? (Select all that apply.)

    A. Grasps a rattle by the handle

    B. Tries building a two-block tower

    C. Uses a crude pincer grasp

    D. Places objects into a container

    E. Walks with one hand held

3. A nurse is conducting a well-baby visit with a 4-month-old infant. Which of the following immunizations should the nurse plan to administer to the infant? (Select all that apply.)

    A. Measles, mumps, rubella (MMR)

    B. Polio (IPV)

    C. Pneumococcal vaccine (PCV)

    D. Varicella

    E. Rotavirus vaccine (RV)

4. A nurse is reinforcing education about introducing new foods to the parents of a 4-month-old infant. The nurse should recommend that the parents introduce which of the following foods first?

    A. Strained yellow vegetables

    B. Iron-fortified cereals

    C. Pureed fruits

    D. Whole milk

5. A nurse is reinforcing teaching about dental care and teething to the parent of a 9-month-old infant. Which of the following statements indicates that the parent understands the information?

    A. "I can give my baby a warm teething ring to relieve discomfort."

    B. "I should clean my baby's teeth with a cool, wet wash cloth."

    C. "I can give ibuprofen for up to 5 days while my baby is teething."

    D. "I should place diluted juice in the bottle my baby drinks while falling asleep."

PRACTICE Active Learning Scenario

A nurse is assisting with the preparation of an educational program for a group of parents of infants. Use the ATI Active Learning Template: Growth and Development to complete this item.

DEVELOPMENTAL STAGE: Identify the infant's developmental stage according to Piaget and Erikson.

COGNITIVE DEVELOPMENT: List two cognitive developmental tasks the infant should accomplish in the first year of life.

AGE-APPROPRIATE ACTIVITIES: List five activities appropriate for infants.

INJURY PREVENTION: Identify two injury prevention methods in each of the following categories.

- Aspiration
- Poisoning
- Drowning
- Suffocation

Application Exercises Key

1. A. By the age of 12 to 18 months, the infant's anterior fontanel should close.

   B. By the age of 12 months, the infant should have six to eight teeth erupted.

   C. **CORRECT:** By the age of 12 months, the infant's birth weight should have tripled. Therefore, the nurse should report this finding to the provider.

   D. By the age of 12 months, the infant's birth length should increase by 50%.

   Ⓝ *NCLEX® Connection: Reduction of Risk Potential, Potential for Alterations in Body Systems*

2. A. **CORRECT:** The infant should be able to grasp a rattle by the handle at the age of 10 months.

   B. The infant should try building a two-block tower at the age of 12 months.

   C. **CORRECT:** The infant should be able to use a crude pincer grasp at the age of 9 months.

   D. The infant should be able to place objects into a container at the age of 11 months.

   E. The infant should be able to walk with one hand held at the age of 12 months.

   Ⓝ *NCLEX® Connection: Health Promotion and Maintenance, Developmental Stages and Transitions*

3. A. The first MMR vaccine is given between the ages of 12 and 15 months.

   B. **CORRECT:** The nurse should administer the IPV vaccine to a 4-month-old infant.

   C. **CORRECT:** The nurse should administer the PCV vaccine to a 4-month-old infant.

   D. The first varicella vaccine is given at a minimum age of 12 months.

   E. **CORRECT:** The nurse should administer the RV vaccine to a 4-month-old infant.

   Ⓝ *NCLEX® Connection: Health Promotion and Maintenance, Health Promotion/Disease Prevention*

4. A. When introducing vegetables to the infant's diet, the nurse should recommend strained yellow vegetables. However, evidence-based practice indicates that the nurse should recommend a different food as the first solid food.

   B. **CORRECT:** According to evidence-based practice, the nurse should recommend iron-fortified cereals as the first solid food to introduce because of the high iron content. The order of introducing solid foods after this is variable.

   C. When introducing fruits to the infant's diet, the nurse should recommend pureed fruits. However, evidence-based practice indicates that the nurse should recommend a different food as the first solid food.

   D. When transitioning the infant to cow's milk, the nurse should recommend whole milk. However, evidence-based practice indicates that the nurse should recommend a different food first.

   Ⓝ *NCLEX® Connection: Basic Care and Comfort, Nutrition and Oral Hydration*

5. A. Teething pain can be relieved using frozen teething rings or an ice cube wrapped in a wash cloth.

   B. **CORRECT:** It is appropriate to use a cool, wet wash cloth for cleaning the infant's teeth.

   C. Ibuprofen should not be used for more than 3 days.

   D. To prevent early childhood caries, infants should not be given bottles of milk or juice while falling asleep.

   Ⓝ *NCLEX® Connection: Basic Care and Comfort, Nonpharmacological Comfort Interventions*

PRACTICE Answer

Using the ATI Active Learning Template: Growth and Development

DEVELOPMENTAL STAGE
- Piaget: Sensorimotor stage
- Erikson: Trust vs. mistrust

COGNITIVE DEVELOPMENT
- Infants progress from reflexive to simple repetitive to imitative activities.
- Separation: Learning to separate themselves from other objects in the environment.
- Object permanence: Understanding that an object still exists when it is out of view.
- Mental representation: Ability to recognize and use symbols.

AGE-APPROPRIATE ACTIVITIES
- Rattles
- Soft stuffed toys
- Teething toys
- Nesting toys
- Playing pat-a-cake
- Playing with balls
- Reading books
- Mirrors
- Brightly colored toys
- Playing with blocks

INJURY PREVENTION
- Aspiration
  - Avoid small objects.
  - Hold infant for feedings; do not prop bottles.
  - Provide age-appropriate toys.
  - Check clothing for hazards such as loose buttons.
- Poisoning
  - Keep toxins and plants out of reach.
  - Place safety locks on cabinets where cleaners/chemicals are stored.
  - Use a carbon monoxide detector in the home.
  - Keep medications in childproof containers and out of reach.
- Drowning
  - Do not leave unattended around any water source.
  - Secure fencing around swimming pool.
  - Keep bathroom door closed.
- Suffocation
  - Avoid plastic bags.
  - Ensure crib mattress fits snugly.
  - Remove crib mobiles by 4 to 5 months of age.
  - Keep pillows out of the crib.
  - Place on back to sleep.

Ⓝ *NCLEX® Connection: Safety and Infection Control, Accident/Error/Injury Prevention*

CHAPTER 4 *Health Promotion of Toddlers (1 to 3 Years)*

EXPECTED GROWTH AND DEVELOPMENT

PHYSICAL DEVELOPMENT

Anterior fontanels close by 18 months of age.
Weight: At 30 months of age, toddlers should weigh four times their birth weight.
Height: Toddlers grow about 7.5 cm (3 in) per year.
Head circumference and chest circumference are usually equal by 1 to 2 years of age.

COGNITIVE DEVELOPMENT

Piaget: Sensorimotor stage transitions to the preoperational stage around age 19 to 24 months. Q_{EBP}
- The concept of object permanence becomes fully developed.
- Toddlers have and demonstrate memories of events that relate to them.
- Domestic mimicry (playing house) is evident.
- Preoperational thought does not allow for toddlers to understand other viewpoints, but it does allow them to symbolize objects and people to imitate previously seen activities.

Language development

- Language increases to about 300 words by the age of 2 years.
- 1 year: using one-word sentences, or holophrases
- 2 years: using multiword sentences by combining two to three words
- 3 years: combining several words to create simple sentences using grammatical rules

PSYCHOSOCIAL DEVELOPMENT

Erikson: Autonomy vs. shame and doubt Q_{EBP}
- Independence is paramount for toddlers, who are attempting to do everything for themselves.
- Toddlers often use negativism, or negative responses, as they begin to express their independence.
- Ritualism, or maintaining routines and reliability, provides a sense of comfort for toddlers as they begin to explore the environment beyond those most familiar to them.

Moral development

- Moral development is closely associated with cognitive development.
- Egocentric: Toddlers are unable to see things from the perspectives of others; they can only view things from their personal points of view.
- Punishment and obedience orientation begin with a sense that good behavior is rewarded and bad behavior is punished.

Self-concept development

Toddlers progressively see themselves as separate from their parents and increase their explorations away from them.

Body-image changes

- Toddlers appreciate the usefulness of various body parts.
- Toddlers develop gender identity by 3 years of age.

4.1 Motor skill development by age

	GROSS MOTOR SKILLS	FINE MOTOR SKILLS
15 MONTHS	Walks without help Creeps up stairs	Uses a cup well Builds a tower of two blocks
18 MONTHS	Runs clumsily; falls often Throws a ball overhand Jumps in place with both feet Pulls and pushes toys	Manages a spoon without rotation Turns pages in a book, two or three at a time Builds tower of three or four blocks
2 YEARS	Walks up and down stairs by placing both feet on each step	Builds a tower of six or seven blocks Turns pages of books one at a time
2.5 YEARS	Jumps across the floor and off a chair or step using both feet Stands on one foot momentarily Takes a few steps on tiptoe	Draws circles Has good hand-finger coordination Builds tower of eight blocks

AGE-APPROPRIATE ACTIVITIES

- Solitary play evolves into parallel play, in which toddlers observe other children and then might engage in activities nearby. Qpcc
- Appropriate activities
  - Filling and emptying containers
  - Water toys and clay
  - Playing with blocks
  - Looking at books
  - Push-pull toys
  - Tossing balls
  - Finger paints
  - Large-piece puzzles
  - Thick crayons
- Temper tantrums result when toddlers are frustrated with restrictions on independence. Providing consistent, age-appropriate expectations helps toddlers to work through frustration.
- Toilet training can begin when toddlers have the sensation of needing to urinate or defecate. Parents should demonstrate patience and consistency in toilet training. Nighttime control might develop last.
- Discipline should be consistent with well-defined boundaries that are established to develop appropriate social behavior.

HEALTH PROMOTION

IMMUNIZATIONS

The Centers for Disease Control and Prevention immunization recommendations for healthy toddlers 12 months to 3 years of age include: QEBP

- 12 to 15 months: inactivated poliovirus (third dose between 6 to 18 months); *Haemophilus influenzae* type B; pneumococcal conjugate vaccine; measles, mumps, and rubella; and varicella
- 12 to 23 months: hepatitis A (Hep A), given in two doses at least 6 months apart
- 15 to 18 months: diphtheria, tetanus, and acellular pertussis (DTaP)
- 12 to 36 months: yearly seasonal trivalent inactivated influenza vaccine; live, attenuated influenza vaccine by nasal spray (must be 2 years or older)

CDC immunization recommendations change periodically; check the CDC's website (http://www.cdc.gov) for its latest recommendations.

NUTRITION

- Children can establish lifetime eating habits during early childhood.
- Toddlers begin developing taste preferences and are generally picky eaters who repeatedly request their favorite foods.
- Physiologic anorexia occurs, resulting in toddlers becoming fussy eaters because of a decreased appetite.
- Toddlers should consume 24 to 28 oz milk per day, and can switch from drinking whole milk to low-fat milk after 2 years of age.

- Juice consumption should be limited to 4 to 6 oz per day.
- Trans fatty acids and saturated fats should be avoided.
- Diet should include 1 cup of fruit daily.
- Food serving size should be 1 tbsp for each year of age, or ¼ to ⅓ of an adult portion.
- Toddlers generally prefer finger foods because of increasing autonomy.
- Regular meal times and nutritious snacks best meet nutrient needs.
- Snacks or desserts that are high in sugar, fat, or sodium should be avoided.
- Foods that are potential choking hazards (nuts, grapes, hot dogs, peanut butter, raw carrots, tough meats, popcorn) should be avoided.
- Adult supervision should always be provided during snack and mealtimes.
- Foods should be cut into bite-size pieces to make them easier to swallow and to prevent choking.
- Toddlers should not be allowed to engage in drinking or eating during play activities or while lying down.
- Parents should follow the U.S. Department of Agriculture's guidelines (www.choosemyplate.gov).

SLEEP AND REST

- Toddlers average 11 to 12 hr of sleep per day, including one nap.
- Naps often are eliminated in older toddlerhood.
- Resistance to bedtime and expression of fears are common in this age group.
- Maintaining a regular bedtime routine and time is helpful to promote sleep.

DENTAL HEALTH

- Children should have an established dental home by the age of 1 year.
- Flossing and brushing should be performed by the adult caregiver and are the best methods of removing plaque.
- Brushing should occur after meals and at bedtime. Nothing to eat or drink, except water, is given to the child after the bedtime cleaning.
- Fluoride is supplemented for children living in areas without adequate levels in drinking water.
- Early childhood caries is a form a tooth decay that develops in toddlers and is more common in children who are put to bed with a bottle of juice or milk.
- Consumption of cariogenic foods should be eliminated if possible. If not, the frequency of consumption should be limited.

INJURY PREVENTION

Aspiration of foreign objects
- Small objects (grapes, coins, candy) that can become lodged in the throat should be avoided. Qs
- Toys that have small parts should be kept out of reach.
- Age-appropriate toys should be provided.
- Clothing should be checked for safety hazards (loose buttons).
- Balloons should be kept away from toddlers.
- Parents should know emergency procedures for choking.

Bodily harm

- Sharp objects should be kept out of reach.
- Firearms should be kept in locked boxes or cabinets.
- Toddlers should not be left unattended with any animals present.
- Toddlers should be taught stranger safety.

Burns

- The temperature of bath water should be checked.
- Thermostats on hot water heaters should be turned down to less than 49° C (120° F).
- Working smoke detectors should be kept in the home.
- Pot handles should be turned toward the back of the stove.
- Electrical outlets should be covered.
- Toddlers should wear sunscreen when outside.

Drowning

- Toddlers should not be left unattended in bathtubs.
- Toilet lids should be kept closed.
- Toddlers should be closely supervised when near pools or any other body of water.
- Toddlers should be taught to swim.

Falls

- Doors and windows should be kept locked.
- Transition from a crib to a bed when the toddler reaches a height of 89 cm (35 in)
- Safety gates should be used across the top and bottom of stairs.

Motor-vehicle injuries

- Infants and toddlers remain in a rear-facing car seat until the age of 2 years or the height and weight recommended by the manufacturer.
- Toddlers older than 2 years, or who exceed the height recommendations for rear-facing car seats, are moved to a forward-facing car seat.
- Safest area for infants and children is the backseat of the car.
- Do not place rear-facing car seats in the front seat of vehicles with deployable passenger airbags.

Poisoning

- Exposure to lead paint should be avoided.
- Safety locks should be placed on cabinets that contain cleaners and other chemicals.
- The phone number for a poison control center should be kept near the phone.
- Medications should be kept in childproof containers, away from the reach of toddlers.
- A working carbon monoxide detector should be placed in the home.

Suffocation

- Plastic bags should be avoided.
- Crib mattresses should fit tightly.
- Crib slats should be no farther apart than 6 cm (2.375 in).
- Pillows should be kept out of cribs.
- Drawstrings should be removed from jackets and other clothing.
- Toy boxes should have removable lids that are lightweight rather than lids that are hinged.
- Avoid latex balloons

Application Exercises

1. A nurse is collecting data from a 2½-year-old toddler at a well-child visit. Which of the following findings should the nurse report to the provider?

   A. Height increased by 7.5 cm (3 in) in the past year.

   B. Head circumference exceeds chest circumference.

   C. Anterior and posterior fontanels are closed.

   D. Current weight equals four times the birth weight.

2. A nurse is assisting with the collection of data for a developmental screening on an 18-month-old. The nurse should expect the toddler to be able to perform which of the following skills? (Select all that apply.)

   A. Builds a tower with six blocks

   B. Throws a ball overhand

   C. Walks up and down stairs

   D. Draws circles

   E. Uses a spoon without rotation

3. A nurse is reinforcing teaching about age-appropriate activities to the parent of a 24-month-old. Which of the following indicates that the parent understands the information?

   A. "I will send my child's favorite stuffed animal when she will be napping away from home."

   B. "My child should be able to stand on one foot for a second."

   C. "The soccer team my child will be playing on starts practicing next week."

   D. "I should expect my child to be able to draw circles."

4. A nurse is reinforcing anticipatory guidance to the parents of a toddler. Which of the following instructions should the nurse include? (Select all that apply.)

   A. Develop food habits that will prevent dental caries.

   B. Meeting caloric needs results in an increased appetite.

   C. Expression of bedtime fears is common.

   D. Expect behaviors associated with negativism and ritualism.

   E. Annual screenings for phenylketonuria are important.

Application Exercises Key

1. A. Toddler height should increase by 7.5 cm (3 in) each year. It is not necessary for the nurse to report this finding to the provider.

   B. **CORRECT:** The head and chest circumference should be equal by 1 to 2 years of age, with the chest circumference continuing to increase in size until it exceeds the head circumference. The nurse should report this finding to the provider.

   C. The posterior fontanel closes by the age of 6 to 8 weeks, and the anterior fontanel closes by 12 to 18 months. It is not necessary for the nurse to report this finding to the provider.

   D. The current weight should be four times the birth weight at the age of 2½ years. It is not necessary for the nurse to report this finding to the provider.

   ℕ *NCLEX® Connection: Reduction of Risk Potential, Potential for Alterations in Body Systems*

2. A. The toddler should build a tower with six blocks at the age of 2 years.

   B. **CORRECT:** An 18-month-old should be able to throw a ball overhand.

   C. The toddler should be able to walk up and down stairs by placing both feet on each step at the age of 2 years.

   D. The toddler should be able to draw circles at the age of 2½ years.

   E. **CORRECT:** An 18-month-old should be able to use a spoon without rotation.

   ℕ *NCLEX® Connection: Health Promotion and Maintenance, Developmental Stages and Transitions*

3. A. **CORRECT:** Transitional objects, such as a favorite stuffed animal, provide a sense of security for toddlers. This is an age-appropriate activity for a 2-year-old.

   B. This is not an age-appropriate activity for a 2-year-old. It requires good gross motor skills and is appropriate for a 2½-year-old.

   C. Toddlers continue to develop gross motor skills and prefer parallel play where they play alongside of, instead of with, other children. This will make the concept of team soccer challenging for the toddler.

   D. This is not an age-appropriate activity for a 2-year-old. It requires good fine motor coordination. Drawing circles is appropriate for a 2½-year-old.

   ℕ *NCLEX® Connection: Health Promotion and Maintenance, Developmental Stages and Transitions*

4. A. **CORRECT:** Because the toddler is developing taste preferences, the development of food habits that will prevent dental caries should be included in the anticipatory guidance.

   B. Toddlers often experience physiologic anorexia and become fussy eaters because of a decreased appetite.

   C. **CORRECT:** Expression of bedtime fears is common for toddlers and should be included in the anticipatory guidance.

   D. **CORRECT:** Negativism and ritualism are exhibited by toddlers as they seek autonomy, and associated behaviors should be included in the anticipatory guidance.

   E. Screening for phenylketonuria occurs in the newborn, not the toddler.

   ℕ *NCLEX® Connection: Health Promotion and Maintenance, Aging Process*

A nurse is conducting a well-child visit with a 2-year-old. Use the ATI Active Learning Template: Growth and Development to complete this item.

DEVELOPMENTAL STAGE: Identify the toddler's developmental stage according to Piaget and Erikson.

NUTRITION: List three concepts to include when reinforcing teaching with the family.

INJURY PREVENTION: Identify two injury prevention methods to include in reinforcement of teaching with the family for each of the following categories.
- Bodily harm
- Drowning
- Burns
- Falls

Using the ATI Active Learning Template: Growth and Development

DEVELOPMENTAL STAGE
- Piaget: Preoperational stage
- Erikson: Autonomy vs. shame and doubt

NUTRITION
- Can switch from whole milk to low-fat milk after the age of 2 years.
- Trans fatty acids and saturated fats should be avoided.
- Diet should include 1 cup of fruit daily.
- Limit fruit juice to 4 to 6 oz per day.
- Cut food into small, bite-size pieces to prevent choking.
- Do not allow drinking or eating during play activities or while lying down.

INJURY PREVENTION
- Bodily harm
  - Keep sharp objects out of reach.
  - Lock firearms in a cabinet or box.
  - Teach toddlers stranger safety.
  - Do not leave toddlers unattended with animals.
- Drowning
  - Do not leave toddlers unattended in the bathtub.
  - Keep toilet lids closed.
  - Begin teaching toddlers water safety and to swim.
  - Keep bathroom doors closed.
- Burns
  - Check bath water temperature prior to toddler contact with water.
  - Set hot water heaters to less than 49° C (120° F).
  - Keep pot handles pointed to back of stove when cooking.
  - Cover electrical outlets.
  - Keep working smoke detectors in the home.
  - Apply sunscreen when toddler will be outside.
- Falls
  - Keep doors and windows locked.
  - Transition from a crib to a bed when the toddler reaches a height of 89 cm (35 in).
  - Use safety gates at the top and bottom of stairs.

ℕ *NCLEX® Connection: Health Promotion and Maintenance, Aging Process*

CHAPTER 5   *Health Promotion of Preschoolers (3 to 6 Years)*

EXPECTED GROWTH AND DEVELOPMENT

PHYSICAL DEVELOPMENT

WEIGHT: Preschoolers should gain about 2 to 3 kg (4.4 to 6.6 lb) per year.

HEIGHT: Preschoolers should grow about 6.5 to 9 cm (2.6 to 3.5 in) per year.

5.1 Average height and weight by age

	3-YEAR-OLD	4-YEAR-OLD	5-YEAR-OLD
WEIGHT	14.5 kg (32 lb)	16.5 kg (36.5 lb)	18.5 kg (41 lb)
HEIGHT	95 cm (37.5 in)	103 cm (40.5 in)	110 cm (43.5 in)

Preschoolers' bodies evolve away from the characteristically unsteady wide stances and protruding abdomens of toddlers into a more graceful postural alignment, allowing more symmetrical movement patterns.

FINE AND GROSS MOTOR SKILLS

Preschoolers should show improvement in fine motor skills, which will be displayed by activities like copying figures on paper and dressing independently.

5.2 Gross motor skills by age

3-YEAR-OLD	4-YEAR-OLD	5-YEAR-OLD
Rides a tricycle	Skips and hops on one foot	Jumps rope
Jumps off bottom step	Throws ball overhead	Walks backward with heel to toe
Stands on one foot for a few seconds	Catches ball accurately	Throws and catches a ball with ease

COGNITIVE DEVELOPMENT

Piaget: preoperational phase Q EBP
The phase of preconceptual thought transitions to intuitive thought around the age of 4 years. The phase of intuitive thought lasts until age of 7 years.
- The preschooler moves from totally egocentric thoughts to social awareness and the ability to consider the viewpoints of others.
- Preschoolers make judgments based on visual appearances. Variations in thinking during this age include the following.
  - **Magical thinking:** Believing thoughts have the power to cause events to take place.
  - **Egocentrism:** Concentrating attention upon oneself, self-centered. Lack of awareness that others have a different point of view.
  - **Animism:** Assigning lifelike qualities to inanimate objects.
  - **Centration:** Focusing on one aspect instead of considering all possible options.
  - **Time:** Beginning to understand the sequence of daily events. Time is best explained to preschoolers in relation to an event. By the end of the preschool years, they have a better comprehension of time-oriented words.

Language development

- The vocabulary of preschoolers increases to more than 2,100 words by the end of the fifth year.
- Preschoolers speak in sentences of three to four words at the ages of 3 and 4 years, and four to five words at the age of 4 to 5 years.
- This age group enjoys talking, and language becomes their primary method of communication.

PSYCHOSOCIAL DEVELOPMENT

Erikson: initiative vs. guilt Q EBP
- Preschoolers become energetic learners, despite not having all of the physical abilities necessary to be successful at everything.
- Guilt can occur when preschoolers believe they have misbehaved or when they are unable to accomplish a task.
- Guiding preschoolers to attempt activities within their capabilities while setting limits is recommended.

Kohlberg: moral development
- Early preschoolers continue in the good-bad orientation of the toddler years, and actions are taken based on whether or not it will result in reward or punishment.
- Older preschoolers primarily take actions based on satisfying their own personal needs, yet are beginning to understand the concepts of justice and fairness.

Self-concept development

Preschoolers feel good about themselves with regard to mastering skills that allow independence (dressing, feeding). During stress, insecurity, or illness, preschoolers can regress to previous immature behaviors or develop unfavorable habits (nose-picking, bedwetting, thumb-sucking).

Body-image changes

- Preschoolers begin to recognize differences in appearances, and identify what is considered acceptable and unacceptable.
- By the age of 5 years, preschoolers begin comparing themselves to their peers.
- Poor understanding of anatomy makes intrusive experiences (injections, cuts) frightening to preschoolers. Therefore, preschoolers believe it is important to use bandages after an injury.

Social development

- Preschoolers generally do not exhibit stranger anxiety and have less separation anxiety.
- Changes in their daily routine are tolerated, but it can cause them to develop more imaginary fears.
- Prolonged separation, such as during hospitalization, can provoke anxiety. Favorite toys and suitable play should be used to help ease preschoolers' fears.
- Pretend play is healthy and allows preschoolers to determine the difference between reality and fantasy.

AGE-APPROPRIATE ACTIVITIES Qpcc

Parallel play shifts to associative play during the preschool years. Play is not highly organized, but cooperation does exist between children.
- Playing with a ball
- Putting puzzles together
- Riding tricycles
- Playing pretend and dress-up activities
- Role-playing
- Hand puppets
- Painting
- Simple sewing
- Reading books
- Wading pools
- Sand boxes
- Skating
- Computer programs
- Musical toys
- Electronic games

HEALTH PROMOTION

IMMUNIZATIONS

The Centers for Disease Control and Prevention (CDC) immunization recommendations for healthy preschoolers 3 to 6 years of age Q EBP

4 TO 6 YEARS: Diphtheria and tetanus toxoids and pertussis (DTaP); measles, mumps, and rubella (MMR); varicella; and inactivated poliovirus (IPV)

3 TO 6 YEARS: Yearly seasonal influenza vaccine; trivalent inactivated influenza vaccine; or quadrivalent inactivated influenza vaccine

> Recommendations for immunizations change periodically. Check the CDC's website (www.cdc.gov) for current recommendations.

NUTRITION

- Preschoolers have a slight decrease in the number of calories required per unit of body weight. Their average daily intake is 1,800 calories or 90 kcal/kg. Fluid requirements also decrease to approximately 100 mL/kg/day, depending on health, environmental conditions, and level of activity.
- Finicky eating remains a common behavior in preschoolers, but they often become more willing to sample different foods by 5 years of age.
- Preschoolers need 13 to 19 g/day (0.46 to 0.67 oz/day) of protein. This amount increases with age. Daily dietary fiber intake should coincide with the preschooler's age plus 5 g. The recommended daily calcium intake for 3-year-olds is 700 mg, and for 4- and 5-year-olds it is 1,000 mg. It is important to ensure the preschooler's diet contains adequate nutrients, iron, folate, vitamin A, and vitamin C.
- Saturated fats should be less than 10% of preschoolers' total caloric intake each day. Total fat over several days should be 20% to 30% of total caloric intake. Cholesterol intake should be less than 300 g/day.
- With obesity rates in young children increasing, the American Academy of Pediatrics recommends that preschoolers have five servings of fruits and vegetables, 2 hr or less of screen time, and 1 hr of physical activity each day, and avoid sugar-sweetened beverages.

> Parents should follow the U.S. Department of Agriculture's healthy diet recommendations (www.choosemyplate.gov).

SLEEP AND REST

- On average, preschoolers need about 12 hr of sleep per day, and infrequently take daytime naps.
- Sleep disturbances frequently occur during early childhood, and problems range from difficulty going to bed to night terrors. Appropriate interventions vary, but can include the following.
  - Keep a consistent bedtime routine.
  - Use a nightlight in the room.
  - Provide the child with a favorite toy.
  - Leave a drink of water by the bed.
  - Reassure preschoolers who are frightened, but discourage sleeping with parents.

DENTAL HEALTH

- Eruption of deciduous (primary) teeth is finalized by the beginning of the preschool years.
- Parents need to assist and supervise brushing and flossing to ensure it is performed correctly to prevent dental caries.
- Trauma to teeth is common in preschoolers and should be immediately assessed by a dentist.

INJURY PREVENTION Qs

Bodily harm
- Firearms should be kept in locked cabinets or containers.
- Preschoolers should be taught stranger safety and awareness.
- Preschoolers should be taught to wear properly fitted protective equipment (helmet, pads, reflective clothing) when riding a bicycle.

Burns
- Hot water thermostats should be set at or less than 49° C (120° F).
- Working smoke detectors should be kept in the home.
- Preschoolers should have sunscreen applied when outside.
- Preschoolers should be taught proper actions in the event of a fire.

Drowning
- Preschoolers should not be left unattended in bathtubs.
- Preschoolers should be closely supervised when near the pool or any other body of water.
- Preschoolers should be taught to swim and basic water safety rules.

Motor-vehicle injuries
- Preschoolers should use a federally approved car restraint according to the manufacturer recommendations.
- When the forward-facing car seat is outgrown, the preschooler transitions to a booster seat.
- Children should use an approved car restraint system until they achieve a height of 145 cm (4 feet, 9 in) or 8 to 12 years old. QEBP
- The safest area for children is the back seat of the vehicle.
- Supervise preschool-age children when playing outside, and do not allow them to play near a curb or parked cars.
- Reinforce pedestrian safety rules to preschoolers.
  - Stand back from curb while waiting to cross the street.
  - Before crossing the street, look left, then right, then left again.
  - Walk on the left, facing traffic, when there are no sidewalks.
  - At night, wear light-colored clothing with fluorescent materials attached.

Application Exercises

1. A nurse is reinforcing teaching with the parent of a preschooler about methods to promote sleep. Which of the following statements by the parent indicates an understanding of the instructions?

   A. "I will sleep in the bed with my child if she wakes up during the night."

   B. "I will allow my child to stay up an additional 2 hours on weekend nights."

   C. "I will let my child watch television for 30 minutes just before bedtime each night."

   D. "I will keep a dim light on in my child's room during the night."

2. A nurse in a provider's office is preparing to administer immunizations to a 5-year-old child. Which of the following immunizations should the nurse plan to administer? (Select all that apply.)

   A. Diphtheria, tetanus, pertussis (DTaP)

   B. Inactivated poliovirus (IPV)

   C. Measles, mumps, rubella (MMR)

   D. Pneumococcal (PCV)

   E. Haemophilus influenzae type B (Hib)

3. A nurse is assisting with a nutrition education program for a group of parents of preschoolers. Which of the following dietary guidelines should the nurse plan to include?

   A. Saturated fats should equal 20% of total daily caloric intake.

   B. Average intake should be 1,800 calories per day.

   C. Daily intake of fruits and vegetables should total 2 servings.

   D. Protein intake should total 8 to 10 g daily.

4. A nurse is assisting the provider with a developmental screening on a 3-year-old child. Which of the following gross motor skills should the nurse expect the child to perform?

   A. Ride a tricycle

   B. Hop on one foot

   C. Jump rope

   D. Throw a ball overhead

5. A nurse is caring for a preschooler who says she needs to leave the hospital because her doll is scared to be at home alone. The nurse recognizes that the child is exhibiting which of the following characteristics of preoperational thought?

   A. Egocentrism

   B. Centration

   C. Animism

   D. Magical thinking

PRACTICE Active Learning Scenario

A nurse is providing anticipatory guidance to the parents of a preschool-age child. Use the ATI Active Learning Template: Growth and Development to complete this item.

PHYSICAL DEVELOPMENT: Identify general expectations for height and weight during the preschool years.

COGNITIVE DEVELOPMENT: List at least two concepts related to language development in preschoolers.

AGE-APPROPRIATE ACTIVITIES: List at least five age-appropriate activities for preschoolers.

INJURY PREVENTION: Identify at least two pedestrian safety rules parents should teach preschoolers.

Application Exercises Key

1. A. The parent should promote a consistent bedtime ritual for the preschooler and ignore attention-seeking behavior. The child should not be allowed to sleep in the same bed as the parent.

   B. The parent should promote a consistent bedtime routine and avoid allowing the child to stay up past a reasonable hour on the weekends.

   C. Watching television prior to bed can cause the child to resist and delay sleep. It can also cause the preschooler to have nightmares, which can lead to difficulty waking in the mornings.

   D. **CORRECT:** Leaving a dim light on in the child's room is a recommended method to promote sleep for a preschool-age child. Other recommended measures include leaving a drink of water on the preschooler's nightstand and allowing the child to sleep with their favorite toy or stuffed-animal.

   Ⓝ *NCLEX® Connection: Basic Care and Comfort, Rest and Sleep*

2. A. **CORRECT:** DTaP is a recommended immunization for 4- to 6-year-old children, and should be administered by the nurse during this visit.

   B. **CORRECT:** IPV is a recommended immunization for 4- to 6-year-old children, and should be administered by the nurse during this visit.

   C. **CORRECT:** MMR is a recommended immunization for 4- to 6-year-old children, and should be administered by the nurse during this visit.

   D. PCV is given as a series of immunizations in the first 15 months of life, and is not recommended for 4- to 6-year-old children.

   E. Hib is given as a series of immunizations in the first 15 months of life, and is not recommended for 4- to 6-year-old children.

   Ⓝ *NCLEX® Connection: Health Promotion and Maintenance, Health Promotion/Disease Prevention*

3. A. Preschoolers' saturated fats should be less than 10% of their total caloric intake each day, and total fat over several days should be 20% to 30%.

   B. **CORRECT:** Preschoolers should consume an average of 1,800 calories or 90 kcal/kg/day.

   C. Preschoolers should consume a total of 5 servings of fruits and vegetables per day.

   D. Preschoolers need to consume 13 to 19 g protein each day, and this amount increases with age.

   Ⓝ *NCLEX® Connection: Basic Care and Comfort, Nutrition and Oral Hydration*

4. A. **CORRECT:** The nurse should expect a 3-year-old child to perform the gross motor skill of riding a tricycle as an indication of expected developmental achievement.

   B. Hopping on one foot is an expected gross motor skill for a 4-year-old child.

   C. Jumping rope is an expected gross motor skill for a 5-year-old child.

   D. Throwing a ball overhead is an expected gross motor skill for a 4-year-old child.

   Ⓝ *NCLEX® Connection: Health Promotion and Maintenance, Developmental Stages and Transitions*

5. A. Egocentrism occurs when the child is unable to see another person's perspective or point of view (self-centered).

   B. Centration occurs when the child focuses on one aspect of something instead of considering the whole.

   C. **CORRECT:** The nurse should recognize that the preschooler is demonstrating the preoperational thought characteristics of animism. This behavior occurs when the child gives living qualities to inanimate objects, such as a doll feeling scared.

   D. Magical thinking occurs when the child believes their thoughts have the power to cause an event to occur.

   Ⓝ *NCLEX® Connection: Health Promotion and Maintenance, Developmental Stages and Transitions*

PRACTICE Answer

Using the ATI Active Learning Template: Growth and Development

PHYSICAL DEVELOPMENT
- Weight: Preschoolers should gain about 2 to 3 kg (4.4 to 6.6 lb) per year.
- Height: Preschoolers should grow about 6.5 to 9 cm (2.6 to 3.5 in) per year.

COGNITIVE DEVELOPMENT
- Vocabulary increases to more than 2,100 words by the end of the fifth year.
- Speak in sentences of three to four words at the ages of 3 and 4 years.
- Speak in sentences of four to five words at the age of 4 to 5 years.
- Enjoy talking, and language becomes their primary method of communication.

AGE-APPROPRIATE ACTIVITIES
- Putting puzzles together
- Playing with a ball
- Playing pretend and dress-up activities
- Painting
- Role-playing
- Riding tricycles
- Simple sewing
- Reading books
- Sandboxes
- Wading pools
- Skating
- Computer programs
- Musical toys
- Electronic games

INJURY PREVENTION
- Stand back from the curb while waiting to cross the street.
- Before crossing the street, look left, then right, then left again.
- Walk on the left, facing traffic, when there are no sidewalks.
- At night, wear light-colored clothing with fluorescent materials attached.

Ⓝ *NCLEX® Connection: Health Promotion and Maintenance, Developmental Stages and Transitions*

CHAPTER 6 **Health Promotion of School-Age Children (6 to 12 Years)**

EXPECTED GROWTH AND DEVELOPMENT

PHYSICAL DEVELOPMENT

Weight: School-age children gain about 2 to 3 kg (4.4 to 6.6 lb) per year.

Height: School-age children grow about 5 cm (2 in) per year.

Prepubescence
- Preadolescence is typically when prepubescence occurs.
- Onset of physiologic changes begins around the age of 9 years, particularly in females.
- Rapid growth in height and weight occurs.
- Differences in the rate of growth and maturation between males and females becomes apparent.
- Visible sexual maturation is minimal in males during preadolescence.
- Permanent teeth erupt.
- Bladder capacity differs with each child, but remains greater in females than males.
- Immune system improves.
- Bones continue to ossify.

COGNITIVE DEVELOPMENT

Piaget: concrete operations Q̃EBP
- Transitions from perceptual to conceptual thinking. The concrete operational stage takes place between the ages of 7 to 11 years old.
- Masters the concept of conservation
  - Realizes that physical elements do not magically appear and disappear.
  - Conservation of mass is understood first, followed by weight, and then volume.
- Learns to tell time
- Develops an awareness of the connection between things and ideas
- Classifies more complex information
- Acquires the ability to read, which expands knowledge base and increases comprehension
- Conventional academic learning starts between 5 and 6 years old
- Able to see the perspective of others
- Able to solve problems

PSYCHOSOCIAL DEVELOPMENT

Erikson: industry vs. inferiority Q̃EBP
- A sense of industry is achieved through the development of skills and knowledge that allows the child to provide meaningful contributions to society.
- A sense of accomplishment is gained through the ability to cooperate and compete with others.
- Children should be challenged with tasks that need to be accomplished, and be allowed to work through individual differences in order to complete the tasks.
- Creating a reward system that offers incentives or benefits for the successful mastery of skills can create a sense of inferiority in children who are unable to complete or acquire the skills.
- Children should be taught that not everyone will master every skill at the same time, and that they may excel at certain activities more than others.

Moral development

EARLY SCHOOL-AGE YEARS
- Do not understand the reasoning behind rules and expectations for behavior.
- Believe what they think is wrong, and what others tell them is right.
- Judgment is guided by rewards and punishment.
- Children 6 to 7 years old might view accidents as discipline for misconduct or misbehavior.

LATER SCHOOL-AGE YEARS
- Able to judge an act by the purpose of it rather than just the ramification of performing it.
- Understands different points of view instead of just whether an act is right or wrong.
- Comprehends and accepts the principle of treating others as they would like to be treated.

Self-concept development

- School-age children develop an awareness of themselves in relation to others, as well as an understanding of personal values, abilities, and physical characteristics.
- Confidence is gained through establishing a positive self-concept, which leads to feelings of worthiness and the perception that they provide significant contributions to society.
- Parents continue to influence the school-age child's self-ideals, but by middle childhood the opinions of peers and teachers become more valuable and beneficial to them.

Body-image changes

- Solidification of body image occurs.
- Curiosity about sexuality should be addressed with education regarding sexual development and the reproductive process.
- School-age children are more modest than preschoolers and place more emphasis on privacy issues.

Social development

- Peer groups play an important part in social development. Peer pressure begins to take effect.
- Social activities and best friends are popular.
- Association with a peer group or clique is an important part of social development with school-age children, and becomes vital to socialization.
- Bullying is unwanted, aggressive behavior among school-age children that involves a real or perceived imbalance of power. These actions are intended to cause harm and are sometimes attributed to poor relationships with peers and difficulty identifying with a group. Bullying can be reduced or prevented through encouragement from family members, involvement and interference of school personnel, and relationships with positive peer groups.
- School-age children prefer the company of same-gender companions, but can begin developing an interest in other genders toward the end of the school-age years.
- Most relationships come from school associations.

AGE-APPROPRIATE ACTIVITIES

Competitive and cooperative play is predominant. Q**pcc**
- Team play
- Clubs and organizations
- Collect objects
- Engage in hobbies
- Simple paintings or drawings
- Make crafts
- Build models
- Read romance or adventure stories
- Play board and card games.
- Join organized, competitive sports for skill-building.

HEALTH PROMOTION

IMMUNIZATIONS

The Centers for Disease Control and Prevention (CDC) immunization recommendations for healthy school-age children 6 to 12 years of age include the following. Q**EBP**
- If not given between 4 and 5 years of age, children should receive the following vaccines by 6 years of age: diphtheria and tetanus toxoids and pertussis (DTaP); inactivated poliovirus; measles, mumps, and rubella (MMR); and varicella.
- Yearly seasonal influenza vaccine: trivalent inactivated influenza vaccine (TIV)
- 11 to 12 years: tetanus and diphtheria toxoids and pertussis vaccine (Tdap); human papillomavirus vaccine (HPV2 or HPV4 in three doses for females, HPV4 for males); and meningococcal (MCV4).

Recommendations for immunizations change periodically. Check the CDC's website (www.cdc.gov) for current recommendations.

HEALTH SCREENINGS

Scoliosis: School-age children should be screened for scoliosis by examining for a lateral curvature of the spine before and during growth spurts. Screening can take place at schools or at health care facilities.

NUTRITION

- By the end of the school-age years, children should be consuming adult portions of food. They also need quality nutritious snacks.
- Obesity is an increasing concern of this age group that predisposes children to low self-esteem, diabetes, heart disease, and high blood pressure. Advise parents to: Q**EBP**
  - Avoid using food as a reward.
  - Encourage physical activity.
  - Ensure that a balanced diet is consumed by following the U.S. Department of Agriculture's healthy diet recommendations (www.choosemyplate.gov).
  - Encourage children to make healthy food selections for meals and snacks.
  - Avoid eating fast food frequently.
  - Discourage skipping meals.
  - Model healthy behaviors.

SLEEP AND REST

- Required sleep is highly variable in the school-age years and dependent on the following.
  - Age
  - Level of activity
  - Health status
- Approximately 9 hr of sleep is needed each night at the age of 11 years.
- Resistance to bedtime is sometimes experienced around the age of 8 and 9 years, and again around the age of 11 years, but is typically resolved by the age of 12 years.

DENTAL HEALTH

- The first permanent teeth erupt around 6 years of age.
- Children should brush after meals and snacks, and at bedtime with a fluoride toothpaste.
- Children should floss daily.
- Children should have regular checkups with a dentist.

INJURY PREVENTION Q**s**

Bodily harm
- Keep firearms in locked cabinets or boxes.
- Identify safe play areas.
- Reinforce stranger safety to children.
- Encourage children to wear helmets and pads (when roller skating, skateboarding, bicycling, riding scooters, skiing, snowboarding).

Burns
- Reinforce fire safety and potential burn hazards.
- Keep working smoke detectors in the home.
- Children should use sunscreen when outside.
- Instruct children to take safety precautions while cooking.

Drowning

- Children should be supervised when swimming or when near a body of water.
- Children should be taught to swim.
- Check depth of water before allowing children to dive.
- Encourage breaks to prevent children from becoming over-tired.

Motor-vehicle injuries

- Children should use an approved car restraint system until they achieve a height of 145 cm (4 feet, 9 inches). Qs
- Reinforce correct seat belt use when no longer using a car restraint system or booster seat.
- The safest area for children is the backseat of the car.
- Never let children ride in the bed of a pickup truck.
- Reinforce safe pedestrian behaviors.

Poisoning/substance abuse Qs

- Cleaners and chemicals should be kept in locked cabinets or out of reach of younger children.
- Children should be instructed and encouraged to say "no" to substance abuse.

PRACTICE Active Learning Scenario

A nurse is providing anticipatory guidance to the parents of a school-age child. Use the ATI Active Learning Template: Growth and Development to complete this item.

DEVELOPMENTAL STAGE: Identify the child's developmental stage according to Piaget and Erikson.

PHYSICAL DEVELOPMENT: Identify three facts relevant to the child's physical development.

NUTRITION: List three strategies the family can implement to reduce the risk of obesity.

Application Exercises

1. A nurse is discussing prepubescence and preadolescence with a group of parents of school-age children. Which of the following information should the nurse include in the discussion?

   A. Initial physiologic changes appear during early childhood.

   B. Changes in height and weight occur slowly during this period.

   C. Growth differences between males and females become evident.

   D. Indications of sexual maturation become highly visible in males.

2. A nurse in a provider's office is preparing to administer immunizations to an 11-year-old child. Which of the following immunizations should the nurse plan to administer? (Select all that apply.)

   A. Trivalent inactivated influenza (TIV)

   B. Pneumococcal (PCV)

   C. Meningococcal (MCV4)

   D. Tetanus and diphtheria toxoids and pertussis (Tdap)

   E. Rotavirus (RV)

3. A nurse is reinforcing teaching about recommended activities with the parents of a school-age child. Which of the following activities should the nurse suggest to the parents?

   A. Team play

   B. Video communication

   C. Join a charitable organization

   D. Follow a sports team

4. A nurse is assisting with an in-service for a group of parents about child safety during the school-age years. Which of the following information should the nurse include? (Select all that apply.)

   A. Placing a gate on stairs at the top and bottom

   B. Wearing helmets when riding bicycles or skateboarding

   C. Riding safely in the bed of pickup trucks

   D. Implementing firearm safety

   E. Wearing seat belts when riding in a vehicle

Application Exercises Key

1. A. Initial physiologic changes appear toward the end of middle childhood, around the age of 9 years.

   B. Changes in height and weight occur rapidly during this time period.

   C. **CORRECT:** The nurse should include in the discussion that growth differences between males and females become evident.

   D. Visible indications of sexual maturation are minimal in males.

   Ⓝ *NCLEX® Connection: Health Promotion and Maintenance, Developmental Stages and Transitions*

2. A. **CORRECT:** TIV is a recommended immunization for 11-year-olds and should be administered by the nurse.

   B. PCV is recommended as a series of immunizations in the first 15 months of life.

   C. **CORRECT:** MCV4 is a recommended immunization for 11-year-olds and should be administered by the nurse.

   D. **CORRECT:** Tdap is a recommended immunization for 11-year-olds and should be administered by the nurse.

   E. RV is recommended as a series of immunizations administered in the first 6 months of life.

   Ⓝ *NCLEX® Connection: Health Promotion and Maintenance, Health Promotion/Disease Prevention*

3. A. **CORRECT:** The nurse should recommend activities such as team play for the school-age child. Team play contributes to skill growth, as well as social and intellectual development.

   B. Video communication is used by adolescents, rather than school-age children, to interact with peers.

   C. Joining a charitable organization is an activity the nurse should recommend for an adolescent, rather than a school-age child.

   D. Following a sports team's wins or losses is an activity the nurse should recommend for an adolescent, rather than a school-age child.

   Ⓝ *NCLEX® Connection: Health Promotion and Maintenance, Developmental Stages and Transitions*

4. A. Gating stairs at the top and bottom should not be included in the in-service. This is important information to include when reinforcing teaching about safety during infant and toddler years.

   B. **CORRECT:** When contributing information about safety in the school-age years, the nurse should include information about wearing helmets when riding bicycles or skateboarding.

   C. The nurse should reinforce that it is never safe to ride in the bed of a pickup truck.

   D. **CORRECT:** The nurse should include information about implementing firearm safety.

   E. **CORRECT:** The nurse should include information about wearing seat belts.

   Ⓝ *NCLEX® Connection: Safety and Infection Control, Accident/Error/Injury Prevention*

PRACTICE Answer

Using the ATI Active Learning Template: Growth and Development

DEVELOPMENTAL STAGE
- Piaget: concrete operations
- Erikson: industry vs. inferiority

PHYSICAL DEVELOPMENT
- Will gain 2 to 3 kg (4.4 to 6.6 lb) per year.
- Will grow about 5 cm (2 in) per year.
- Bladder capacity differs with each child, but generally remains greater in females rather than males.
- Immune system improves.
- Bones continue to ossify.

NUTRITION
- Avoid using food as a reward.
- Encourage physical activity.
- Ensure a balanced diet is consumed.
- Encourage children to select healthy foods and snacks.
- Avoid eating fast food frequently.
- Discourage skipping meals.
- Model healthy behaviors.

Ⓝ *NCLEX® Connection: Health Promotion and Maintenance, Developmental Stages and Transitions*

UNIT 1   FOUNDATIONS OF NURSING CARE OF CHILDREN

SECTION: PERSPECTIVES OF NURSING CARE OF CHILDREN

CHAPTER 7   *Health Promotion of Adolescents (12 to 20 Years)*

EXPECTED GROWTH AND DEVELOPMENT

PHYSICAL DEVELOPMENT

- The final 20% to 25% of height is achieved during puberty.
- Acne can appear during adolescence.
- Females stop growing about 2 to 2.5 years after the onset of menarche. They grow 5 to 20 cm (2 to 8 in) and gain 7 to 25 kg (15.4 to 55.1 lb).
- Males stop growing at around 18 to 20 years of age. They grow 10 to 30 cm (4 to 12 in) and gain 7 to 30 kg (15.4 to 66.1 lb).
- In females, sexual maturation occurs in the following order.
  - Breast development
  - Pubic hair growth (some females experience hair growth before breast development)
  - Axillary hair growth
  - Menstruation
- In males, sexual maturation occurs in the following order.
  - Testicular enlargement
  - Pubic hair growth
  - Penile enlargement
  - Growth of axillary hair
  - Facial hair growth
  - Vocal changes

COGNITIVE DEVELOPMENT

Piaget: formal operations
- Able to think through more than two categories of variables concurrently
- Capable of evaluating the quality of their own thinking
- Able to maintain focus and are attentive for longer periods of time
- Highly imaginative and idealistic
- Increasingly capable of using formal logic to make decisions
- Think beyond current circumstances
- Able to understand how the actions of an individual influence others

PSYCHOSOCIAL DEVELOPMENT

Erikson: identity vs. role confusion
- Adolescents develop a sense of personal identity and come to view themselves as unique individuals.
- Group identity: Adolescents become part of a peer group that greatly influences behavior.

Sexual identity

- Begins with close, same-sex friendships during early adolescence, which sometimes involve sexual experimentation driven by curiosity.
- Self-exploration occurs through masturbation.
- Transition from friendships to intimate relationships during adolescence.
- In late adolescence, sexual identity typically is formed through the integration of sexual experiences, feelings, and knowledge.

Health perceptions

Adolescents can view themselves as invincible to bad outcomes of risky behaviors.

Moral development

- Solves moral dilemma using internalized moral principles.
- Questions relevance of existing moral values to society and individuals.

Self-concept development

- View themselves in relation to similarities with peers during early adolescence.
- View themselves according to their unique characteristics as the adolescent years progress.

Body-image changes

- Base their own characteristics on comparisons with peers.
- The image established during adolescence is retained throughout life.

Social development

- Peer relationships develop. These relationships act as a support system for adolescents.
- Best-friend relationships are more stable and longer-lasting than they were in previous years.
- Parent-child relationships change to allow for a greater sense of independence.

HEALTH PROMOTION

IMMUNIZATIONS

Centers for Disease Control and Prevention (CDC) recommendations for healthy adolescents 13 to 18 years old include catch-up doses of any recommended immunizations not received at 11 to 12 years old. **Q**EBP

- Yearly seasonal influenza vaccine
- 16 to 18 years: Meningococcal (MCV4) booster is recommended if first dose was received between the ages of 13 and 15 years. A booster dose is not needed if the first dose is received at age 16 or older.

> Recommendations for immunizations change periodically. Check the CDC's website (www.cdc.gov) for current recommendations.

HEALTH SCREENINGS

Screenings for scoliosis should continue during the adolescent years. These screenings should include an examination for a lateral curvature of the spine before and during growth spurts. Screenings can take place at school or at a health care facility.

NUTRITION

- Rapid growth and high metabolism require increases in quality nutrients and make adolescents unable to tolerate caloric restrictions.
  - During times of rapid growth, additional calcium, iron, protein, and zinc are needed.
  - Inadequate intake of folic acid, vitamin B_6, vitamin A, iron, calcium, and zinc is common. Combined with other factors, this can result in the adolescent developing chronic diseases later in life, and increases the risk of obesity.
- Overeating and undereating present challenges during the adolescent years. Yearly checks of height, weight, and BMI for age are needed to identify nutritional issues and intervene early.
- Advise parents to:
  - Avoid using food as a reward.
  - Emphasize physical activity.
  - Ensure that a balanced diet is consumed by following the U.S. Department of Agriculture's healthy diet recommendations (www.choosemyplate.gov).
  - Encourage adolescents to make healthy food selections for meals and snacks.

SLEEP AND REST

- Adolescents should get about 9 hr of sleep each night.
- Sleep habits change with puberty due to increased metabolism and rapid growth.
- Adolescents tend to stay up late, sleep in later in the morning, and sleep more than during the school-age years.
- During periods of active growth, the need for sleep increases.

DENTAL HEALTH

- Corrective appliances are most common with this age group.
- Adolescents should brush after meals and snacks, and at bedtime using a toothpaste that contains fluoride.
- Adolescents should floss daily.
- Adolescents should have regular checkups.
- Fluoridated water is recommended to promote growth of tooth enamel.

SEXUALITY

- Provide adolescents with accurate information, and discuss what is heard from peers.
- Emphasize abstinence and practicing safe sex.
- Provide information about preventing sexually transmitted infections and pregnancy.
- Promote an atmosphere where adolescents are comfortable asking questions.
- Assist adolescents with problem-solving and decision-making skills.

INJURY PREVENTION Qs

Bodily harm
- Keep firearms unloaded and in a locked cabinet or box.
- Reinforce proper use of sporting equipment prior to use.
- Insist on use of a helmet and pads when roller skating, skateboarding, bicycling, riding scooters, skiing, and snowboarding.
- Be aware of changes in mood. Monitor for self-harm in adolescents who are at risk. Watch for the following.
  - Poor school performance
  - Lack of interest in things that were of interest to the adolescent in the past
  - Social isolation
  - Disturbances in sleep or appetite
  - Expression of suicidal thoughts

Burns
- Reinforce fire safety.
- Adolescents should apply sunscreen when outside.
- Adolescents should avoid tanning beds.

Drowning
- Encourage adolescents to learn how to swim.
- Advise adolescents not to swim alone.

Motor-vehicle injuries
- Encourage attendance at drivers' education courses. Emphasize the need for adherence to seat belt use.
- Insist on helmet use with motorcycles
- Discuss the dangers of using cell phones or texting while driving and enforce laws regarding use.
- Reinforce the dangers of combining substance use with driving.
- Role model desired behavior.

Substance use
- Monitor for indications of substance use disorders in adolescents who are at risk.
- Encourage adolescents to say "no" to harmful substances and alcohol.
- Present a no-tolerance attitude.

Application Exercises

1. A nurse is reinforcing teaching with a group of parents of early adolescent females about expected changes during puberty. Which of the following parent statements indicates an understanding of the teaching?

   A. "Females usually stop growing about 2 years after menarche."

   B. "Females are expected to gain about 65 pounds during puberty."

   C. "Females experience menstruation prior to breast development."

   D. "Females typically grow more than 10 inches during puberty."

2. A nurse is reinforcing teaching about health promotion with the parent of a 13-year-old adolescent. Which of the following screenings should the nurse recommend? (Select all that apply.)

   A. Body mass index

   B. Blood lead level

   C. 24-hr dietary recall

   D. Weight

   E. Scoliosis

3. A nurse is caring for an adolescent whose mother expresses concerns about her adolescent sleeping long hours on weekends. The nurse should inform the mother that which of the following issues require additional sleep?

   A. Sleep terrors

   B. Rapid growth

   C. Elevated zinc levels

   D. Slowed metabolism

4. A school nurse is preparing a class about male puberty. Which of the following manifestations should the nurse identify as occurring first when sexual maturation begins?

   A. Pubic hair growth

   B. Vocal changes

   C. Testicular enlargement

   D. Facial hair growth

PRACTICE Active Learning Scenario

A nurse is assisting with the preparation of an educational program for a group of parents of adolescents. Use the ATI Active Learning Template: Growth and Development to complete this item.

DEVELOPMENTAL STAGE: Identify adolescent developmental stages according to Piaget and Erikson.

COGNITIVE DEVELOPMENT: List five cognitive developmental tasks the adolescent should accomplish.

INJURY PREVENTION: Identify three injury prevention methods in each of the following categories.

- Bodily harm
- Motor vehicle injuries

Application Exercises Key

1. A. **CORRECT:** Females usually stop growing about 2 to 2 ½ years after menarche. This statement indicates that the parent understands the teaching.

   B. Females are expected to gain 7 to 25 kg (15.5 to 55 lb) during puberty.

   C. Breast development is usually the first manifestation of sexual maturity in females, and appears before menstruation.

   D. Females typically grow 5 to 20 cm (2 to 8 in) during puberty.

   Ⓝ *NCLEX® Connection: Health Promotion and Maintenance, Developmental Stages and Transitions*

2. A. **CORRECT:** The nurse should recommend that the adolescent have a body mass index screening annually to provide for early identification of and intervention for nutritional issues.

   B. Blood lead level screenings are recommended for children at the age of 1 and 2 years, and for children between the ages of 3 and 6 years who have not previously been screened.

   C. A 24-hr dietary recall is not a routine screening for an adolescent.

   D. **CORRECT:** The nurse should recommend that the adolescent have a weight screening annually to provide for early identification of and intervention for nutritional issues.

   E. **CORRECT:** The nurse should recommend that the adolescent have a scoliosis screening to check for lateral curvature of the spine.

   Ⓝ *NCLEX® Connection: Health Promotion and Maintenance, Health Promotion/Disease Prevention*

3. A. Sleep terrors occur most often in preschool-age children and do not contribute to the adolescent's need for additional sleep.

   B. **CORRECT:** Rapid growth during the adolescent years results in the need for additional sleep. Adolescents should get about 9 hr of sleep each night.

   C. Zinc levels do not typically elevate during the adolescent years and do not contribute to the adolescent's need for additional sleep. Zinc is often identified as deficient due to inadequate dietary intake during adolescence.

   D. An increased metabolism contributes to the adolescent's need for additional sleep.

   Ⓝ *NCLEX® Connection: Basic Care and Comfort, Rest and Sleep*

4. A. The nurse should identify pubic hair growth as a manifestation of sexual maturation in males. However, evidence-based practice indicates that another manifestation occurs first.

   B. The nurse should identify vocal changes as a manifestation of sexual maturation in males. However, evidence-based practice indicates that another manifestation occurs first.

   C. **CORRECT:** According to evidence-based practice the nurse should identify testicular enlargement as the first manifestation of sexual maturation in males.

   D. The nurse should identify facial hair growth as a manifestation of sexual maturation in males. However, evidence-based practice indicates that another manifestation occurs first.

   Ⓝ *NCLEX® Connection: Health Promotion and Maintenance, Developmental Stages and Transitions*

PRACTICE Answer

Using the ATI Active Learning Template: Growth and Development

DEVELOPMENTAL STAGE
- Piaget: formal operations
- Erikson: identity vs. role confusion
  - Adolescents develop a sense of personal identity and come to view themselves as unique individuals.
  - Group identity: Adolescents become part of a peer group that greatly influences behavior.

COGNITIVE DEVELOPMENT
- Able to think through more than two categories of variables concurrently
- Capable of evaluating the quality of own thinking
- Able to maintain attention for longer periods of time
- Highly imaginative and idealistic
- Increasingly capable of using formal logic to make decisions
- Think beyond current circumstances
- Understand how the actions of an individual influence others

INJURY PREVENTION
- Bodily injury
  - Keep firearms unloaded and in a locked cabinet or box.
  - Reinforce proper use of sporting equipment prior to use.
  - Insist on use of a helmet and pads when roller skating, skateboarding, bicycling, riding scooters, skiing, and snowboarding.
  - Be aware of changes in mood. Continuously monitor adolescents at risk for self-harm.
- Motor vehicle injuries
  - Encourage attendance at drivers' education courses.
  - Emphasize the need for adherence to seat belt use.
  - Discourage use of cell phones while driving and enforce laws regarding use.
  - Reinforce the dangers of combining substance abuse with driving.
  - Role-model desired behavior.

Ⓝ *NCLEX® Connection: Health Promotion and Maintenance, Developmental Stages and Transitions*

ⓝ NCLEX® Connections

When reviewing the following chapters, keep in mind the relevant topics and tasks of the NCLEX outline, in particular:

Health Promotion and Maintenance

AGING PROCESS: Provide care that meets the needs of the preschool, school-age, and adolescent client ages 3 through 17 years.

DEVELOPMENTAL STAGES AND TRANSITIONS
Identify occurrence of expected body image changes.

Compare the client's development to norms.

Modify approaches to care in accordance with the client's development stage.

HEALTH PROMOTION/DISEASE PREVENTION: Provide assistance for screening examinations (scoliosis, breast and testicular self-examinations, blood pressure check).

Psychosocial Integrity

CULTURAL AWARENESS: Identify importance of client culture/ethnicity when planning/providing/monitoring care.

END-OF-LIFE CONCEPTS: Provide care or support for the client/family at end-of-life.

Basic Care and Comfort

NONPHARMACOLOGICAL COMFORT INTERVENTIONS
Assist in planning comfort interventions for the client with impaired comfort.

Monitor client nonverbal signs of pain/discomfort.

Evaluate pain using standardized rating scales.

Pharmacological Therapies

EXPECTED ACTIONS/OUTCOMES: Apply knowledge of pathophysiology when addressing client pharmacological agents.

MEDICATION ADMINISTRATION
Administer medication by oral route.

Administer a subcutaneous, intradermal, or intramuscular medication.

Administer medication by ear, eye, nose, inhalation, rectum, vagina, or skin route.

CHAPTER 8 **Safe Administration of Medication**

Growth and organ system maturity affect the metabolism and excretion of medications in infants and children. Administration of medications to the pediatric population can be challenging and requires critical thinking, nursing patience, and creativity. Pediatric dosages are based on age, body weight, and body surface area.

DATA COLLECTION

- Medication and food allergies
- Appropriateness of medication dose for age and weight
- Child's developmental age
- Child's physiological and psychological condition
- Tissue and skin integrity when administering intramuscular (IM), subcutaneous, and topical medications
- Intravenous (IV) patency when administering IV medications
- Compatibility with other prescribed medications

NURSING INTERVENTIONS

MEDICATION ADMINISTRATION

- Calculate the safe dosage for medication. **Qs**
- Notify the charge nurse and provider if medication dosage is determined to be outside the safe dosage range, and for any questions about medication preparation or route.
- Double-check high-risk and facility-regulated medications with another nurse.
- Use two client identifiers prior to administration (client name, date of birth). Use parent(s) for verification of infants or nonverbal children. Two identifiers from the ID band must be confirmed (client name, date of birth, hospital identification number).
- Determine parental involvement with administration.
- Allow the child to make appropriate choices regarding administration (choosing the left or right leg, whether the parent or nurse will administer the medication).
- Prepare the child according to age and developmental stage.

Oral

This route of medication administration is preferred for children.
- Determine the child's ability to swallow pills.
- Use the smallest measuring device for doses of liquid medication. Use an oral medication syringe for smaller amounts, and a medication cup for larger amounts.
- Avoid measuring liquid medication in a teaspoon or tablespoon.
- Avoid mixing medication with formula or putting it in a bottle of formula because the infant might not take the entire feeding, and the medication can alter the taste of the formula.
- Hold infants in a semireclining position similar to a feeding position.
- Hold small children in an upright position to prevent aspiration.
- Administer the medication in the side of the mouth in small amounts. This allows the infant or child to swallow.
- Only use the droppers that come with the medication for measurement.
- Stroke infants under the chin to promote swallowing while holding cheeks together.
- Reinforce teaching with the child to swallow tablets that aren't available in liquid form and can't be crushed. Instruct in short sessions using verbal instruction, demonstration, and positive reinforcement.
- Provide atraumatic care.
  ○ Mix the medication in a small amount of nonessential food (applesauce, sherbet).
  ○ Offer juice or a snack after administration if not contraindicated.
  ○ Add flavoring to medications as available.
  ○ Use a nipple to allow the infant to suck the medication.
- Administer medications via a feeding tube.
  ○ Confirm placement.
  ○ Use liquid formulation.
  ○ Do not add medication to the formula bag.
  ○ Flush with water to clear tubing of residual medication.

Optic

- Place the child in a supine or sitting position.
- Extend the child's head and ask the child to look up.
- Pull the lower eyelid downward and apply medication in the pocket.
- Administer ointments before nap or bedtime.
- Provide atraumatic care.
  ○ If an infant clenches his eyes closed, place the drops in the nasal corner. When the infant opens his eyes, the medication will enter the eye.
  ○ Apply light pressure to the lacrimal punctum for 1 min to prevent unpleasant taste.
  ○ Play games with younger children.

Otic

- Place the child in a prone or supine position with the affected ear upward.
- Children younger than 3 years: Pull the pinna downward and straight back.
- Children older than 3 years: Pull the pinna upward and back.
- Provide atraumatic care.
  - Allow refrigerated medications to warm to room temperature prior to administration.
  - Massage the outer area for a few minutes following administration.
  - Play games with younger children.

Nasal

- Position the child with the head extended.
- Use a football hold for infants.
- Provide atraumatic care.
  - Insert the tip into the naris vertically, then angle it prior to administration.
  - Play games with younger children.

Aerosol

- Use a mask for younger children.
- Provide atraumatic care.
  - Allow parents to hold the child during treatment.
  - Use distraction.

Rectal

- Insert beyond both rectal sphincters.
- Hold the buttocks gently together for 5 to 10 min.
- Halve the medication lengthwise, if necessary.
- Provide atraumatic care.
  - Perform the procedure quickly.
  - Use distraction.

Injection

- Change needle if it pierced a rubber stopper on a vial.
- Secure the infant or child prior to injections.
- Determine the need for assistance.
- Avoid tracking (leaking) of medication.
- When selecting sites, consider the following.
  - Medication amount, viscosity, and type
  - Muscle mass, condition, access of site, and potential for contamination
  - Treatment course and number of injections
  - Age and size of child

Intradermal

- Administer on the inside surface of the forearm.
- Use a TB syringe with 26- to 30-gauge needle with an intradermal bevel.
- Insert needle at 15° angle.
- Do not aspirate.

Subcutaneous

Give in areas of adequate subcutaneous tissue. Common sites are the lateral aspect of the upper arm, abdomen, and anterior thigh.
- Inject volumes of less than 0.5 mL.
- Use a 1 mL syringe with a 26- to 30-gauge needle.
- Insert at a 90° angle. Use a 45° angle for children who are thin.
- Check policy for aspiration practices.

Intramuscular

Use a 22- to 25-gauge, ½- to 1-inch needle.

Vastus lateralis
- This is the recommended site in infants and small children.
- Position the child supine, side-lying, or sitting.
- Inject up to 0.5 mL for infants.
- Inject up to 2 mL for children.

Ventrogluteal
- Position the child supine, side-lying, or prone.
- Inject 0.5 to 1 mL, depending on muscle size of infant.
- Inject up to 2 mL in children.

Deltoid
- Position the child sitting or standing.
- Inject up to 1 mL.
- Provide atraumatic care
  - Apply eutectic mixture of lidocaine and prilocaine (EMLA) to the site for 60 min prior to injection.
  - Change needle after puncturing a rubber stopper. Q EBP
  - Use the smallest gauge of needle possible.
  - Use therapeutic hugging.
  - Secure the child firmly to decrease movement of the needle while injecting.
  - Use distraction.
  - Encourage parents to hold the child after.
  - Offer praise.
  - Use play therapy.
  - Offer sucrose pacifiers to infants.

Intravenous

- Inspect venipuncture site per facility protocol and prior to administration of medications.
- Provide atraumatic care.
  - Discuss with the charge nurse the possible need for a peripherally inserted central catheter (PICC) before multiple peripheral attempts. Qtc
  - Use a transilluminator to assist in vein location.
  - Avoid terminology such as a "bee sting" or "stick."
  - Attach an extension tubing to decrease movement of the catheter.
  - Use play therapy.
  - Apply EMLA to the site for 60 min prior to attempt.
  - Keep equipment out of site until procedure begins.
  - Perform procedure in a treatment room. Qpcc
  - Use nonpharmacologic therapies.
  - Allow parents to stay if they prefer.
  - Use therapeutic holding.
  - Avoid using the dominant or sucking hand.
  - Cover site with a colorful wrap.
  - Swaddle infants.
  - Offer nonnutritive sucking to infants before, during, and after the procedure.

Peripheral venous access devices

- Use a 24- to 20-gauge catheter.
- Use for continuous and intermittent IV medication administration.
- Short-term IV therapy can be completed at home with the assistance of a home health nurse.

Central venous access devices

- Short term: nontunneled catheter or PICC
- Long term: tunneled catheter or implanted infusion ports

PRACTICE Active Learning Scenario

A nurse is caring for a toddler who requires insertion of an IV access. What actions should the nurse plan to take? Use the ATI Active Learning Template: Basic Concept to complete this item.

NURSING INTERVENTIONS: Describe 10 atraumatic care interventions.

Application Exercises

1. A nurse is planning to administer the influenza vaccine 0.5 mL IM to a toddler. Which of the following actions should the nurse take?
   - A. Administer the medication in the abdomen.
   - B. Use a 20-gauge needle.
   - C. Divide the medication into two injections.
   - D. Place the child in the supine position.

2. A nurse is preparing to administer an intramuscular (IM) injection to a child. Which of the following muscle groups is contraindicated?
   - A. Deltoid
   - B. Ventrogluteal
   - C. Vastus lateralis
   - D. Dorsogluteal

3. A nurse is reinforcing teaching with the parent of an infant about administration of oral medications. Which of the following information should the nurse include in the teaching? (Select all that apply.)
   - A. Use a universal dropper for medication administration.
   - B. Ask the pharmacy to add flavoring to the medication.
   - C. Add the medication to a formula bottle before feeding.
   - D. Use the nipple of a bottle to administer the medication.
   - E. Hold the infant in a semireclining position.

4. A nurse is preparing to administer medication to a toddler. Which of the following actions should the nurse take? (Select all that apply.)
   - A. Identify the toddler by asking the parent.
   - B. Tell the parent to administer the medication.
   - C. Calculate the safe dosage.
   - D. Ask the toddler what toy he wants to hold during administration.
   - E. Offer juice after the medication.

5. A nurse is caring for an infant who needs otic medication. Which of the following actions should the nurse take?
   - A. Hold the infant in an upright position.
   - B. Pull the pinna downward and straight back.
   - C. Hyperextend the infant's neck.
   - D. Ensure that the medication is cool.

Application Exercises Key

1. A. The abdomen is an appropriate site for a subcutaneous injection.

    B. A 22- to 25-gauge needle is recommended for IM injections.

    C. The nurse can safely administer a volume of 0.5 mL of medication to the toddler using the IM route.

    D. **CORRECT:** The vastus lateralis is recommended for administering IM medications. Placing the toddler in a supine position is the appropriate action for the nurse to take.

    (N) *NCLEX® Connection: Pharmacological Therapies, Medication Administration*

2. A. The deltoid muscle can be used once developed in children for IM injections for medication containing up to 1 mL fluid.

    B. The ventrogluteal muscle can be used for IM injections in children for medication containing up to 2 mL fluid.

    C. The vastus lateralis muscle can be used for intramuscular injections in children for medication containing up to 2 mL fluid.

    D. **CORRECT:** The dorsogluteal site has major nerves and blood vessels and is not a recommended site for IM injections for children.

    (N) *NCLEX® Connection: Reduction of Risk Potential, Potential for Complications of Diagnostic Tests/Treatments/Procedures*

3. A. Medication has different viscosities, and droppers do not have a standard opening. A universal dropper is not an accurate way to measure medications.

    B. **CORRECT:** Multiple flavorings are available to add to medications and can assist in masking the taste.

    C. Because an infant might not finish an entire bottle of formula, it is not recommended to add medication to the bottle.

    D. **CORRECT:** Administering medications through an empty nipple can assist with successful administration of the medication.

    E. **CORRECT:** For successful medication administration, the infant should be held in a semireclining position, similar to when feeding.

    (N) *NCLEX® Connection: Pharmacological Therapies, Medication Administration*

4. A. For safe medication administration, confirm two identifiers by looking at the identification band or having the toddler state his name and date of birth.

    B. The nurse should identify the preferred level of involvement of the parents prior to medication administration.

    C. **CORRECT:** For safe medication administration, the nurse should calculate the safe dosage prior to administering medication.

    D. **CORRECT:** Offering choices to the toddler is an example of atraumatic care.

    E. **CORRECT:** Offering juice after the medication, if not contraindicated, is an example of atraumatic care.

    (N) *NCLEX® Connection: Pharmacological Therapies, Medication Administration*

5. A. The nurse should position the infant supine or prone for administration of otic medication.

    B. **CORRECT:** Pulling the pinna downward and straight back will straighten the ear canal to allow medication to flow into the ear.

    C. Hyperextending the infant's neck could occlude the airway.

    D. Allowing the otic medication to warm up to room temperature is recommended to provide atraumatic care.

    (N) *NCLEX® Connection: Pharmacological Therapies, Medication Administrations*

PRACTICE Answer

Using the ATI Active Learning Template: Basic Concept

NURSING INTERVENTIONS

- Discuss insertion of a peripherally inserted catheter with the charge nurse before multiple peripheral attempts.
- Use a transilluminator to assist in vein location.
- Avoid terminology such as a "bee sting" or "stick."
- Attach extension tubing to decrease movement of the catheter.
- Use play therapy.
- Apply eutectic mixture of lidocaine and prilocaine (EMLA) to the site for 60 min prior to the procedure.

- Keep equipment out of sight until procedure begins.
- Perform the procedure in a treatment room.
- Use nonpharmacologic therapies.
- Allow parents to stay if they prefer.
- Use therapeutic holding.
- Avoid using the dominant or sucking hand.
- Cover site with a colorful wrap.
- Swaddle infants.
- Offer nonnutritive sucking to infants before, during, and after the procedure.

(N) *NCLEX® Connection: Pharmacological and Parenteral Therapies, Parenteral/Intravenous Therapies*

CHAPTER 9 # Pain Management

Determination of pain depends on the child's cognitive, emotional, and physical development. Pain is managed by atraumatic, nonpharmacological, and pharmacological interventions. Atraumatic care is the use of interventions that minimize or eliminate physical and psychological distress.

INFLUENTIAL FACTORS

Factors that can have a positive or negative effect on pain perception
- Age
- Development stage
- Chronic or acute disease
- Prior experiences with pain
- Personality
- Family dynamics
- Culture
- Socioeconomic status

DATA COLLECTION

EXPECTED FINDINGS

Developmental characteristics

Young infant (birth to 5 months)
- Loud cry
- Rigid body or thrashing
- Local reflex withdrawal from pain stimulus
- Expressions of pain (eyes tightly closed, mouth open in a squarish shape, eyebrows lowered and drawn together)
- Lack of association between stimulus and pain

Older infant (6 months to 12 months)
- Loud cry
- Deliberate withdrawal from pain
- Facial expression of pain

Toddler
- Loud cry or screaming
- Verbal expressions of pain
- Thrashing of extremities
- Attempt to push away or avoid stimulus
- Noncooperation
- Clinging to a significant person
- Behaviors occur in anticipation of painful stimulus
- Requests physical comfort

School-age child
- Stalling behavior
- Muscular rigidity
- Any behaviors of the toddler, but less intense in the anticipatory phase and more intense with painful stimulus

Adolescent
- More verbal expressions of pain with less protest
- Muscle tension with body control

Pain intensity (9.1)

- Data collection is multidimensional and includes behavioral measures and self-report.
- Self-report is the method used for children 4 years or older. Children younger than 4 cannot accurately or verbally report their pain.
- Multiple tools are reliable are available for the nurse to use when evaluating a child's pain.
- A nurse should choose a pain tool that will adequately determine the severity of the infant or child's pain.
- Include the parent or caregiver in rating the child's pain.
- Determine the location, quality, and severity of pain.

PATIENT-CENTERED CARE

NURSING CARE

- Recheck the child's pain level frequently.
- Use nonpharmacological and/or pharmacological approaches to manage pain.
- Ask a parent or caregiver to monitor the child's pain level.
- Ask the parent or caregiver their satisfaction of the pain management.
- Monitor the child for adverse reactions to pain medications.
- Review laboratory reports.
- Monitor the child's physical functioning following pain management intervention.
- Monitor for negative effects or distress the child might experience related to pain (anxiety, withdrawal, sleep disruption, fear, depression, unhappiness).

ATRAUMATIC MEASURES

- Use a private treatment room for painful procedures.
- Avoid procedures in "safe places" (play room, the child's bed).
- Use developmentally suitable terminology when explaining procedures.
- Offer choices to the child.
- Allow parents to stay with the child during painful procedures.
- Use play therapy to explain procedures, allowing the child to perform the procedure on a doll or toy.

PHARMACOLOGICAL MEASURES

- A two-step approach for pharmacological management of pain in children is recommended.
  - For children older than 3 months of age who have mild pain, the first step is to administer a nonopioid. Nonsteroidal anti-inflammatory drugs (NSAIDs) are frequently used for mild pain.
  - The second step for children who have moderate or severe pain is to administer a strong opioid. Morphine is the medication of choice.
- Administer an optimal dosage of medication to control pain without causing severe adverse effects.
- Select the least traumatic route for medication administration.
- Give medications routinely (vs. PRN) to manage pain that is expected to last for an extended period of time.
- Combine adjuvant medications (steroids, antidepressants, sedatives, antianxiety medications, muscle relaxants, anticonvulsants) with analgesics.

- Use nonopioid and opioid medications.
  - Acetaminophen and NSAIDs are indicated for mild to moderate pain.
  - Opioids are indicated for moderate to severe pain. Medications used include morphine sulfate, oxycodone, and fentanyl.
  - Combining a nonopioid and an opioid medication treats pain peripherally and centrally. This offers greater analgesia with fewer adverse effects (respiratory depression, constipation, nausea).
- IM injections are not recommended for pain control in children.
- Intranasal medications are not recommended for children younger than 18 years.
- Rectal medications have variable absorption rates, and children dislike them.
- Intradermal medications are used for skin anesthesia prior to procedures.

9.1 Pain assessment tool for evaluation by age

FLACC: 2 months to 7 years

Pain rated on a scale of 0 to 10.
Observe behaviors of the child.

FACE (F)
0: Smile or no expression
1: Occasional frown or grimace, withdrawn
2: Frequent or constant frown, clenched jaw, quivering chin

LEGS (L)
0: Relaxed or expected position
1: Uneasy, restless, tense
2: Kicking or legs drawn up

ACTIVITY (A)
0: Lying quietly, moves easily, expected position
1: Squirming, shifting, tense
2: Arched, ridged, or jerking

CRY (C)
0: No cry
1: Moans or whimpers, occasional complaints
2: Crying, screaming, sobbing, frequent complaints

CONSOLABILITY (C)
0: Content or relaxed
1: Reassured by occasional touching or hugging. Able to distract
2: Difficult to console or comfort

Numeric scale: 5 years and older

Pain rated on a scale of 0 to 10.
Explain to the child that 0 means "no pain" and 10 means "worst pain."
Have the child verbally report a number or point to their level of pain on a visual scale.

FACES: 3 years and older

Pain rated on a scale of 0 to 5 using a diagram of six faces.
Explain each face to the child; ask the child to choose a face that best describes how they are feeling.

0: No hurt
1: Hurts a bit
2: Hurts a little more
3: Hurts even more
4: Hurts a whole lot
5: Hurts the worst

Noncommunicating children's pain checklist: 3 to 18 years

Intended for use with children who are unable to communicate due to postoperative status, cognitive impairment, or disabilities.
Behaviors are observed for 10 min.
Six subcategories are each scored on a 0 to 3 scale.

0: Not at all
1: Just a little
2: Fairly often
3: Very often
NA: Not applicable

SUBCATEGORIES

Vocal	Facial	Body and limbs
Social	Activity	Physiological

CUTOFF SCORES
11 or higher indicates moderate to severe pain.
6 to 10 indicates mild pain.

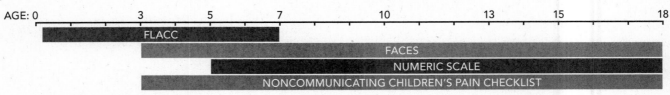

AGE: 0   3   5   7   10   13   15   18

FLACC
FACES
NUMERIC SCALE
NONCOMMUNICATING CHILDREN'S PAIN CHECKLIST

ROUTES OF ADMINISTRATION

Oral

- Route is preferred due to convenience, cost, and ability to maintain steady blood levels.
- Takes 1 to 2 hr to reach peak analgesic effects. Oral medications are not suited for children experiencing pain that requires rapid relief or pain that is fluctuating in nature.

Topical/transdermal

NURSING ACTIONS

Lidocaine is available in a cream or gel.

- Used for any procedure in which the skin will be punctured (IV insertion, biopsy) 60 min prior to a superficial puncture and 2.5 hr prior to a deep puncture.
- Place an occlusive dressing over the cream after application.
- Prior to procedure, remove the dressing and clean the skin.
- Demonstrate to the child that the skin is not sensitive by tapping or scratching lightly.

Transdermal fentanyl

- Use for children older than 12 years of age.
- Use to provide continuous pain control. Onset of 12 to 24 hr and a duration of 72 hr.
- Use an immediate-release opioid for breakthrough pain.
- Monitor for respiratory depression and assist with the administration of naloxone if this adverse effect occurs. Qs

NONPHARMACOLOGICAL MEASURES

Distraction

- Use play, music, a computer game, or a movie. Qpcc
- Tell jokes or a story to the child.

Relaxation

- Hold or rock the infant or young child.
- Assist older children into a comfortable position.
- Assist with breathing techniques.

Guided imagery

- Assist the child in an imaginary experience.
- Have the child describe the details.

Positive self-talk: Have the child say positive things during a procedure or painful episode.

Behavioral contracting

- Use stickers or tokens as rewards.
- Give time limits for the child to cooperate.
- Reinforce cooperation with a reward.

Containment

- Swaddle the infant.
- Place rolled blankets around the child.
- Maintain proper positioning.

Nonnutritive sucking

- Offer pacifier with sucrose before, during, and after painful procedures.
- Offer nonnutritive sucking during episodes of pain.

Kangaroo care: skin-to-skin contact between infants and parents

Complementary and alternative medicine

- Offer foods, vitamins, or supplements.
- Offer massage or chiropractic options.
- Review energy-based treatments such as magnets.
- Discuss mind-body techniques (hypnosis, homeopathy, naturopathy).

COMPLICATIONS

Chronic pain syndromes: Poorly controlled pain predisposes children to chronic pain conditions.

NURSING ACTIONS

- Monitor pain thoroughly and adequately.
- Administer medications in a timely manner.
- Evaluate and monitor the child's response to treatments.
- Titrate analgesic medications to achieve optimal dosing.
- Recommend alternate medications if needed.

Application Exercises

1. A nurse is caring for a preschooler who is experiencing mild pain. Which of the following types of medication should the nurse administer first?

   A. Opioid analgesic

   B. Antianxiety medication

   C. Nonsteroidal anti-inflammatory drug

   D. Sedative

2. A nurse is contributing to the plan of care for a child following a surgical procedure. Which of the following interventions should the nurse recommend?

   A. Administer NSAIDs for pain greater than 7 on a scale of 0 to 10.

   B. Administer intranasal analgesics PRN.

   C. Administer IM analgesics for pain.

   D. Administer analgesics on a schedule.

3. A nurse is collecting data from an infant. The nurse should identify that which of the following findings indicates that the infant is experiencing pain? (Select all that apply.)

   A. Pursed lips

   B. Loud cry

   C. Lowered eyebrows

   D. Rigid body

   E. Pushes away stimulus

4. A nurse is contributing to the plan of care for an infant who is experiencing pain. Which of the following interventions should the nurse recommend? (Select all that apply.)

   A. Offer a pacifier.

   B. Use guided imagery.

   C. Use swaddling.

   D. Initiate a behavioral contract.

   E. Encourage kangaroo care.

5. A nurse is preparing a toddler for insertion of an IV catheter. Using atraumatic care, which of the following actions should the nurse take? (Select all that apply.)

   A. Explain the procedure using the child's favorite toy.

   B. Ask the parents to leave during the procedure.

   C. Plan to assist with the procedure with the child in his bed.

   D. Allow the child to make one choice regarding the procedure.

   E. Apply lidocaine cream to three potential insertion sites.

PRACTICE Active Learning Scenario

A nurse is reviewing pain evaluation tools with a group of newly licensed nurses. What should the nurse include in the discussion? Use the ATI Active Learning Template: Nursing Skill to complete this item.

DESCRIPTION OF SKILL: Describe four pain tools used with pediatric clients.

Application Exercises Key

1. A. The nurse should administer an opioid analgesic if the preschooler's pain becomes moderate to severe. However, evidence-based practice indicates that the nurse should take a different action first.

   B. The nurse should administer an adjuvant medication, such as an antianxiety medication, along with an analgesic if an analgesic alone is ineffective. However, the nurse should take a different action first.

   C. **CORRECT:** According to evidence-based practice, the nurse should first administer a nonopioid such as a nonsteroidal anti-inflammatory drug or acetaminophen for children older than 3 months of age who have mild pain.

   D. The nurse should administer an adjuvant medication, such as a sedative, along with an analgesic if an analgesic alone is ineffective. However, the nurse should take a different action first.

   Ⓝ *NCLEX® Connection: Pharmacological Therapies, Pharmacological Pain Management*

2. A. NSAIDs are used for mild to moderate pain.

   B. Intranasal analgesics are used for clients older than 18 years.

   C. IM analgesics are not recommended for pain management in children.

   D. **CORRECT:** The nurse should administer analgesics on a schedule to achieve optimal pain management.

   Ⓝ *NCLEX® Connection: Pharmacological Therapies, Expected Actions/Outcomes*

3. A. Infants who are experiencing pain have their mouth open in a squarish shape.

   B. **CORRECT:** Infants who are experiencing pain exhibit a loud cry.

   C. **CORRECT:** Infants who are experiencing pain lower and draw together their eyebrows.

   D. **CORRECT:** Infants who are experiencing pain exhibit a rigid body.

   E. Infants who are experiencing pain exhibit a local reflex to withdraw from the stimulus.

   Ⓝ *NCLEX® Connection: Health Promotion and Maintenance, Data Collection Techniques*

4. A. **CORRECT:** The nurse should provide nonnutritive sucking as a nonpharmacological strategy for infants who are experiencing pain.

   B. Guided imagery is a nonpharmacological strategy used with children.

   C. **CORRECT:** The nurse should use swaddling as a nonpharmacological pain management strategy for infants who are experiencing pain.

   D. Behavioral contracts are a nonpharmacological strategy used with children.

   E. **CORRECT:** The nurse should encourage skin-to-skin touch as a relaxation technique for infants who are experiencing pain.

   Ⓝ *NCLEX® Connection: Basic Care and Comfort, Nonpharmacological Comfort Interventions*

5. A. **CORRECT:** The nurse should explain the procedure using the toddler's favorite toy to manage fears and provide atraumatic care.

   B. The nurse should allow the toddler's parents to remain for procedures to offer comfort to the toddler.

   C. The nurse should avoid the use of safe places, such as the toddler's bed, for procedures.

   D. **CORRECT:** The nurse should allow the toddler to make choices when possible to offer a sense of control over the situation and to provide atraumatic care.

   E. **CORRECT:** The nurse should apply a topical analgesic, such as lidocaine cream, prior to IV insertion to decrease pain and to provide atraumatic care.

   Ⓝ *NCLEX® Connection: Health Promotion and Maintenance, Developmental Stages and Transitions*

PRACTICE Answer

Using the ATI Active Learning Template: Nursing Skill

DESCRIPTION OF SKILL
- FLACC (2 months to 7 years)
  - Pain rated on a scale of 0 to 10.
  - Observe behaviors of the child.
  - Face (F)
    - 0: Smile or no expression
    - 1: Occasional frown or grimace, withdrawn
    - 2: Frequent or constant frown, clenched jaw, quivering chin
  - Legs (L)
    - 0: Relaxed or expected position
    - 1: Uneasy, restless, tense
    - 2: Kicking or legs drawn up
  - Activity (A)
    - 0: Lying quietly, moves easily, expected position
    - 1: Squirming, shifting, tense
    - 2: Arched, ridged, or jerking
  - Cry (C)
    - 0: No cry
    - 1: Moans or whimpers, occasional complaints
    - 2: Crying, screaming, sobbing, frequent complaints
  - Consolability (C)
    - 0: Content or relaxed
    - 1: Reassured by occasional touching or hugging. Able to distract
    - 2: Difficult to console or comfort
- FACES (3 years and older)
  - Pain rated on a scale of 0 to 5 using a diagram of six faces.
  - Explain each face to the child.
    - 0: No hurt
    - 1: Hurts a bit
    - 2: Hurts a little more
    - 3: Hurts even more
    - 4: Hurts a whole lot
    - 5: Hurts the worst
  - Ask the child to choose a face that best describes how they are feeling
- Numeric scale (5 years and older)
  - Pain rated on a scale of 0 to 10.
  - Explain to the child that 0 means "no pain" and 10 means "worst pain."
  - Have the child verbally report a number or point on a visual scale their pain level.
- Noncommunicating children's pain checklist (3 to 18 years)
  - Intended for us with children who are unable to communicate due to postoperative status, cognitive impairment, or disabilities.
  - Behaviors are observed for 10 min.
  - Six subcategories are scored on a scale 0 to 3.
  - Subcategories are vocal, social, facial, activity, body and limbs, and physiological, each with observable behaviors to be scored.
    - 0: Not at all
    - 1: Just a little
    - 2: Fairly often
    - 3: Very often
    - NA: Not applicable
  - Cutoff scores:
    - 11 or more indicates moderate to severe pain.
    - 6 to 10 indicates mild pain.

Ⓝ *NCLEX® Connection: Pharmacological and Parenteral Therapies, Pharmacological Pain Management*

CHAPTER 10 *Hospitalization, Illness, and Play*

Nurses encounter children who are ill or hospitalized. When caring for these children, it is important to know what play activities are considered appropriate.

Hospitalization and illness

- Families and children can experience major stress related to hospitalization. The nurse should monitor for evidence of stress and intervene as needed for the child's age and developmental level as well as the family's individual needs.
- Families should be considered clients when children are ill.
- Separation anxiety manifests in three behavioral responses.
  ○ **Protest:** screaming, clinging to parents, verbal and physical aggression toward strangers (this stage is expected during hospitalization)
  ○ **Despair:** withdrawal from others, depression, decreased communication, developmental regression (this stage is expected during hospitalization)
  ○ **Detachment:** interacting with strangers, forming new relationships, happy appearance (this stage is rarely observed during hospitalization)
- Each child's understanding of illnesses and hospitalization is dependent on the child's stage of development and cognitive ability.

EFFECT BASED ON DEVELOPMENT

Infant

LEVEL OF UNDERSTANDING
- Inability to describe illness and follow directions
- Lack of understanding of the need of therapeutic procedures

EFFECT OF HOSPITALIZATION
- Experiences stranger anxiety between 6 and 18 months of age
- Displays physical behaviors as expressions of discomfort due to inability to verbalize
- Can experience sleep deprivation due to strange noises, monitoring devices, and procedures
- Can experience anxiety due to the unfamiliar environment and fear of the unknown

Toddler

LEVEL OF UNDERSTANDING
- Limited ability to describe illness
- Poorly developed sense of body image and boundaries
- Limited understanding of the need for therapeutic procedures
- Limited ability to follow directions

EFFECT OF HOSPITALIZATION
- Experiences separation anxiety
- Can exhibit an intense reaction to any type of procedure due to the intrusion of boundaries
- Behavior can regress

Preschooler

LEVEL OF UNDERSTANDING
- Limited understanding of the cause of illness but knows what illness feels like
- Limited ability to describe manifestations
- Fears related to magical thinking
- Ability to understand cause and effect inhibited by concrete thinking

EFFECT OF HOSPITALIZATION
- Can experience separation anxiety
- Can harbor fears of bodily harm
- Might believe illness and hospitalization are a punishment

School-age child

LEVEL OF UNDERSTANDING
- Beginning awareness of body functioning
- Ability to describe pain
- Increasing ability to understand cause and effect

EFFECT OF HOSPITALIZATION
- Fears loss of control
- Seeks information as a way to maintain a sense of control
- Can sense when not being told the truth
- Can experience stress related to separation from peers and regular routine

Adolescent

LEVEL OF UNDERSTANDING
- Increasing ability to understand cause and effect
- Perceptions of illness severity are based on the degree of body image changes

EFFECT OF HOSPITALIZATION
- Develops body image disturbance
- Attempts to maintain composure but is embarrassed about losing control
- Experiences feelings of isolation from peers
- Worries about outcome and impact on school/activities
- Might not adhere to treatments/medication regimen due to peer influence

Family responses

- Fear and guilt regarding not bringing the child in for care earlier
- Frustration due to the perceived inability to care for the child
- Altered family roles
- Worry regarding finances if work is missed
- Worry regarding care of other children within the household
- Fear related to lack of knowledge regarding illness or treatments
- Siblings can experience loneliness, jealousy, guilt, fear, or anger
- Caregiver role strain, related to the effect of hospitalization on family processes

DATA COLLECTION

- Child's and family's understanding of the illness or the reason for hospitalization
- Stressors unique to the child and family (needs of other children in the family, socioeconomic situation, health of extended family members)
- Past experiences with hospitalization and illness
- Developmental level and needs of child/family
- Parenting role and the family's perception of role changes
- Support available to the child/family
- Coping strategies for periods of crisis

NURSING INTERVENTIONS

- Discuss with the child and family what to expect during hospitalization. Qᴘᴄᴄ
- Encourage family members to stay with the child during the hospital experience to reduce the stress.
- Maintain routine as much as possible.
- Encourage independence and choices.
- Explain treatments, procedures, and cares to the child.
- Provide developmentally appropriate activities.

Infants

- Place infants whose parents are not in attendance close to nurses' stations so that their needs can be quickly met.
- Provide consistency in assigning caregivers.

Toddlers

- Encourage parents to provide routine care for the child, such as changing diapers and feeding.
- Encourage the child's autonomy by offering appropriate choices.
- Provide consistency in assigning caregivers.

Preschoolers

- Explain procedures using simple, clear language. Avoid medical jargon and terms that can be misinterpreted.
- Encourage independence by letting the child provide self-care.
- Encourage the child to express feelings.
- Validate the child's fears and concerns.
- Provide toys that allow for emotional expression, such as a pounding board to release feelings of protest.
- Provide consistency in assigning caregivers.
- Give choices when possible, such as, "Do you want your medicine in a cup or a spoon?"
- Allow younger children to handle equipment if it is safe.

School-age children

- Provide factual information.
- Encourage the child to express feelings.
- Try to maintain a normal routine for long hospitalizations, including time for school work.
- Encourage contact with peer group.

Adolescents

- Provide factual information.
- Allow the adolescent to contribute to the plan of care to relieve feelings of powerlessness and lack of control.
- Encourage contact with peer group.

Play

- Allows children to express feelings and fears.
- Facilitates mastery of developmental stages and assists in the development of problem solving abilities.
- Allows children to learn socially acceptable behaviors.
- A means of protection from everyday stressors.
- The nurse should select play activities that are specific to each child's stage of development.
- The nurse can use play to reinforce teaching with children.

CONTENT OF PLAY

Social affective: taking pleasure in relationships

Sense-pleasure: objects in the environment catching the child's attention

Skill: demonstrating new abilities

Unoccupied behavior: focusing attention on something of interest

Dramatic: pretending and fantasizing Qᴇʙᴘ

Games: imitative, formal, or competitive

SOCIAL CHARACTER OF PLAY

Onlooker: A child observes others.

Solitary: A child plays alone.

Parallel: Children play independently but among other children, which is characteristic of toddlers.

Associative: Children play together without organization, which is characteristic of preschoolers.

Cooperative play: Organized playing in groups, which is characteristic of school-age children.

FUNCTIONS OF PLAY

Play helps in the development of various types of skills.
- Intellectual
- Sensorimotor
- Social
- Self-awareness
- Creativity
- Therapeutic and moral values

PLAY ACTIVITIES RELATED TO AGE

Infants

Birth to 3 months: colorful moving mobiles, music/sound boxes

3 to 6 months: noise-making objects, soft toys

6 to 9 months: teething toys, social interaction

9 to 12 months: large blocks, toys that pop apart, push-and-pull toys

Toddlers

- Cloth books, puzzles with large pieces
- Large crayons and paper
- Push-and-pull toys, balls
- Tricycles
- Educational media programs

Preschoolers

- Imitative and imaginative play
- Drawing, painting, riding a tricycle, swimming, jumping, running
- Educational media programs

School-age children

- Games that can be played alone or with another person
- Team sports
- Musical instruments
- Arts and crafts
- Collections

Adolescents

- Team sports
- School activities
- Reading, listening to music
- Technology-based games and activities
- Peer interactions through in-person visits, phone calls, and social media

THERAPEUTIC PLAY

- Encourages the acting out of feelings of fear, anger, hostility, and sadness
- Enables the child to learn coping strategies in a safe environment
- Assists in gaining cooperation for medical treatment

DATA COLLECTION

- Developmental level of the child
- Motor skills
- Level of activity tolerance
- Child's preferences

NURSING INTERVENTIONS

- Select toys that are safe for the child. Q̲s̲
- Consider isolation precautions and the child's illness in relation to toy selection.
- Select activities that enhance development.
- Observe the child's play for clues to the child's fears or anxieties.
- Encourage parents to bring one favorite toy from home.
- Use dolls or stuffed animals to demonstrate a procedure before it is performed.
- Provide play opportunities that meet the child's level of activity tolerance.
- Allow the child to go to the play room if able.
- Encourage the adolescent's peers to visit.
- Consult with a child life specialist about recommendations for activities. Q̲ᴛᴄ

Application Exercises

1. A nurse is caring for a preschooler. Which of the following should the nurse identify as an expected behavior for preschoolers?

   A. Describing manifestations of illness

   B. Relating fears to magical thinking

   C. Understanding cause of illness

   D. Awareness of body functioning

2. A nurse on a pediatric unit is caring for a toddler. The nurse should identify which of the following behaviors as expected effects of hospitalization for a toddler? (Select all that apply.)

   A. Believes the experience is a punishment

   B. Experiences separation anxiety

   C. Displays intense emotions

   D. Exhibits regressive behaviors

   E. Manifests disturbance in body image

3. A nurse is reinforcing teaching with a parent about parallel play in children. Which of the following statements should the nurse include?

   A. "The child sits and observes others playing."

   B. "The child exhibits organized play when in a group."

   C. "The child plays alone."

   D. "The child plays independently when in a group."

4. A nurse is reinforcing teaching with a group of parents about separation anxiety. Which of the following information should the nurse include?

   A. Separation anxiety is commonly observed in the school-age child.

   B. The detachment stage of separation anxiety is expected during hospitalization.

   C. Separation anxiety begins with the child withdrawing from others.

   D. The child might kick health care staff during the protest stage of separation anxiety.

PRACTICE Active Learning Scenario

A nurse working in a pediatric unit is assisting with the planning of play activities for a group of children of different ages. What activities should the nurse recommend? Use the ATI Active Learning Template: Basic Concept to complete this item.

RELATED CONTENT: Identify appropriate toys and activities for children in three age groups.

Application Exercises Key

1. A. Preschoolers have limited ability to describe manifestations of illness.

    B. **CORRECT:** The nurse should expect preschoolers to be egocentric and relate fears to magical thinking.

    C. Preschoolers have limited understanding of cause-and-effect relationships but understand what illness feels like.

    D. Awareness of body functioning is a behavior of an adolescent.

    Ⓝ *NCLEX® Connection: Health Promotion and Maintenance, Developmental Stages and Transitions*

2. A. Belief that hospitalization is a punishment is an expected effect of hospitalization in a preschoolers.

    B. **CORRECT:** The nurse should expect separation anxiety as a potential effect of hospitalization in a toddler.

    C. **CORRECT:** The nurse should expect intense emotions as a potential effect of hospitalization in a toddler.

    D. **CORRECT:** The nurse should expect regressive behaviors as a potential effect of hospitalization in a toddler.

    E. Body image disturbances are an expected effect of hospitalization in adolescents.

    Ⓝ *NCLEX® Connection: Health Promotion and Maintenance, Developmental Stages and Transitions*

3. A. Onlooker play is when a child sits and observes others playing.

    B. Cooperative play is when a child exhibits organized play in a group.

    C. Solitary play is when a child plays alone.

    D. **CORRECT:** Parallel play is when a child plays independently but is among other children in a group.

    Ⓝ *NCLEX® Connection: Health Promotion and Maintenance, Aging Process*

4. A. Separation anxiety is commonly observed in toddlers.

    B. The detachment stage is rarely observed in the hospital setting.

    C. Withdrawing from others is expected as the child moves from the protest stage to the despair stage of separation anxiety.

    D. **CORRECT:** Children can demonstrate aggression toward health care staff during as an expected behavior during the protest stage of separation anxiety.

    Ⓝ *NCLEX® Connection: Health Promotion and Maintenance, Developmental Stages and Transitions*

PRACTICE Answer

Using the ATI Active Learning Template: Basic Concept

RELATED CONTENT

Infants
- Birth to 3 months: colorful moving mobiles, music/sound boxes
- 3 to 6 months: noise-making objects, soft toys
- 6 to 9 months: teething toys, social interaction
- 9 to 12 months: large blocks, toys that pop apart, push-and-pull toys

Toddlers
- Cloth books
- Large crayons and paper
- Push-and-pull toys
- Tricycles
- Balls
- Puzzles with large pieces
- Educational television
- Videos for children

Preschoolers
- Imitative and imaginative play
- Drawing, painting, riding a tricycle, swimming, jumping, running
- Educational television and videos

School-age children
- Games that can be played alone or with another person
- Team sports
- Musical instruments
- Arts and crafts
- Collections

Adolescents
- Team sports
- School activities
- Reading, listening to music
- Technology based games and activities
- Peer interactions through visits, phone calls, and social media

Ⓝ *NCLEX® Connection: Health Promotion and Maintenance, Developmental Stages and Transitions*

CHAPTER 11   *Death and Dying*

A nurse must meet the physical, psychological, spiritual, and emotional needs of a client and family during illness and at the time of death.

Palliative care is an interprofessional approach that focuses on the process of dying rather than prolonging life when cures are not possible. Focus is managing the client's manifestations and offering supportive care.

Hospice care specializes in the care of a client who is dying. Family members are often the primary caregivers. Nursing focus is on pain control, comfort, and allowing the client to die with dignity. Family and client needs are equal. Provide support for the family's grieving process, which can continue after the client's death.

End-of-life decisions require honest information regarding prognosis, disease progression, treatment options, and effects of treatments. These decisions are made during a highly stressful time. It is important that all health care personnel be aware of the client's and family's decisions.

Nurses can experience personal grief when caring for children with whom they have developed a therapeutic relationship.

FACTORS INFLUENCING LOSS, GRIEF, AND COPING ABILITY

- Interpersonal relationships and social support networks
- Type and significance of loss
- Culture and ethnicity
- Spiritual and religious beliefs and practices
- Prior experience with loss
- Socioeconomic status

GRIEF AND MOURNING

Anticipatory grief: when death is expected or a possible outcome

Complicated grief: extends for more than 1 year following the loss
- Intense thoughts
- Distressing yearning
- Feelings of loneliness
- Distressing emotions and feelings
- Disturbances in personal activities, such as sleep
- Can require referral to an expert in grief counseling

Parental grief
- Intense, long-lasting, and complex
- Secondary losses related to the death of the child (absence of hope and dreams, disruption of the family unit, loss of identity as a parent)
- Differences in maternal and paternal grief

Sibling grief
- Differs from adult/parental grief
- Reactions depend on age and developmental stage

CURRENT STAGE OF DEVELOPMENT

INFANTS/TODDLERS (BIRTH TO 3 YEARS)
- Have little to no concept of death.
- Egocentric thinking prevents toddlers from understanding death.
- Mirror parental emotions (sadness, anger, depression, anxiety).
- React in response to the changes brought about by being in the hospital (change of routine, painful procedures, immobilization, less independence, separation from family).
- Can regress to an earlier stage of behavior.

PRESCHOOL CHILDREN (3 TO 6 YEARS)
- Egocentric thinking.
- Magical thinking allows for the belief that thoughts can cause an event such as death. As a result, the child can feel guilt and shame.
- Interpret separation from parents as punishment for bad behavior.
- View dying as temporary because of the lack of a concept of time. To the toddler, the dead person can still have attributes of the living (sleeping, eating, breathing).

SCHOOL-AGE CHILDREN (6 TO 12 YEARS)

- Start to respond to logical or factual explanations.
- Begin to have an adult concept of death (inevitable, irreversible, universal), which generally applies to older school-age children (9 to 12 years).
- Experience fear of the disease process, death process, the unknown, and loss of control.
- Fear often displayed through uncooperative behavior.
- Can be curious about funeral services and what happens to the body after death.

ADOLESCENTS (12 TO 20 YEARS)

- Can have an adult-like concept of death.
- Can have difficulty accepting death because they are discovering who they are, establishing an identity, and dealing with issues of puberty.
- Rely more on peers than the influence of parents, which can result in the reality of a serious illness causing adolescents to feel isolated.
- Can be unable to relate to peers and communicate with parents.
- Can become increasingly stressed by changes in physical appearance due to medications or illness more than the prospect of death.
- Can experience guilt and shame.

Factors that can increase the family's potential for dysfunctional grieving following the death of a child

- Lack of a support system
- Presence of inadequate coping skills
- Association of violence or suicide with the death
- Sudden and unexpected death of a child
- Lack of hope or presence of pre-existing mental health issues

DATA COLLECTION

- Knowledge regarding diagnosis, prognosis, and care
- Perceptions and desires regarding diagnosis, prognosis, and care
- Nutritional status, as well as growth and development patterns
- Activity and energy level of the child
- Parents' wishes regarding the child's end-of-life care
- Presence of a do-not-resuscitate (DNR) order
- Family coping and available support
- Stage of grief the child and family are experiencing

PHYSICAL MANIFESTATIONS OF DEATH

- Sensation of heat when the body feels cool
- Decreased sensation and movement in lower extremities
- Loss of senses (hearing is the last to be lost)
- Confusion or loss of consciousness
- Decreased appetite and thirst
- Swallowing difficulties
- Loss of bowel and bladder control
- Bradycardia, hypotension
- Cheyne-Stokes respirations

NURSING INTERVENTIONS

- Allow an opportunity for anticipatory grieving, which affects the way a family will cope with the death of a child.
- Provide consistency among nursing personnel who are caring for the child/family.
- Encourage parents to remain with the child.
- Attempt to maintain a normal environment.
- Communicate with the child and family honestly and respectfully.
- Encourage independence.
- Stay with the child as much as possible.
- Administer analgesics to control pain.
- Provide privacy.
- Soften lights.
- Offer soft music if desired.
- Assist with arranging religious or cultural rituals desired by the child and family.
- Assist the child with unfinished tasks.
- Provide support for the family and child.

PALLIATIVE CARE

- Consider the child, siblings, and parents as the units of care.
- Provide an environment that is as close to being like home as possible.
- Consult with the child and family for desired measures.
- Respect the family's cultural and religious preferences and rituals. Qᴘᴄᴄ
- Provide and clarify information and explanations.
- Encourage physical contact; address feelings; and show concern, empathy, and support.
- Provide comfort measures (warmth, quiet, noise control, dry linens).
- Provide adequate nutrition and hydration.
- Collaborate with the RN and provider to control the child's pain.
  - Give medications on a regular schedule.
  - Treat breakthrough pain.
  - Increase doses as necessary to control pain.
  - Encourage use of relaxation, imagery, and distraction to help manage pain.

CARE FOR GRIEVING FAMILIES DURING THE DYING PROCESS

- Reinforce information with the child and family about the disease, medications, procedures, and expected events.
- Encourage and support parents to participate in caring for the child.
- Encourage parents to remain near the child as much as possible.
- Encourage the child's independence and control as developmentally and physically appropriate.
- Allow for visitation of family and friends as desired.
- Emphasize open, honest communication among the child, family, and health care team.

- Provide support to the child and family with decision-making.
- Provide opportunities for the child and family to ask questions.
- Assist parents to cope with their feelings and help them to understand the child's behaviors.
- Use books, movies, art, music, and play therapy to stimulate discussions and provide an outlet for emotions.
- Provide and encourage professional support and guidance from a trusted member of the health care team. Qᴛᴄ
- Remain neutral and accepting.
- Give reassurance that all efforts are being made to maintain comfort and support of the child's life.
- Recognize and support the individual differences of grieving. Advise families that each member can react differently on any given day.
- Give families privacy, unlimited time, and opportunities for any cultural or religious rituals. Respect the family's decisions regarding care of the child.
- Encourage discussion of special memories and people, reading of favorite books, providing favorite toys/objects, physical contact, sibling visits, and continued verbal communication, even if the child seems unconscious.

AFTER DEATH

- Allow family to stay with the body as long as they desire.
- Allow family to rock the infant/toddler.
- Remove tubes and equipment.
- Offer to allow family to assist with preparation of the body.
- Assist with preparations involving the death ritual.
- Encourage parents to prepare siblings for the funeral and related death rituals.
- Remain with the family and offer support.
- Allow family to share stories about the child's life.
- Refer to the child by name.
- Allow all family members to communicate feelings.

SELF-CARE FOR NURSES

- Express personal feelings of loss to someone who can offer support.
- Maintain good general health.
- Develop the ability for empathy.
- Take time off from work as needed.
- Develop a variety of interests and hobbies.
- Develop professional and social support systems.
- Focus on the positive aspects of caring for children who are dying.
- Attend funeral services if desired.
- Maintain contact with the family.

Application Exercises

1. A nurse is caring for a child who is dying. The nurse should identify which of the following findings as indications of impending death? (Select all that apply.)

   A. Heightened sense of hearing

   B. Tachycardia

   C. Difficulty swallowing

   D. Sensation of being cold

   E. Cheyne-Stokes respirations

2. A nurse is reinforcing teaching with a parent about complicated grief. Which of the following statements should the nurse make?

   A. "It is considered complicated grief if you are still grieving 6 months after your loss."

   B. "Personal activities are affected when experiencing complicated grief."

   C. "Parents will experience complicated grief together."

   D. "Complicated grief self-resolves in 12 months."

3. A nurse is reinforcing teaching with a parent of a preschooler about the child's perception of death. Which of the following should the nurse include?

   A. Preschoolers can understand a logical explanation of death.

   B. Preschoolers perceive death as temporary.

   C. Preschoolers are very curious about what happens to the body after death.

   D. Preschoolers experience fear related to the disease process.

4. A nurse is caring for a child who is dying. Which of the following actions should the nurse take to provide self-care? (Select all that apply.)

   A. Remain in contact with the family after their loss.

   B. Develop a professional support system.

   C. Take time off from work.

   D. Suggest that a hospital representative attend the funeral.

   E. Demonstrate feelings of sympathy toward the family.

5. A nurse is caring for a child who has a terminal illness and reviews palliative care with an assistive personnel (AP). Which of the following statements by the AP indicates understanding of this review?

   A. "I'm sure the family is hopeful that the new medication will stop the child's illness."

   B. "I'll miss working with this child now that only nurses will be caring for him."

   C. "I will get all the child's personal objects out of his room."

   D. "I will listen and respond as the family talks about their child's life."

Application Exercises Key

1. A. A decrease in the senses of smell, sight, and hearing are manifestations of impending death.

   B. Bradycardia is a manifestation of impending death.

   C. **CORRECT:** Difficulty swallowing is a manifestation of impending death.

   D. A client's sensation of heat when the body feels cool is a manifestation of impending death.

   E. **CORRECT:** Cheyne-Stokes respirations are an abnormal breathing pattern with periods of apnea and a manifestation of impending death.

   Ⓝ *NCLEX® Connection: Physiological Adaptation, Basic Pathophysiology*

2. A. A parent who is still experiencing intense grieving after 1 year should be evaluated for complicated grief.

   B. **CORRECT:** A parent who is experiencing complicated grief experiences intense emotions that affect personal activities.

   C. Parents grieve differently, and not all parents experience complicated grief.

   D. A nurse should refer the parent to an expert in grief counseling if complicated grief is identified.

   Ⓝ *NCLEX® Connection: Psychosocial Integrity, Support Systems*

3. A. School-age children are beginning to understand the concept of death and start to respond to logical or factual explanations.

   B. **CORRECT:** Preschoolers do not yet understand the concept of death and perceive death as temporary because they lack a concept of time.

   C. School-age children are beginning to understand the concept of death and become curious about what happens to the body after death.

   D. School-age children are beginning to understand the concept of death and experience fear related to the disease process.

   Ⓝ *NCLEX® Connection: Health Promotion and Maintenance, Developmental Stages and Transitions*

4. A. **CORRECT:** Maintaining contact with the family after their loss is an act of support for the family and a strategy to provide self-care.

   B. **CORRECT:** Developing professional support systems is a strategy the nurse can use to provide self-care and maintain effectiveness when working with the child who is dying and their family.

   C. **CORRECT:** Taking time off from work is a strategy the nurse can use to provide self-care and maintain effectiveness when working with the child who is dying.

   D. Nurses should be encouraged to participate in funeral rituals as a strategy to provide self-care and to show support for the family.

   E. A nurse should develop empathy, rather than sympathy, as a strategy to provide self-care when dealing with a child who is dying.

   Ⓝ *NCLEX® Connection: Psychosocial Integrity, End-of-Life Concepts*

5. A. Palliative care is provided when there is no longer hope for a disease cure.

   B. Palliative care focuses on providing consistency among the interprofessional team to offer supportive care and a normal environment.

   C. Palliative care focuses on offering support and a normal environment as the dying process occurs.

   D. **CORRECT:** Palliative care focuses on the process of dying and grieving, which includes using therapeutic communication.

   Ⓝ *NCLEX® Connection: Basic Care and Comfort, Nonpharmacological Comfort Interventions*

PRACTICE Active Learning Scenario

A nurse is contributing to the plan of care for a child who is nearing the end of life. What interventions should the nurse recommend? Use the ATI Active Learning Template: Basic Concept to complete this item.

NURSING INTERVENTIONS: Provide at least eight nursing interventions to recommend.

PRACTICE Answer

Using the ATI Active Learning Template: Basic Concept

NURSING INTERVENTIONS
- Allow an opportunity for anticipatory grieving, which affects the way a family will cope with the death of a child.
- Provide consistency among nursing staff caring for the child and family.
- Encourage parents to remain with the child.
- Attempt to maintain a normal environment.
- Communicate with the child honestly and respectfully.
- Encourage independence.
- Stay with the child as much as possible.
- Administer analgesics to control pain.
- Provide privacy.
- Soften lights.
- Offer soft music if desired.
- Assist with arranging religious or cultural rituals desired by the child and family.
- Assist the child with unfinished tasks.
- Provide support for the family and child.

Ⓝ *NCLEX® Connection: Psychosocial Integrity, Grief and Loss*

NCLEX® Connections

When reviewing the following chapters, keep in mind the relevant topics and tasks of the NCLEX outline, in particular:

Health Promotion and Maintenance

DEVELOPMENTAL STAGES AND TRANSITIONS
Identify and report client deviations from expected growth and development.

Identify barriers to communication.

Reduction of Risk Potential

LABORATORY VALUES: Monitor diagnostic or laboratory test results.

POTENTIAL FOR ALTERATIONS IN BODY SYSTEMS
Compare current client clinical data to baseline information.

Perform neurological checks.

Reinforce client teaching on methods to prevent complications associated with activity level/diagnosed illness/disease (foot care for client with diabetes mellitus).

THERAPEUTIC PROCEDURES: Reinforce client teaching on treatments and procedures.

Physiological Adaptation

ALTERATIONS IN BODY SYSTEMS: Provide care to the client who has experienced a seizure.

MEDICAL EMERGENCIES: Respond/intervene to a client's life-threatening situation (cardiopulmonary resuscitation).

CHAPTER 12 *Acute Neurological Disorders*

Meningitis is an inflammation of the cerebrospinal fluid (CSF) and meninges, which are the connective tissues that cover the brain and spinal cord.

Reye syndrome is a life-threatening disorder that involves acute encephalopathy and fatty changes of the liver.

Meningitis and Reye syndrome have similar manifestations and are both sometimes preceded by viral infections. Testing is necessary to differentiate between them.

Meningitis

Viral (aseptic) meningitis usually requires only supportive care for recovery.

Bacterial (septic) meningitis is a contagious infection. Prognosis depends on how quickly care is initiated.

DATA COLLECTION

RISK FACTORS

VIRAL MENINGITIS: Many viral illnesses (enterovirus, cytomegalovirus, adenovirus, mumps, herpes simplex virus, arbovirus, human immunodeficiency virus)

BACTERIAL MENINGITIS
- Infections caused by bacterial agents: *Neisseria meningitidis* (meningococcal), *Streptococcus pneumoniae* (pneumococcal), *Haemophilus influenzae* type B (Hib), *Escherichia coli*
  - Incidence of bacterial meningitis has decreased in all age groups except infants under 2 months since the introduction of the Hib and pneumococcal conjugate vaccines (PCV). Qᴇʙᴘ
  - Injuries that provide direct access to CSF (skull fracture, penetrating head wound)
- Crowded living conditions

EXPECTED FINDINGS
- Photophobia
- Nausea
- Irritability
- Headache

PHYSICAL FINDINGS: Manifestations of viral and bacterial meningitis are similar.
- **Birth to 3 months**
  - No illness is present at birth, but it progresses within a few days.
  - Manifestations are vague and difficult to diagnose.
    - Poor muscle tone, weak cry, poor suck, refuses feeding, vomiting, diarrhea
    - Possible fever, hypothermia
  - Neck is supple without nuchal rigidity.
  - Bulging fontanels are a late manifestation.
- **3 months to 2 years**
  - Seizures with a high-pitched cry
  - Fever and irritability
  - Bulging fontanels
  - Possible nuchal rigidity
  - Poor feeding
  - Vomiting
  - Brudzinski's and Kernig's signs are not reliable for diagnosis. **(12.1, 12.2)**
- **2 years through adolescence**
  - Seizures (often initial manifestation)
  - Nuchal rigidity
  - Positive Brudzinski's sign (flexion of extremities occurring with deliberate flexion of the child's neck)
  - Positive Kernig's sign (resistance to extension of the child's leg from a flexed position)
  - Fever and chills
  - Headache
  - Vomiting
  - Irritability and restlessness that can progress to drowsiness, delirium, stupor, and coma
  - Petechial or purpuric-type rash (with meningococcal infection)
  - Involvement of joints (with meningococcal and Hib)
  - Chronic draining ear (with pneumococcal infection)

LABORATORY TESTS
- Blood cultures are sometimes positive when the CSF culture is negative.
- Collect complete blood counts.

CSF analysis indicative of meningitis
- BACTERIAL
  - Cloudy color
  - Elevated WBC count
  - Elevated protein content
  - Decreased glucose content
  - Positive Gram stain
- VIRAL
  - Clear color
  - Slightly elevated WBC count
  - Normal or slightly elevated protein content
  - Normal glucose content
  - Negative Gram stain

DIAGNOSTIC PROCEDURES

Lumbar puncture

This is the definitive diagnostic test for meningitis.
- The provider inserts a spinal needle into the subarachnoid space between L3 and L4, or L4 and L5 vertebral spaces.
- The provider measures spinal fluid pressure and collects CSF for analysis.

NURSING ACTIONS
- Have the child empty his bladder.
- Assist the provider with the procedure.
- A topical anesthetic (EMLA cream) can be applied over the biopsy area at least 1 hr prior to the procedure. Qpcc
- Place the child in the side-lying position with the head flexed and knees drawn up toward the chest, and assist in maintaining the position. Use distraction methods as necessary.
- The provider can sedate the child with fentanyl and midazolam.
- The provider cleans the skin and injects a local anesthetic.
- The provider takes pressure readings and collects three to five test tubes of CSF.
- Apply pressure and an elastic bandage to the puncture site after the needle is removed.
- Label specimens appropriately, and deliver them to the laboratory.
- Monitor the site for bleeding, hematoma, or infection.

CLIENT EDUCATION: Remain in bed in a flat position to prevent leakage and a resulting spinal headache. This might not be possible for an infant, toddler, or preschooler. Time required for bed rest depends on facility protocol and amount of fluid collected. Qpcc

CT scan or MRI

Performed to identify increased intracranial pressure (ICP) or an abscess.

NURSING ACTIONS
- Assist with positioning.
- Administer sedatives.

PATIENT-CENTERED CARE

NURSING CARE
- The presence of petechial or a purpuric-type rash requires immediate medical attention. QEBP
- Isolate the client as soon as meningitis is suspected, and maintain transmission-based precautions per facility protocol.
  - Maintain respiratory isolation for a minimum of 24 hr after initiation of antibiotic therapy.
  - Providers and visitors should wear a mask.
  - Droplet precautions require a private room or a room with clients who have the same infectious disease, ensuring that each client has designated equipment.
- Monitor vital signs, urine output, fluid status, pain level, and neurologic status.
- For newborns and infants, monitor head circumference and fontanels for presence of or changes in bulging.
- Correct fluid volume deficits and then restrict fluids until no evidence of increased ICP and serum sodium levels are within the expected range.
- Maintain NPO status if the client has a decreased level of consciousness. As the client's condition improves, advance to clear liquids and then a diet the client can tolerate.
- Decrease environmental stimuli.
  - Provide a quiet environment.
  - Minimize exposure to bright light (natural and artificial).
- Provide comfort measures.
  - Keep the room cool.
  - Position the client without a pillow, and slightly elevate the head of the bed. The client can also be positioned side-lying to reduce neck discomfort.
- Maintain safety. (Keep the bed in a low position. Implement seizure precautions.) Qs
- Keep the family informed of the client's condition.

MEDICATIONS

Antibiotics

Assist with administration of IV antibiotics for bacterial infections. Length of therapy is determined by the client's condition and CSF results (normal blood glucose levels, negative culture). Therapy can last up to 10 days.

NURSING ACTIONS
- Check for allergies.
- Provide support for the client and family.

CLIENT EDUCATION: Complete the entire course of medication.

Corticosteroids (dexamethasone)

- Not indicated for viral meningitis
- Assists with initial management of increased ICP, but might not be effective for long-term complications
- Most effective for reducing neurologic complications in children who have infections caused by Hib

NURSING ACTIONS
- Monitor for effectiveness of medication.
- Provide support for the client and family.
- Reinforce teaching with the client about administration and adverse effects of the medication.

Analgesics

Acetaminophen with codeine can be used to relieve discomfort.

NURSING ACTIONS
- Check temperature prior to administering acetaminophen or ibuprofen, which can mask a fever.
- Monitor respiratory status.
- Monitor level of consciousness.
- Provide support for the client and family.

CLIENT EDUCATION

- Early and complete treatment is necessary for upper respiratory infections.
- Maintain appropriate immunizations. Children should receive the Hib and PCV vaccines at 2, 4, and 6 months of age, and again between 12 and 15 months of age.

> Recommendations for immunizations change periodically. Check the CDC's website (www.cdc.gov) for current recommendations.

COMPLICATIONS

Increased intracranial pressure

Could lead to neurological dysfunction

NURSING ACTIONS
- Monitor for indications of increased ICP. Qs
  - **Newborns and infants:** bulging or tense fontanels, increased head circumference, high-pitched cry, distended scalp veins, irritability, bradycardia, respiratory changes
  - **Children:** increased irritability, headache, nausea, vomiting, diplopia, seizures, bradycardia, respiratory changes
- Provide interventions to reduce ICP (positioning; avoidance of coughing, straining, and bright lights; minimizing environmental stimuli).

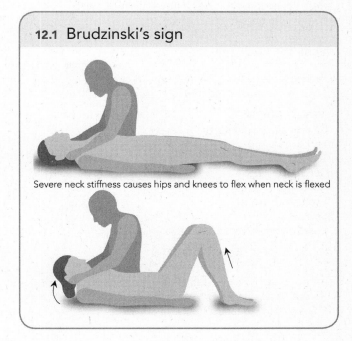

12.1 Brudzinski's sign

Severe neck stiffness causes hips and knees to flex when neck is flexed

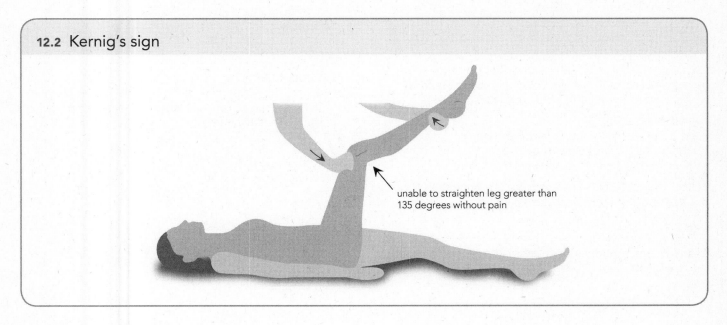

12.2 Kernig's sign

unable to straighten leg greater than 135 degrees without pain

Reye syndrome

- Reye syndrome is a life-threatening disorder involving acute encephalopathy and fatty changes of the liver.
- The cause is not understood but is associated with a viral illness (influenza, varicella) that is treated with salicylates.
- Peak incidence occurs when influenza is most common, typically January through March.
- The prognosis is best with early recognition and treatment.

DATA COLLECTION

RISK FACTORS

- There is an association between using aspirin (salicylate) products for treating fevers caused by viral infections and the development of Reye syndrome. Q_{EBP}
- Reye syndrome typically follows a viral illness (influenza, gastroenteritis, varicella).

EXPECTED FINDINGS

Recent viral illness and use of aspirin or aspirin-containing products.

PHYSICAL FINDINGS
- Changes in personality
- Lethargy
- Irritability
- Combativeness
- Confusion
- Profuse vomiting
- Seizures
- Loss of consciousness progressing to coma

LABORATORY TESTS
- Liver enzymes (alanine aminotransferase [ALT], aspartate aminotransferase [AST]): elevated
- Serum ammonia level: elevated
- Coagulation times can be extended

DIAGNOSTIC PROCEDURES

Liver biopsy

A liver biopsy consists of taking a piece of liver tissue via a large-bore needle, and sending this tissue to the pathology department. Ensure that clotting studies are within normal limits prior to the procedure.

NURSING ACTIONS
- Maintain NPO status prior to the procedure.
- Monitor for hemorrhage postprocedure.
- Monitor vital signs frequently postprocedure.

CLIENT EDUCATION: Limit postprocedure activities to decrease the risk of hemorrhage.

CSF analysis

A lumbar puncture should be performed to collect CSF and rule out meningitis.

PATIENT-CENTERED CARE

NURSING CARE

- Maintain hydration while preventing cerebral edema.
  - Assist with the administration of IV fluids.
  - Maintain accurate I&O.
  - Insert indwelling urinary catheter.
- Position the client. Q_s
  - Avoid extreme flexion, extension, or rotation.
  - Maintain the head in a midline neutral position.
  - Keep the head of the bed elevated 30°.
- Monitor coagulation and prevent hemorrhage.
  - Note unexplained or prolonged bleeding.
  - Apply pressure after procedures that cause bleeding.
- Monitor pain status and response to painful stimuli. Administer pain medications when appropriate.
- Monitor respiratory status. Intubation and mechanical ventilation can be necessary.
- Implement seizure precautions.
- Keep the family informed of the client's status.
- Provide private time for the family to be with the client if death is imminent.
- Assist with referrals to support resources for family.

CLIENT EDUCATION

- Avoid salicylates for pain or fever in children.
- Read labels of over-the-counter medications to check for the presence of salicylates.
- Clients regain full liver function, but can have some neurological deficits.
- Refer to the National Reye's Syndrome Foundation.

COMPLICATIONS

Neurologic sequelae

Neurologic complications vary by degree of severity.

NURSING ACTIONS
- Explain the client's condition and needs to the family.
- Help the family identify support services for home care if needed.

Death

NURSING ACTIONS
- Support the family in grief.
- Make referrals to spiritual support depending on the family's individual needs.

Application Exercises

1. A nurse is assisting with the care of a client who has suspected meningitis and a decreased level of consciousness. Which of the following actions should the nurse take?

   A. Place the client on NPO status.

   B. Prepare the client for a liver biopsy.

   C. Position the client dorsal recumbent.

   D. Put the client in a protective environment.

2. A nurse is reviewing cerebrospinal fluid analysis for a client who has suspected meningitis. Which of the following findings indicate viral meningitis? (Select all that apply.)

   A. Negative Gram stain

   B. Blood glucose level within the expected reference range

   C. Cloudy cerebrospinal fluid

   D. Decreased WBC count

   E. Protein level within the expected reference range

3. A nurse is collecting data from a 4-month-old infant who has meningitis. Which of the following findings should the nurse expect?

   A. Depressed anterior fontanel

   B. Constipation

   C. Presence of the rooting reflex

   D. High-pitched cry

4. A nurse is reviewing the medical history of a school-age client who possibly has Reye syndrome. The nurse should identify which of the following findings as a risk factor for Reye syndrome?

   A. Recent history of infectious cystitis caused by candida

   B. Recent history of bacterial otitis media

   C. Recent episode of varicella

   D. Recent episode of *Haemophilus influenzae* meningitis

5. A nurse is assisting with the development of an in-service about viral and bacterial meningitis. The nurse should include that the introduction of which of the following immunizations decreased the incidence of bacterial meningitis in children? (Select all that apply.)

   A. Inactivated polio vaccine (IPV)

   B. Pneumococcal conjugate vaccine (PCV)

   C. Diphtheria and tetanus toxoids and acellular pertussis vaccine (DTaP)

   D. *Haemophilus influenzae* type B (Hib) vaccine

   E. Trivalent inactivated influenza vaccine (TIV)

PRACTICE Active Learning Scenario

A nurse is assisting with the admission of a school-age child who has Reye syndrome. Use the ATI Active Learning Template: System Disorder to complete this item.

ALTERATION IN HEALTH (DIAGNOSIS)

EXPECTED FINDINGS: Identify five.

LABORATORY TESTS: List two results that indicate Reye syndrome.

Application Exercises Key

1. A. **CORRECT:** To prevent aspiration, the nurse should place the client on NPO status due to the decreased level of consciousness.

   B. The nurse should expect a client who has Reye syndrome to require a liver biopsy.

   C. The nurse should position the client without a pillow and slightly elevate the head of the bed to prevent increasing intracranial pressure.

   D. Clients who are immunocompromised require a protective environment. The nurse should place a client who has suspected meningitis on respiratory isolation for at least 24 hr after the initiation of antibiotic therapy.

   (N) *NCLEX® Connection: Physiological Adaptation, Basic Pathophysiology*

2. A. **CORRECT:** The nurse should expect a client who has viral meningitis to have a negative Gram stain.

   B. **CORRECT:** The nurse should expect a client who has viral meningitis to have a blood glucose level within the expected reference range.

   C. The nurse should expect the cerebrospinal fluid to be clear for a client who has viral meningitis.

   D. The nurse should expect a slightly elevated WBC count for a client who has viral meningitis.

   E. **CORRECT:** The nurse should expect a client who has viral meningitis to have a protein level within the expected reference range.

   (N) *NCLEX® Connection: Physiological Adaptation, Alterations in Body Systems*

3. A. The nurse should expect a 4-month-old infant who has meningitis to have a bulging anterior fontanel.

   B. Vomiting is an expected finding of meningitis.

   C. The rooting reflex is expected in infants until the age of 3 to 4 months, and can remain until the age of 12 months.

   D. **CORRECT:** A high-pitched cry is a finding associated with meningitis between ages 3 months to 2 years.

   (N) *NCLEX® Connection: Reduction of Risk Potential, Diagnostic Tests*

4. A. Candida is a fungal infection and is therefore not a risk factor for Reye syndrome.

   B. A bacterial infection is not a risk factor for Reye syndrome.

   C. **CORRECT:** Varicella is a viral illness, which is a risk factor for developing Reye syndrome. Reye syndrome typically follows a viral illness, such as influenza, gastroenteritis, or varicella.

   D. *Haemophilus influenzae* is a bacteria and is therefore not a risk factor for Reye syndrome.

   (N) *NCLEX® Connection: Reduction of Risk Potential, Potential for Alterations in Body Systems*

5. A. IPV does not decrease the incidence of bacterial meningitis.

   B. **CORRECT:** The introduction of the PCV decreased the incidence of bacterial meningitis in children, as it provides immunity against bacteria that causes the illness.

   C. The DTaP vaccine does not decrease the incidence of bacterial meningitis.

   D. **CORRECT:** The introduction of the Hib vaccine decreased the incidence of bacterial meningitis in children, as it provides immunity against bacterium that cause the illness.

   E. TIV does not decrease the incidence of bacterial meningitis.

   (N) *NCLEX® Connection: Reduction of Risk Potential, Therapeutic Procedures*

PRACTICE Answer

Using the ATI Active Learning Template: System Disorder

ALTERATION IN HEALTH (DIAGNOSIS): Reye syndrome is a life-threatening disorder involving acute encephalopathy and fatty changes of the liver.

EXPECTED FINDINGS
- Recent viral illness
- Recent use of aspirin or aspirin-containing products
- Changes in personality
- Lethargy
- Irritability
- Combativeness
- Confusion
- Profuse vomiting
- Seizures
- Loss of consciousness progressing to coma

LABORATORY TESTS
- Elevated liver enzymes
- Elevated serum ammonia levels
- Extended coagulation times

(N) *NCLEX® Connection: Physiological Adaptation, Pathophysiology*

CHAPTER 13 *Seizures*

Seizures are abnormal, excessive electrical discharges of neurons within the brain caused by a disease process.

Seizures are classified according to their type and etiology.

Epilepsy is chronic, recurring, and diagnosed after two or more unprovoked seizures and all other possible etiologies for the seizures have been ruled out.

DATA COLLECTION

RISK FACTORS FOR SEIZURES

- Some seizures have no known etiology
- Febrile episode
- Cerebral edema
- Intracranial infection or hemorrhage
- Brain tumors or cysts
- Anoxia
- Toxins or medications
- Lead poisoning
- Tetanus, shigella, or salmonella
- Hypoglycemia, hypocalcemia, alkalosis, hyponatremia, hypernatremia, or hypomagnesemia

RISK FACTORS FOR EPILEPSY

- Trauma
- Hemorrhage
- Congenital defects
- Anoxia
- Infection
- Toxins
- Hypoglycemic injury
- Uremia
- Migraine
- Cardiovascular dysfunction

EXPECTED FINDINGS

Generalized

Tonic-clonic seizure (previously referred to as grand mal)
- Onset without warning. Q EBP
- Tonic phase (10 to 30 seconds)
  - Eyes roll upward
  - Loss of consciousness
  - Tonic contraction of entire body, with arms flexed and legs, head, and neck extended
  - Mouth snaps shut and tongue can be bitten
  - Thoracic and abdominal muscles contract
  - Possible piercing cry
  - Increased salivation
  - Flushing
  - Blood pressure and heart rate increases
  - Loss of swallowing reflex
  - Apnea leading to cyanosis
- Clonic phase (30 to 50 seconds)
  - Violent jerking movements of the body
  - Trunk and extremities experience rhythmic contraction and relaxation
  - Can having foaming in the mouth
  - Can be incontinent of urine and feces
  - Gradual slowing of movements until cessation
- Postictal state (30 min)
  - Remains semiconscious but arouses with difficulty
  - Confused for several hours
  - Impairment of fine motor movements
  - Lack of coordination
  - Possible vomiting, headache, visual or speech difficulties
  - Sleeps for several hours
  - Feels tired and can complain of sore muscles
  - No recollection of the seizure

Absence seizure (previously referred to petit mal or lapses)
- Onset between ages of 5 to 8 years and ceases by the teenage years
- Loss of consciousness lasting 5 to 10 seconds
- Minimal or no change in behavior
- Resembles daydreaming or inattentiveness
- Can drop items being held, but the child seldom falls
- Lip smacking, twitching of eyelids or face, or slight hand movements
- Unable to recall episodes, but can be momentarily confused
- Can immediately resume previous activities

Myoclonic seizure
- Variety of seizure episodes
- Symmetric or asymmetric involvement
- Brief contractions of muscle or groups of muscle
- Can involve only the face and trunk or one or more extremities
- No postictal drowsiness

Atonic or akinetic seizure
- Onset between 2 and 5 years of age
- Muscle tone is lost for a few seconds
- Loss of muscle tone frequently results in falling
- Able to quickly get up and resume previous activity
- If seizures are frequent, child should wear a helmet to prevent injury Qs

Partial (focal/local)

Simple partial seizures with motor manifestations
- Aversive seizure (most common): Eyes and head turn away from the side of focus, with or without loss of consciousness
- Rolandic (Sylvan) seizure: Tonic-clonic movements involving the face, salivation, arrested sleep, and most common during sleep

Simple partial seizure with sensory manifestations
- Tingling, numbness or pain in one area of the body then spreading to other parts
- Visual sensations
- Motor development (hypertonia, posturing)

Complex partial seizures (psychomotor seizures)
- Altered behavior
- Inability to respond to the environment
- Impaired consciousness
- Confusion and unable to recall event
- Complex sensory aura
  - Strange feeling in stomach that rises to the throat
  - Olfactory, auditory, or visual hallucinations
  - Feelings of fear
  - Distorted sense of time and self

LABORATORY TESTS

Depend on age, history, and physical condition
- Lead level
- WBC
- Blood glucose
- Serum electrolytes
- Metabolic panel
- Chromosomal analysis
- Toxicology screen

DIAGNOSTIC PROCEDURES

Electroencephalogram (EEG)

Records electrical activity and can identify the origin of seizure activity
- Can be monitored during sleep, when awake, and with stimulation and hyperventilation
- Can last 1 hr to multiple periods and days of monitoring
- Can be performed with video monitoring

CLIENT EDUCATION
- Provide the child's usual oral intake of food prior to the procedure to prevent hypoglycemia during the EEG.
- Abstain from caffeine the morning of the procedure.
- Wash hair (no oils or sprays) before and after the procedure to remove electrode gel.
- The child can be asked to take deep breaths and exposed to flashes of light (photostimulation) during the procedure.
- If prescribed, withhold sleep from child prior to the test.
- The child may be allowed to sleep during the test.
- The test will not be painful.

Magnetic resonance imaging (MRI)

Used to detect malformations, cortical dysplasia, or tumors.

Lumbar puncture

Measures spinal fluid pressure and detects infection

Computed tomography (CT) scan

Detects hemorrhage, infarction, or malformations

PATIENT-CENTERED CARE

NURSING CARE

Initiate seizure precautions for any child at risk.
- Pad side rails of bed, crib, and wheelchair.
- Keep bed free of objects that could cause injury.
- Have suction and oxygen equipment available.

During a seizure
- Protect from injury (move furniture away, place folded blanket or pillow under the child's head).
- Maintain a position to provide a patent airway.
- Be prepared to suction oral secretions.
- Turn child to a side-lying position (decreases risk of aspiration).
- Loosen restrictive clothing.
- Do not attempt to restrain the child.
- Do not attempt to open the jaw or insert an airway during seizure activity. (This can damage teeth, lips, or tongue). Do not put anything in the child's mouth.
- Remove the child's glasses.
- Administer oxygen.
- Remain with the child.
- Note onset, time, and characteristics of seizure.
- Allow the seizure to end spontaneously.

Postseizure
- Maintain the child in a side-lying position to prevent aspiration and to facilitate drainage of oral secretions.
- Check for breathing, check vital signs, and check position of head and tongue.
- Check for injuries, including the mouth (tongue, teeth).
- Perform neurologic checks.
- Allow for rest if necessary.
- Reorient and calm the child (due to agitation or confusion).
- Maintain seizure precautions (placing the bed in the lowest position, padding the side rails to prevent future injury).
- Check inside the mouth to see if tongue or lips have been bitten.
- Note the time of the postictal period.
- Remain with the child.
- Do not offer food or liquids until completely awake and swallowing reflex has returned.

- Encourage the child to describe the period before, during, and after the seizure activity.
- Determine if the child experienced an aura, which can indicate the origin of seizure in the brain.
- Try to determine the possible trigger (fatigue, stress).
- Document the onset and duration of seizure and manifestations prior to, during, and following the seizure (level of consciousness, apnea, cyanosis, motor activity, incontinence).

> ! Call emergency medical services
> if any of the following occur.
> · Child stops breathing.
> · Seizure lasts more than 5 min.
> · Status epilepticus occurs.
> · Pupils are not equal following seizure.
> · Child vomits 30 min continually after end of seizure.
> · Child is unresponsive to pain or cannot be awakened.
> · Seizure occurs in water.
> · This is the child's first seizure.

MEDICATIONS

Antiepileptic drugs (AEDs)

Diazepam, phenytoin, carbamazepine, valproic acid, fosphenytoin sodium, topiramate, lamotrigine, clonazepam
- Medication selection is based on the child's age, type of seizure, and other factors.
- A single medication is initiated at low dosage and gradually increased until seizures are controlled.
- A second medication can be added to achieve seizure control.

NURSING ACTIONS
- Monitor for seizure control.
- Check for allergies.
- Monitor for adverse effects.
- Monitor therapeutic serum medication levels for required medications.
- Instruct the child and family about adverse effects of the medications.

CLIENT EDUCATION
- Medications should be taken at the same time every day to enhance effectiveness.
- Be aware of medication and food interactions that are specific to each medication.
- Dosage might need to be increased as the child grows.
- Blood cell counts, urinalysis, and liver function tests will need to be obtained at frequent intervals to determine effect on organ function.

INTERPROFESSIONAL CARE

- The school nurse should be involved in providing for the child's safety in the school setting. This can include implementation of an Individualized Education Plan or another specialized program. Qpcc
- Referral to nutrition services if a ketogenic diet (high-fat, low-carbohydrate, adequate protein) is prescribed. Qtc

THERAPEUTIC PROCEDURES

Surgical removal and separation

- Removal of a tumor, lesion, or hematoma
- **Focal resection** of an area of the brain to remove epileptogenic zone
- **Hemispherectomy:** removal of one hemisphere of the brain
- **Corpus callosotomy:** separation of the two hemispheres in the brain

Vagal nerve stimulator

- Under general anesthesia, the stimulator is implanted into the left chest wall and connected to an electrode that is placed at the left vagus nerve. The device is then programmed to administer intermittent vagal nerve stimulation at a rate specific to the child's needs.
- Treatment is adjunctive therapy for clients 12 years and older with partial onset seizures, which are not manageable with antiepileptic medications.
- In addition to routine stimulation, the child can initiate vagal nerve stimulation by holding a magnet over the implantable device at the onset of seizure activity. This will either abort the seizure or lessen its severity.

CLIENT EDUCATION

- Monitor AED levels through periodic laboratory testing.
- Do not stop medications without provider approval.
- Adhere to medication regimen.
- Possible medication interactions include decreased effectiveness of oral contraceptives.
- Wear a medical alert bracelet or necklace at all times.
- Refer to the state's Department of Motor Vehicles to determine laws regarding driving for adolescents who have seizure disorders.
- The child should wear safety devices, such as helmets, while participating in activities.
- Do not to leave the child unattended in water.
- Encourage older children to use a shower, rather than a bathtub, and leave the bathroom door unlocked while showering.
- Avoid triggering factors (emotional stress, sleep deprivation, fatigue, physical maltreatment).

COMPLICATIONS

Status epilepticus

Status epilepticus is prolonged seizure activity that lasts longer than 30 min or continuous seizure activity in which the child does not enter a postictal phase. This acute condition requires immediate treatment to prevent loss of brain function, which can become permanent.

NURSING ACTIONS
- Maintain airway.
- Administer oxygen.
- Assist in obtaining IV access.
- Monitor ECG, pulse oximetry and ABG results.
- Assist with administration of a loading dose of diazepam or lorazepam. If seizures continue after the loading dose is given, fosphenytoin followed by phenobarbital should be administered.
- Provide support for the child and family.

Developmental delays

NURSING ACTIONS
- Promote optimal development.
- Provide support for the family.
- Assist with referrals depending on the child and family's individual needs.

Application Exercises

1. A nurse is caring for a child who has absence seizures. Which of the following findings should the nurse expect? (Select all that apply.)
   - A. Loss of consciousness
   - B. Appearance of daydreaming
   - C. Dropping held objects
   - D. Falling to the floor
   - E. Having a piercing cry

2. A nurse is caring for a child who just experienced a generalized seizure. Which of the following is the priority action for the nurse to take?
   - A. Maintain the child in a side-lying position.
   - B. Check to see if the child bit his tongue.
   - C. Reorient the child to the environment.
   - D. Document the time and characteristics of the child's seizure.

3. A nurse is reinforcing teaching with the parent of a child who is to have an electroencephalogram (EEG). Which of the following responses should the nurse include?
   - A. "Offer decaffeinated beverages the morning of the procedure."
   - B. "Do not wash your child's hair the night before the procedure."
   - C. "Withhold all foods the morning of the procedure."
   - D. "Promote extra hours of sleep the night before the procedure."

4. A nurse is reinforcing teaching with a group of parents about the risk factors for seizures. Which of the following factors should the nurse include? (Select all that apply.)
   - A. Febrile episodes
   - B. Hypoglycemia
   - C. Sodium imbalances
   - D. Low serum lead levels
   - E. Presence of diphtheria

5. A nurse is reviewing treatment options with the parent of a child who has worsening seizures. Which of the following treatment options should the nurse include in the discussion? (Select all that apply.)
   - A. Vagal nerve stimulator
   - B. Additional antiepileptic medications
   - C. Corpus callosotomy
   - D. Focal resection
   - E. Radiation therapy

PRACTICE Active Learning Scenario

A nurse is contributing to the plan of care for a child who has tonic-clonic seizures. What actions should the nurse recommend? Use the ATI Active Learning Template: System Disorder to complete this item.

NURSING CARE: Describe nursing actions during and after a seizure.

Application Exercises Key

1. A. **CORRECT:** Loss of consciousness for 5 to 10 seconds is a manifestation of an absence seizure.

   B. **CORRECT:** Behavior that resembles daydreaming is a manifestation of an absence seizure.

   C. **CORRECT:** A child who is having absence seizures might drop a held object.

   D. It is rare for a child who has absence seizures to fall to the floor. However, this is a common manifestation of a tonic-clonic seizure.

   E. A piercing cry is a manifestation of an atonic-akinetic seizure.

   Ⓝ *NCLEX® Connection: Physiological Adaptation, Basic Pathophysiology*

2. A. **CORRECT:** The greatest risk to this client is aspiration from vomiting. Therefore the priority intervention the nurse should take is to place the child in a side-lying position to maintain a patent airway and prevent aspiration of secretions.

   B. The nurse should check to see if child has bitten his tongue to provide appropriate treatment and make appropriate dietary modifications. However, another intervention is the priority.

   C. The nurse should reorient the child to the environment following a generalized seizure because confusion is expected during the postseizure period. However, another intervention is the priority.

   D. The nurse should document the time and characteristics of the child's seizure in the child's medical record. However, another intervention is the priority.

   Ⓝ *NCLEX® Connection: Physiological Adaptation, Alterations in Body Systems*

3. A. **CORRECT:** Caffeine can alter the results of an EEG and should be avoided prior to the test. However, the child should maintain an adequate food and fluid intake prior to the EEG to prevent hypoglycemia during the procedure.

   B. The child's hair should be washed to remove oils that permit adherence of the EEG electrodes.

   C. Foods are not withheld prior to an EEG. Fasting can cause hypoglycemia during the procedure.

   D. Children are often required to be sleep deprived the night prior to the procedure.

   Ⓝ *NCLEX® Connection: Reduction of Risk Potential, Diagnostic Tests*

4. A. **CORRECT:** Febrile episodes are a risk factor for seizures.

   B. **CORRECT:** Hypoglycemia is a risk factor for seizures.

   C. **CORRECT:** Hypernatremia and hyponatremia are risk factors for seizures.

   D. High serum lead levels are a risk factor for seizure activity.

   E. Diphtheria is a respiratory illness causing difficulty breathing and is not a risk factor for seizures.

   Ⓝ *NCLEX® Connection: Health Promotion and Maintenance, Health Promotion/Disease Prevention*

5. A. **CORRECT:** The implantation of a vagal nerve stimulator is an option to provide seizure control.

   B. **CORRECT:** Additional antiepileptic medication can be added to the current medication regime to control seizures.

   C. **CORRECT:** A corpus callosotomy can be performed for uncontrolled seizures.

   D. **CORRECT:** A focal resection can be performed for uncontrolled seizures.

   E. Radiation therapy is used in cancer treatment and is not indicated for the management or treatment of seizures.

   Ⓝ *NCLEX® Connection: Reduction of Risk Potential, Therapeutic Procedures*

PRACTICE Answer

Using the ATI Active Learning Template: System Disorder

NURSING CARE

- During a seizure
  - Protect the child from injury. (Move furniture away. Place folded blanket or pillow under the child's head.)
  - Position the child to maintain a patent airway.
  - Be prepared to suction oral secretions.
  - Turn the child to the side (decreases risk of aspiration).
  - Loosen restrictive clothing.
  - Do not attempt to restrain the child.
  - Do not attempt to open the jaw or insert an airway during seizure activity. (This can damage teeth, lips, or tongue.) Do not use tongue blades.
  - Remove glasses.
  - Administer oxygen.
  - Remain with the child.
  - Note the onset, time, and characteristics of the seizure.
  - Allow the seizure to end spontaneously.

- Postseizure
  - Maintain the child in a side-lying position to prevent aspiration and to facilitate drainage of oral secretions.
  - Check for breathing, check vital signs, and check position of head and tongue.
  - Check for injuries, including the mouth.
  - Perform neurologic checks.
  - Allow the child to rest if necessary.
  - Reorient and calm the child, who might be agitated or confused.
  - Maintain seizure precautions (placing the bed in the lowest position, padding the side rails to prevent future injury).
  - Check inside the mouth to see if the lips and tongue have been bitten.
  - Note the time of the postictal period.
  - Remain with the child.
  - Do not offer food or liquids until completely awake and has a swallowing reflex has returned.
  - Encourage the child to describe the period before, during, and after the seizure activity.
  - Determine if the child experienced an aura, which can indicate the origin of seizure in the brain.
  - Try to determine the possible trigger, such as fatigue or stress.
  - Document the onset and duration of seizure and manifestations prior to, during, and following the seizure (level of consciousness, apnea, cyanosis, motor activity, incontinence).

Ⓝ *NCLEX® Connection: Physiological Adaptation, Alterations in Body Systems*

CHAPTER 14

Cognitive and Sensory Impairments

Sensory impairments in children most commonly affect the eyes and ears. Vision and hearing affect growth and development. Therefore, it is important to identify any impairments early in life.

Down syndrome is a common chromosomal abnormality that affects growth and development, and results in cognitive and sensory impairments.

Visual impairments

- Visual impairments include partial sight and legal blindness.
- Common visual impairments in children include myopia, hyperopia, astigmatism, anisometropia, amblyopia, strabismus, cataracts, and glaucoma.

HEALTH PROMOTION AND DISEASE PREVENTION

- Encourage the family to work with the child's school to meet educational needs.
- Screen children for visual impairments yearly.

DATA COLLECTION

RISK FACTORS

- Prenatal or postnatal conditions (retinopathy of prematurity, trauma, postnatal infections)
- Perinatal infections (herpes, rubella, syphilis, chlamydia, gonorrhea, toxoplasmosis)
- Chronic illness (sickle cell disease, rheumatoid arthritis, retinoblastoma, albinism, Tay-Sachs disease)

EXPECTED FINDINGS

Visual impairment manifestations

Myopia (nearsightedness)
- Sees close objects clearly, but not objects in the distance
- Headaches and vertigo
- Eye rubbing
- Difficulty reading
- Clumsiness (frequently walking into objects)
- Poor school performance

Hyperopia (farsightedness)
- Sees distant objects clearly, but not objects that are close
- Because of accommodation, not usually detected until age 7

Astigmatism (curvature of the cornea or lens impairs the ability for light to focus on the retina)
- Uneven vision in which only parts of letters on a page can be seen
- Headache and vertigo
- Appearance of normal vision because tilting the head enables all letters to be seen

Anisometropia (each eye has a different refractive strength)
- Headache and vertigo
- Excessive eye rubbing
- Poor school performance
- Can progress to amblyopia

Amblyopia (lazy eye)
- Reduced visual acuity in one eye
- Can progress to functional blindness in the weaker eye

Strabismus: Esotropia (inward deviation of eye); **exotropia** (outward deviation of eye)
- Abnormal corneal light reflex or cover test
- Misaligned eyes
- Frowning or squinting
- Difficulty seeing print clearly
- One eye closed to enable better vision
- Head tilted to one side
- Headache, dizziness, diplopia, photophobia, crossed eyes

Cataracts (opacity of the lens)
- Decreased ability to see clearly
- Decreased peripheral vision
- Nystagmus
- Strabismus
- Gray opacity of the lens
- Absence of red reflex

Glaucoma (increased intraocular pressure)
- Loss of peripheral vision
- Perception of halos around objects
- Red eye
- Excessive tearing (epiphora)
- Photophobia
- Spasmodic winking (blepharospasm)
- Corneal haziness
- Enlargement of the eyeball (buphthalmos)
- Possible pain

DIAGNOSTIC PROCEDURES

Visual acuity screening
- This is completed using the Snellen letter, tumbling E, or picture chart.
  - Place the client 10 feet from the chart with heels on the 10-foot mark.
  - Client should be wearing glasses, if appropriate, and keep both eyes open during the screening.
  - While covering one eye, the client reads each line on the chart, starting at the bottom of the chart, until he can pass a line. The client needs to identify four of the six characters in the line correctly to pass.
  - The client is then asked to start at the top and move down until he can no longer pass a line.
  - The procedure is repeated with the other eye.
  - Some facilities vary in procedure regarding distance and order of lines to read.
- **Partial visual impairment** is classified as visual acuity of 20/70 to 20/200.
- **Legal blindness** is classified as visual acuity of 20/200 or worse or a visual field of 20° or less in the child's better eye.

Ocular alignment: Observed using the corneal light reflex test
- A flashlight is shone directly into the client's eye, from a distance of 16 inches.
- Reflected light should be observed in the same location on both corneas.

Cover test: Client is asked to cover each eye and observe an object at a distance of 13 inches. The cover is removed and the eye is observed for movement, which should not occur.

Peripheral vision: Evaluated by having the client fixate on an object
- A pencil is moved from beyond the field of vision into the range of peripheral vision.
- The client is asked to say stop when the object is noted in the peripheral vision. This angle is then measured.
- Each quadrant of peripheral vision is tested. The test is repeated in the other eye.
- Normal findings are 50° upward, 70° downward, 60° nasalward, and 90° temporally.

Color vision
- The client is shown a set of cards and asked to identify the number embedded in the confusion of colors.
- The client should identify all of the numbers on the cards with correct color vision.

PATIENT-CENTERED CARE

NURSING CARE
- Maintain normal to bright lighting for the child when reading, writing, or participating in any activity that requires close vision.
- Check infants and children for visual impairments, and identify children that are high-risk.
- Observe for behaviors that suggest a decrease or loss of vision.
- Promote child's optimal development and parent-child attachment.
- Identify safety hazards, and prevent injury to the eyes (helmets, safety glasses). Qs
- Reinforce information regarding laser surgery for clients who have myopia, hyperopia, or astigmatism.
- Inform the child and family about corrective measures.
  - Myopia, hyperopia, astigmatism, anisometropia: Prescribed lenses, laser surgery
  - Amblyopia: Treat primary visual defect
  - Strabismus: Occlusion therapy (patch stronger eye), surgery
  - Cataracts and glaucoma: Surgery

CARING FOR A CHILD WHO HAS A VISION IMPAIRMENT
- Reassure the child and family.
- Orient the child to the surroundings and provide a safe environment.
- Promote independence and meeting developmental milestones while assisting with play and socialization. Qpcc
- Assist with referral to educational services for visual impairment (braille, audio tapes, specialized computers).

Hearing impairments

Hearing impairments affect speech and the ability to clearly process linguistic sounds.
- **Conductive losses** involve interference of sound transmission, which can result from otitis media, external ear infection, foreign bodies, or excessive ear wax.
- **Sensorineural losses** involve interference of the transmission along the nerve pathways, which can result from congenital defects or secondary to acquired conditions (infection, ototoxic medication, exposure to constant noise [as in a NICU]).
- **Central auditory imperception** involves all other hearing losses (aphasia, agnosia [inability to interpret sounds]).

HEALTH PROMOTION AND DISEASE PREVENTION

- Screen for hearing impairments.
- Help families identify community resources for children who have hearing loss.
- Prevent further damage and hearing loss.
  - Avoid exposing children to hazardous noise.
  - Encourage children to wear ear protection if loud environmental noise cannot be avoided.

DATA COLLECTION

RISK FACTORS

- Exposure to loud environmental sounds.
- Hearing defects can be caused by a variety of conditions (anatomic malformation, maternal ingestion of toxic substances during pregnancy, perinatal asphyxia, perinatal infection, chronic ear infection, ototoxic medications).
- Hearing defects can be associated with chronic conditions (Down syndrome, cerebral palsy).

EXPECTED FINDINGS

INFANTS
- Lack of startle reflex
- Failure to respond to noise
- Absence of vocalization by 7 months
- Lack of response to the spoken word

OLDER CHILDREN
- Using gestures rather than talking after 15 months
- Failure to develop understood speech by 24 months
- Yelling to express emotions
- Irritability due to inability to gain attention
- Seeming shy or withdrawn
- Inattentive to surroundings
- Speaking in monotone
- Need for repeated conversation

PATIENT-CENTERED CARE

NURSING CARE

- Check for hearing impairment.
- Promote speech development, lip reading, and use of cued speech (hand gestures with verbal communication).
- Encourage socialization and use of aids to promote independence (flashing light when the doorbell or phone rings, telecommunication devices, closed captioning).
- Assist with referral for child and family to community support groups.
- Use sign language or an interpreter if appropriate. Always talk to the child, not the interpreter.
- Monitor gait/balance for instability.
- Identify safety hazards and adjust environment as needed. Qs
- Assist with the use of hearing aids.

COMPLICATIONS

Delayed growth and development

Visual and hearing impairments can affect the child's speech and motor development. Identifying the impairment early can minimize this.

NURSING ACTIONS
- Encourage self-care and optimal independence.
- Assist with interprofessional referrals as needed (social services, speech therapy, physical therapy, occupational therapy, teachers). Qrc
- Assist the family to obtain and access appropriate assistive devices.

Down syndrome

- The most common chromosomal abnormality of a generalized syndrome, trisomy 21 is seen in 97% of cases of Down syndrome.
- Many medical conditions accompany Down syndrome (congenital heart malformation, hypotonicity, dysfunction of the immune system, thyroid dysfunction, leukemia).

DATA COLLECTION

RISK FACTORS

- The cause is unclear but might be multicausal.
- Maternal age greater than 35 years
- Paternal age greater than 55 years

EXPECTED FINDINGS

- Separated sagittal suture
- Enlarged anterior fontanel
- Small, round head
- Flattened forehead
- Upward, outward slant to eyes
- Small nose with depressed nasal bridge (saddle nose)
- Small ears with short pinna
- Epicanthal folds
- High-arched narrow palate
- Protruding tongue
- Short, broad neck
- Shortened rib cage
- Possible congenital heart defect
- Protruding abdomen
- Incurved fifth finger (clinodactyly)
- Broad, short feet and hands with stubby toes and fingers
- Transverse palmar crease
- Large space between big and second toes with plantar crease
- Short stature
- Hyperflexibility, muscle weakness, and hypotonia
- Dry skin that cracks easily

DIAGNOSTIC PROCEDURES

PRENATAL: Testing for alpha-fetoprotein in maternal serum

INFANT: Chromosome analysis and echocardiography

PATIENT-CENTERED CARE

NURSING CARE

- Swaddle the infant to prevent heat loss due to limp, extended body position.
- Assist family with feeding difficulties, and monitor dietary intake.
- Promote good skin care.
- Monitor developmental progress at regular intervals.
- Support family at the time of diagnosis.
- Assist with appropriate referrals.
- Assist the parents in holding and bonding with the infant.

THERAPEUTIC PROCEDURES

Surgical interventions depend on the associated congenital anomalies. These can include cardiac defects or strabismus.

INTERPROFESSIONAL CARE

Social work, home health, school early intervention, genetic counseling, speech therapy, physical therapy, occupational therapy

NURSING ACTIONS

- Listen to the concerns of the parents and discuss ethical dilemmas regarding treatment for physical defects.
- Assist in providing standard postoperative care with emphasis on wound care, respiratory care, and pain management.
- Reinforce postoperative and home-care management.
- Reinforce the therapeutic plan of care.
- Advise the family how to prevent complications.

CLIENT EDUCATION

- Aspirate nasal secretions.
- Rinse the mouth after feedings.
- Use cool mist in the room to assist in moistening secretions.
- Change the infant's position frequently.
- Use feeding strategies to accommodate for the protruding tongue.
- Provide skin care and use moisturizing creams daily.
- Provide a diet high in fiber and fluid to prevent constipation. Monitor calorie intake to prevent obesity.
- Schedule regular health care visits.
- Monitor developmental milestones.
- Monitor height and weight by plotting growth on National Center for Health Statistics or World Health Organization charts.
- Prepare for surgery for cardiac problems or strabismus if indicated.
- Evaluate eyesight and hearing frequently.
- Schedule frequent thyroid functioning tests.
- Monitor for atlantoaxial instability (neck pain, weakness, torticollis).

COMPLICATIONS

INTELLIGENCE: Mental capacity varies typically from mild to moderate cognitive impairment

SOCIAL DEVELOPMENT: Development can be 2 to 3 years beyond the mental age.

CONGENITAL ANOMALIES: About 40% to 45% have congenital heart disease. Other possible anomalies include hip subluxation, patella dislocation, duodenal atresia, tracheoesophageal fistula, and Hirschsprung's disease.

SENSORY PROBLEMS
- **Ocular problems** include strabismus, nystagmus, astigmatism, myopia, hyperopia, head tilt, excessive tearing, and cataracts.
- **Hearing loss** occurs in a large percentage of children who have Down syndrome. Frequent otitis media, narrow canals, and impacted cerumen can contribute to the hearing problems.

OTHER PHYSICAL DISORDERS
- Frequent respiratory tract infections
- Increased incidence of leukemia
- Impaired thyroid function.

GROWTH: Both height and weight are reduced. Weight gain is more rapid than growth in height and can result in excessive weight by 36 months.

SEXUAL DEVELOPMENT: Genitalia can be underdeveloped and delayed.

Respiratory infections

Respiratory infections are common due to decreased muscle tone and poor drainage of mucus because of hypotonicity and associated underdeveloped nasal bone.

NURSING ACTIONS

- Rinse the child's mouth with water after feeding and at other times of the day when it is dry. Mucous membranes are dry due to constant mouth breathing, which also increases the risk for respiratory infection.
- Provide cool mist humidification and clearing of the nasal passages with a bulb syringe as needed.
- Encourage physical activity and exercise.

CLIENT EDUCATION
- Use good hand hygiene.
- Reposition the child frequently to promote respiratory function.
- Get routine immunizations.
- Seek health care at the earliest indication of infection.
- Follow the antibiotic schedule if prescribed.

Application Exercises

1. A nurse is preparing to perform a peripheral vision test on a child. Which of the following actions should the nurse take?

   A. Place the child 10 feet away from a Snellen chart.

   B. Show a set of cards to the child one at a time.

   C. Cover the child's eye while performing the test on the other eye.

   D. Have the child focus on an object while performing the test.

2. A nurse is reinforcing teaching with a group of parents about possible manifestations of Down syndrome. Which of the following findings should the nurse include? (Select all that apply.)

   A. A large head with bulging fontanels

   B. Larger ears that are set back

   C. Protruding abdomen

   D. Broad, short feet and hands

   E. Hypotonia

3. A nurse is collecting data from a child who has myopia. Which of the following findings should the nurse expect? (Select all that apply.)

   A. Headaches

   B. Photophobia

   C. Difficulty reading

   D. Difficulty focusing on close objects

   E. Poor school performance

4. A nurse is screening a toddler for hearing loss. Which of the following findings are indications of a hearing impairment? (Select all that apply.)

   A. Uses monotone speech

   B. Yells to express emotions

   C. Wants to repeat conversations

   D. Appears shy

   E. Is overly attentive to the surroundings

5. A nurse is reinforcing teaching with the parent of an infant who has Down syndrome. Which of the following statements by the parent indicates an understanding of the information?

   A. "I should expect him to have frequent diarrhea."

   B. "I should place a cool mist humidifier in his room."

   C. "I should avoid the use of lotion on his skin."

   D. "I should expect him to grow faster in length than other infants."

PRACTICE Active Learning Scenario

A nurse is preparing to perform a visual acuity screening test on a child. What nursing actions should the nurse include? Use the ATI Active Learning Template: Nursing Skill to complete this item.

DESCRIPTION OF SKILL: Explain the procedure.

OUTCOMES/EVALUATION: Describe findings that indicate visual impairment.

Application Exercises Key

1. A. The nurse should place the child 10 feet away from a Snellen chart when performing a visual acuity test.

   B. The nurse should show a set of cards to the child one at a time when performing a color test.

   C. The nurse should cover the child's eye while testing the other eye when performing a cover test.

   D. **CORRECT:** When performing a peripheral vision test, the nurse asks the child to focus on an object while bringing a pencil into the child's peripheral vision.

   Ⓝ *NCLEX® Connection: Health Promotion and Maintenance, Health Promotion/Disease Prevention*

2. A. A child who has hydrocephalus will exhibit a large head with bulging fontanels due to the increased cerebrospinal fluid in the head.

   B. A child who has Down syndrome will exhibit small features, such as small ears with a short pinna.

   C. **CORRECT:** A child who has Down syndrome will exhibit a protruding abdomen.

   D. **CORRECT:** A child who has Down syndrome will exhibit small features, such as broad, short feet and hands.

   E. **CORRECT:** A child who has Down syndrome will exhibit hyperflexibility and hypotonia.

   Ⓝ *NCLEX® Connection: Physiological Adaptation, Basic Pathophysiology*

3. A. **CORRECT:** Headaches are a manifestation of myopia.

   B. Photophobia is a manifestation of strabismus.

   C. **CORRECT:** Difficulty reading is a manifestation of myopia.

   D. Difficulty focusing on close objects is a manifestation of hyperopia.

   E. **CORRECT:** Poor school performance is a manifestation of myopia.

   Ⓝ *NCLEX® Connection: Physiological Adaptation, Basic Pathophysiology*

4. A. **CORRECT:** Monotone speech is a manifestation of a hearing impairment.

   B. **CORRECT:** Yelling to express emotions is a manifestation of a hearing impairment.

   C. **CORRECT:** Need for repeated conversation is a manifestation of a hearing impairment.

   D. **CORRECT:** Shyness and withdrawn behavior are manifestations of a hearing impairment.

   E. Inattentiveness to surroundings is a manifestation of a hearing impairment.

   Ⓝ *NCLEX® Connection: Health Promotion and Maintenance, Developmental Stages and Transitions*

5. A. Down syndrome increases the risk for constipation, resulting in the need for additional fluid and fiber in the diet.

   B. **CORRECT:** Down syndrome increases the risk for respiratory infections. Using a cool mist humidifier in the infant's room helps prevent respiratory infections.

   C. Down syndrome causes dry skin that cracks easily. The parent should practice good skin care, including the application of lotion.

   D. Down syndrome results in reduced growth in length for infants and height for children.

   Ⓝ *NCLEX® Connection: Physiological Adaptation, Alterations in Body Systems*

PRACTICE Answer

Using the ATI Active Learning Template: Nursing Skill

DESCRIPTION OF SKILL
- Choose appropriate chart: Snellen Letter, tumbling E, or picture chart.
- Place the child 10 feet from the chart with heels on the 10-foot mark.
- Screen the child wearing glasses, if appropriate.
- Child keeps both eyes open and covers one eye.
- First have the child start at the bottom and read each line, continuing up until the child can pass a line.
- Then have the child start at the top and move down until the child can no longer pass a line.
- To pass, the child needs to identify four of the six characters correctly.
- Repeat the procedure with the other eye.

OUTCOMES/EVALUATION
- Partial visual impairment is classified as visual acuity of 20/70 to 20/200.
- Legal blindness is classified as visual acuity of 20/200 or worse or a visual field of 20° or less in the child's better eye.

Ⓝ *NCLEX® Connection: Health Promotion and Maintenance, Health Screening*

When reviewing the following chapters, keep in mind the relevant topics and tasks of the NCLEX outline, in particular:

Pharmacological Therapies

EXPECTED ACTIONS/OUTCOMES
Apply knowledge of pathophysiology when addressing client pharmacological agents.

Reinforce education to client regarding medications.

Reduction of Risk Potential

DIAGNOSTIC TESTS: Perform diagnostic testing (blood glucose, oxygen saturation, testing for occult blood).

POTENTIAL FOR COMPLICATIONS OF DIAGNOSTIC TESTS/ TREATMENTS/PROCEDURES: Evaluate client oxygen (O_2) saturation.

POTENTIAL FOR COMPLICATIONS FROM SURGICAL PROCEDURES AND HEALTH ALTERATIONS: Identify the client's response to surgery or health alterations.

THERAPEUTIC PROCEDURES: Reinforce client teaching on treatments and procedures.

Physiological Adaptation

ALTERATIONS IN BODY SYSTEMS
Intervene to improve client respiratory status (breathing treatment, suctioning, repositioning).

Reinforce education to the client regarding care and condition.

BASIC PATHOPHYSIOLOGY
Identify signs and symptoms related to an acute or chronic illness.

Consider general principles of client disease process when providing care (injury and repair, immunity, cellular structure).

Apply knowledge of pathophysiology to monitoring client for alterations in body systems.

MEDICAL EMERGENCIES: Respond/intervene to a client's life-threatening situation (cardiopulmonary resuscitation).

UNIT 2 **NURSING CARE OF CHILDREN WHO HAVE SYSTEM DISORDERS**
SECTION: RESPIRATORY DISORDERS

CHAPTER 15 # Oxygen and Inhalation Therapy

Oxygen is used to maintain adequate cellular oxygenation. It is used in the treatment of many acute and chronic respiratory problems (hypoxemia, cystic fibrosis, asthma). Supplemental oxygen is delivered using a variety of methods, depending on individual circumstances.

Pulse oximetry is used to monitor the effectiveness of inhalation therapies.

Nebulized aerosol therapy, metered-dose inhaler (MDI), dry powder inhaler (DPI), chest physiotherapy (CPT), oxygen therapy, suctioning, and artificial airway are common treatment methods used for children who have acute or chronic respiratory problems.

Pulse oximetry

- Pulse oximetry is a noninvasive measurement of the percentage of oxygen saturation in hemoglobin.
- A pulse oximeter is a device that is operated by battery or electricity and has a sensor probe that is attached securely to the child's fingertip, toe, earlobe, or around the foot with a clip or band.

INDICATIONS

Pulse oximetry is used for a variety of situations in which quick data collection of a child's respiratory status is needed.

CONSIDERATIONS

PREPROCEDURE NURSING ACTIONS

- Find an appropriate probe site. The probe site must be dry and have adequate circulation. Remove polish from nails or remove earrings if using the earlobe.
- Be sure the child is in a comfortable position and that the arm is supported if a finger is used as a probe site.

INTRAPROCEDURE NURSING ACTIONS

- Note the pulse reading and compare it with the child's radial pulse. Any discrepancy between the values warrants further data collection.
- If continuous monitoring is required, make sure the alarms are set for a low and a high limit, the alarms are functioning, and the sound is audible. Move the probe every 4 to 8 hr or per facility policy to prevent pressure necrosis in infants who have disrupted skin integrity or poor perfusion. Qs

POSTPROCEDURE NURSING ACTIONS

Report unexpected findings to the charge nurse and provider.

If a child's SaO₂ is less than the expected range
- Confirm that the sensor probe is properly placed with the LED placed on the top of the nail when digits are used.
- Confirm that the oxygen delivery system is functioning and that the child is receiving the prescribed oxygen flow rate. Increase oxygen rate as prescribed.
- Place the child in a semi-Fowler's or Fowler's position to maximize ventilation.
- Encourage deep breathing.
- Remain with the child and provide emotional support to decrease anxiety.

INTERPRETATION OF FINDINGS

- The expected reference range for SaO₂ is 95% to 100%, although adequate levels can range from 91% to 100%. Some illnesses can cause SaO₂ of 85% to 89%.
- Results of 90% or less require nursing intervention to assist the child to regain adequate SaO₂ levels. SaO₂ less than 86% is a life-threatening emergency. The lower the SaO₂ level, the less accurate the value.

Nebulized aerosol therapy

The process of nebulization breaks up medications into minute particles that are then dispersed throughout the respiratory tract. These droplets are much finer than those created by inhalers.

INDICATIONS

Respiratory conditions that necessitate bronchodilators, corticosteroids, mucolytics, or antibiotics

CONSIDERATIONS

PREPARATION OF THE CLIENT

- Instruct the child and family that the treatment can take 10 to 15 min.
- Determine if the child should use a mouthpiece, mask, or blow-by.
- Collect preprocedure data, including vital signs, oxygen saturation, breath sounds, and effort of breathing.
- Pour the medication into the small container and attach the device to an air or oxygen source.

ONGOING CARE

- Encourage the child to take slow, deep breaths by mouth. If using a mask, instruct the child to breathe with an open mouth to avoid inhalation of medication into the nose and pharynx.
- Monitor the child during the treatment, watching carefully for indications of local tracheal or bronchial effects (spasms, edema).
- Check vital signs, oxygen saturation, and lung sounds at the completion of treatment.
- Assist the family with obtaining a nebulizer for home use if needed.
- Reinforce recommendations for aerosolized medications.
- Monitor for adverse reactions to medications.
- Reinforce teaching with the family on how to operate a home nebulizer.
- Discuss adverse effects of medications with the family.

Metered-dose inhaler or dry powder inhaler

These are handheld devices that allow children to self-administer medications on an intermittent basis.

INDICATIONS

Respiratory conditions that necessitate bronchodilators or corticosteroids

CONSIDERATIONS

Instructions for use of an MDI (15.1)

- Remove the cap from the inhaler.
- Shake the inhaler five to six times.
- Attach the spacer. (The use of a spacer allows for particles of medication to remain suspended for longer periods. Encourage the use of a spacer for children to facilitate effective inhalation of the medication.)
- Hold the inhaler with the mouthpiece at the bottom.
- Hold the inhaler with the thumb near the mouthpiece, and the index and middle fingers at the top.
- Instruct the child on an MDI placement technique.
  - **Open-mouth method:** Hold the inhaler approximately 3 to 4 cm (1.2 to 1.6 in) away from the front of the mouth.
  - **Closed-mouth method:** Place the inhaler between the lips and instruct the child to form a seal around the MDI.
- Take a deep breath and then exhale.
- Tilt the head back slightly, and press the inhaler. While pressing the inhaler, begin a slow, deep breath that lasts for 3 to 5 seconds to facilitate delivery to the air passages.
- Hold the breath for approximately 5 to 10 seconds to allow the medication to deposit in the airways.
- If an additional puff is needed, wait 1 min between puffs.
- Take the inhaler out of the mouth and slowly exhale through the nose.
- Resume normal breathing.
- Rinse mouth after inhaler use.

Instructions for the use of a DPI

- Do not shake the device.
- Take the cover off the mouthpiece.
- Follow the directions of the manufacturer for preparing the medication, such as turning the wheel of the inhaler.
- Exhale completely.
- Place the mouthpiece between the lips and take a deep breath through the mouth.
- Hold breath for 5 to 10 seconds.
- Take the inhaler out of the mouth and slowly exhale through pursed lips.
- Resume normal breathing.
- If more than one puff is prescribed, wait the length of time directed before administering the second puff.
- Remove the canister and rinse the inhaler, cap, and spacer once a day with warm running water. Dry the inhaler before reuse.

COMPLICATIONS

Improper medication dosage related to improper use

- Inhalation is too rapid.
- Inability to coordinate inhalation with spray.
- Not holding breath for adequate period.

NURSING ACTIONS
- Ensure the child uses the inhaler with proper technique.
- Reinforce proper technique with client and family.

Fungal infections

Fungal infections of the oral cavity can occur with corticosteroid use.

NURSING ACTIONS
- Inspect mouth for indications of infections.
- Assist the child with rinsing his mouth after administration.

CLIENT EDUCATION: Clean the MDI and spacer after each use and have the child rinse his mouth and expectorate. Qpcc

Chest physiotherapy

Chest physiotherapy is a set of techniques that includes manual or mechanical percussion, vibration, cough, forceful expiration (or huffing), and breathing exercises. Gravity and positioning loosen respiratory secretions and move them into the central airways, where they can be eliminated by coughing or suctioning to rid excessive secretions from specific areas of the lungs.

INDICATIONS

CLIENT PRESENTATION: Thick secretions with an inability to clear the airway

CONTRAINDICATIONS: Decreased cardiac reserves, pulmonary embolism, pulmonary hemorrhage, end-stage kidney disease, osteogenesis imperfecta, increased intracranial pressure

CONSIDERATIONS

PREPROCEDURE NURSING ACTIONS

- Schedule treatments before meals or at least 1 hr after meals and at bedtime to decrease the likelihood of vomiting or aspirating.
- Offer the child an emesis basin and facial tissues.
- Administer a bronchodilator medication or nebulizer treatment prior to postural drainage.
- Recombinant human deoxyribonuclease can also be used to decrease the viscosity of the mucus.

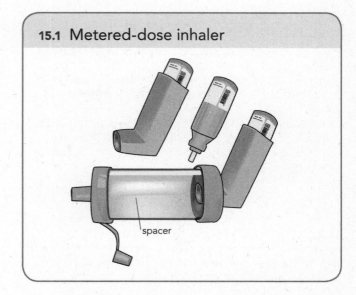

15.1 Metered-dose inhaler

spacer

INTRAPROCEDURE NURSING ACTIONS

- Perform hand hygiene, provide privacy, and explain the procedure to the child and parents.
- Ensure proper positioning to promote drainage of specific areas of the lungs. Qebp
  - **Apical sections of the upper lobes:** Fowler's position
  - **Posterior sections of the upper lobes:** Sitting position with child leaning forward curled over pillows
  - **Anterior segments of both upper lobes:** Supine and rotated slightly away from side being drained
  - **Superior segments of both lower lobes:** Prone with hips elevated on pillows
- Avoid head-down position if history of GERD
- Apply manual percussion by using cupped hand or a special device to clap rhythmically on the chest wall to break up secretions.
- Electronic percussion is applied by a vest device worn by the child.
- Have the child remain in each postural drainage position for 20 to 30 min to allow time for percussion, vibration, and postural drainage. Older children can tolerate longer periods.
- Individualize the position used and the duration and frequency of treatment.
- Discontinue the procedure if the child reports faintness or dizziness.

POSTPROCEDURE NURSING ACTIONS

- Perform lung auscultation and inspect the amount, color, and character of the expectorated secretions.
- Document interventions and repeat the procedure as prescribed (typically three or four times per day).

COMPLICATIONS

Hypoxia (decrease in SaO₂)

NURSING ACTIONS
- Monitor respiratory status during the procedure.
- Discontinue the procedure if dyspnea occurs.

Oxygen therapy

- Oxygen therapy increases the oxygen concentration of the air that is being breathed.
- Oxygen can be delivered via nasal cannula, face mask, face tent, CPAP, BiPAP, tent, hood, or mechanical ventilator. **(15.2)**
- Humidification of oxygen moistens the airways, which promotes loosening and mobilization of pulmonary secretions and prevents drying and injury of respiratory structures.

INDICATIONS

Hypoxemia

Hypoxemia develops when there is an inadequate level of oxygen in the blood. Hypovolemia, hypoventilation, and interruption of arterial flow can lead to hypoxemia.

EXPECTED FINDINGS
- Tachypnea
- Tachycardia
- Restlessness
- Anxiety
- Pallor of the skin and mucous membranes
- Evidence of respiratory distress (use of accessory muscles, nasal flaring, tracheal tugging, adventitious lung sounds)
- Infant: inability to suck

As hypoxemia worsens
- Confusion and stupor
- Cyanosis of skin and mucous membranes
- Bradypnea
- Bradycardia
- Hypotension or hypertension
- Chronic hypoxemia: clubbing of fingers and polycythemia

CONSIDERATIONS

PREPARATION OF THE CLIENT

- Warm oxygen to prevent hypothermia.
- Use a calm, nonthreatening approach.
- Explain all procedures to the child and parents.
- Place the client in semi-Fowler's or Fowler's position to facilitate breathing and to promote chest expansion.
- Ensure that equipment is working properly.
- Inspect nostrils if using nasal cannula for oxygen administration.

ONGOING CARE

- Provide oxygen therapy at the lowest flow that corrects hypoxemia.
- Monitor lung sounds and respiratory rate, rhythm, and effort to determine the need for supplemental oxygen.
- Do not allow oxygen to blow directly onto the infant's face.
- Change linens and clothing frequently.
- Monitor the child's temperature closely in an oxygen tent for hypothermia.
- Monitor oxygenation status with pulse oximetry and ABGs.
- Apply the oxygen delivery device.
- Provide oral hygiene as needed.
- Promote turning, coughing, deep breathing, and use of incentive spirometry and suctioning.
- Promote rest and decrease environmental stimuli.
- Provide emotional support for children who appear anxious.
- Evaluate nutritional status and provide supplements.
- Inspect skin integrity closely for pressure ulcers. Move devices and inspect the skin several times daily. Provide moisture and pressure-relief devices as indicated.
- Monitor and document response to oxygen therapy.
- Titrate oxygen to maintain the prescribed oxygen saturation.
- Discontinue oxygen gradually.

COMPLICATIONS

Combustion

Oxygen is combustible. **Qs**

NURSING ACTIONS
- Place "No Smoking" or "Oxygen in Use" signs to alert others of the combustion hazard.
- Know where the closest fire extinguisher is located.
- Have the child wear a cotton gown, because synthetics or wools can create sparks of static electricity.
- Ensure that all electric machinery (monitors, suction machines) are grounded.
- Avoid toys that can induce a spark.
- Do not use volatile, flammable materials (alcohol, acetone) near children who are receiving oxygen.
- Educate the child and others about the fire hazards of smoking with oxygen use. **Qpcc**

Oxygen toxicity

- Oxygen toxicity can result from high concentrations of oxygen, long duration of oxygen therapy, and the degree of lung disease.
- Hypoventilation and increased $PaCO_2$ levels allow for rapid progression into unconscious state.

NURSING ACTIONS
- Use the lowest level of oxygen necessary to maintain an adequate SaO_2.
- Monitor ABGs and notify the charge nurse and provider if $PaCO_2$ levels rise outside of the expected reference range.
- Decrease the oxygen flow rate gradually.

15.2 Oxygen therapy delivery systems

DELIVERY SYSTEM	NURSING CONSIDERATIONS
Oxygen hood Small plastic hood that fits over the infant's head	• Use a minimum flow rate of 4 to 5 L/min to prevent carbon dioxide buildup. • Ensure that neck, chin, or shoulders do not rub against the hood. • Secure a pulse oximeter for continuous SaO_2 monitoring.
Nasal cannula Disposable plastic tube with two prongs for insertion into the nostrils that delivers an oxygen concentrations of 24% to 40% FiO_2 at a flow rate of 1 to 6 L/min	• Nasal cannulas are safe, easy to apply, and well tolerated. • The child is able to eat, talk, and ambulate while wearing a cannula. • Cannulas can be used by infants and older children who are cooperative. • Determine the patency of the nares. • Ensure that the prongs fit in the nares properly. • A nasal cannula can cause skin breakdown and dry mucous membranes. • Supply the child with a water-soluble gel if the nares are dry. • Provide humidification for flow rates greater than 4 L/min. • Prongs can become dislodged easily. Monitor the child frequently.
Pediatric face mask Pediatric-size mask that covers the nose and mouth	• Used for short-term therapy • Used at a flow rate of 5 to 10 L/min to minimize carbon dioxide rebreathing. • Face masks require a snug fit and might not be tolerated. • Used for supplying high oxygen flow rate or for children who are mouth breathers.

Suctioning

Suctioning can be accomplished orally, nasally, endotracheally, or through a tracheostomy tube.

INDICATIONS

To remove mucus plugs and excessive secretions

CLIENT PRESENTATION: Manifestations of hypoxemia (restlessness, tachypnea, tachycardia, decreased SaO_2 levels), adventitious breath sounds, visualization of secretions, cyanosis, absence of spontaneous cough

CONSIDERATIONS

Nasal suctioning

• Use clean technique.
• Use a mushroom tip catheter.
• Use bulb syringe for infants.

Oral suctioning

• Use clean technique.
• Use a hard catheter tip.
• Insert in sides of mouth.

Endotracheal and tracheal suctioning

PREPROCEDURE NURSING ACTIONS
• Perform hand hygiene, provide privacy, and explain the procedure to the child.
• Don the required personal protective equipment. Assist the child to a high-Fowler's or Fowler's position for suctioning if possible.
• Perform through a tracheostomy or an endotracheal tube. Select a catheter with a diameter half the diameter of the tracheostomy tube.

• Ask for assistance if necessary.
• Hyperoxygenate and hyperventilate the child (before and after suctioning) using a bag–valve–mask resuscitator or specialized ventilator function with an FiO_2 of 100%.
• Obtain baseline breath sounds and vital signs, including oxygen saturation (SaO_2) by pulse oximeter. Monitor oxygen saturation continually during the procedure.

INTRAPROCEDURE NURSING ACTIONS
• Use correct surgical aseptic technique as identified in appropriate resources.
• Maintain ongoing monitoring of oxygen status while performing the procedure.
• Limit suction time to less than 5 seconds for infants and less than 10 seconds for children.
• Allow the child to rest 30 to 60 seconds after each aspiration for oxygen saturation to return to normal.
• Ensure vacuum pressure is set accordingly.
  ○ 60 to 100 mm Hg for infants and children
  ○ 40 to 60 mm Hg for preterm infants

POSTPROCEDURE NURSING ACTIONS
• Hyperoxygenate with 100% oxygen.
• Auscultate lung sounds.
• Monitor oxygen saturation level.
• Evaluate and document the child's response.

COMPLICATIONS

Hypoxia

NURSING ACTIONS
• Stop the procedure.
• Hyperoxygenate the child.

Artificial airways

- A tracheotomy is a sterile surgical incision into the trachea through the skin and muscles for the purpose of establishing an airway.
- A tracheotomy can be performed as an emergency procedure for epiglottitis, croup, or foreign-body aspiration, or as a scheduled surgical procedure.
- A tracheostomy is the stoma/opening that results from a tracheotomy to provide and secure a patent airway. A tracheostomy can be permanent or temporary.
- Artificial airways can be placed orotracheally, nasotracheally, or through a tracheostomy to assist with respiration.
- Pediatric tracheostomy tubes made of plastic or silicone rubber and have a more acute angle than adult tubes. Pediatric tracheostomy tubes soften with body temperature to shape to the contour of the child's trachea. No inner cannula is necessary, because this material resists the accumulation of dried secretions.

INDICATIONS

CLIENT PRESENTATION: Obstruction of the upper airway requiring the use of artificial ventilation

CONSIDERATIONS

- Monitor the following.
  - Oxygenation, ventilation (respiratory rate, effort, SaO_2), and vital signs hourly
  - Thickness, quantity, odor, and color of mucous secretions
  - The stoma and skin surrounding the stoma for indications of inflammation or infection (redness, swelling, drainage)
- Provide adequate humidification and hydration to thin secretions and decrease the risk of mucus plugging.
- Suction only as often as necessary to maintain patency of the tube. Do not suction routinely, as this can cause mucosal damage, bleeding, hypoxemia, infection and bronchospasm.
- Monitor the need for suctioning. Suction as necessary when findings indicate the need to do so (audible/noisy secretions, crackles, restlessness, tachypnea, tachycardia, mucus in the airway).
- Maintain surgical aseptic technique when suctioning to prevent infection.
- Provide emotional support to the child and parents.

- Provide oral hygiene, usually every 2 hr.
- For cuffed tubes, keep the pressure less than 20 mm Hg to reduce the risk of tracheal necrosis due to prolonged compression of tracheal capillaries.
- Provide tracheostomy care every 8 hr.
- Change nondisposable tracheostomy tubes every 6 to 8 weeks or per protocol.
- Reposition the client every 2 hr to prevent atelectasis and pneumonia.
- Keep an emergency tracheostomy tube (one size smaller), suction source, sterile gauze, and obturator at the bedside.
- Reinforce discharge teaching regarding the following.
  - Tracheostomy care
  - Inspecting skin at the tracheostomy site for drainage or breakdown (this area should be cleaned with soap and water)
  - Findings that the family should immediately report to the provider (indications of infection or copious secretions)
  - Ways to promote improved nutrition
- Provide written material for parents to reinforce instructions. Qᴘᴄᴄ

COMPLICATIONS

Accidental decannulation

Accidental decannulation in the first 72 hr after surgery is an emergency because the tracheostomy tract has not matured and replacement can be difficult.

NURSING ACTIONS: Always have an additional staff member present when moving the tube or during any situation in which decannulation can occur. Qᴛᴄ

CLIENT EDUCATION
- When caring for the tube at home, have a second tube available in the event of dislodgement.
- Have scissors available to cut the old strings in an emergency. Qs

Occlusion

Occlusion is a life-threatening situation in which the tube is clogged with secretions and prevents adequate air exchange.

NURSING ACTIONS
- Maintain a patent airway with suctioning.
- Instruct the parents about the need to suction to prevent occlusion.

Application Exercises

1. A nurse is reinforcing teaching with an adolescent about how to self-administer a corticosteroid medication using a dry powder inhaler (DPI). Which of the following instructions should the nurse include? (Select all that apply.)

    A. Shake the device prior to use.

    B. Rinse and expectorate after administration.

    C. Inhale slowly with medication administration.

    D. Exhale quickly after medication administration.

    E. Use an alcohol swab to clean the cannister twice a day.

2. A nurse is caring for a child who is receiving oxygen therapy and is on a continuous oxygen saturation monitor that is reading 89%. Which of the following actions should the nurse take first?

    A. Increase the oxygen flow rate.

    B. Encourage the child to take deep breaths.

    C. Ensure proper placement of the sensor probe.

    D. Place the child in the Fowler's position.

3. A nurse is collecting data from an infant who has a respiratory infection. Which of the following findings should the nurse identify as an indication of acute hypoxemia?

    A. Productive cough

    B. Emesis

    C. Pallor of mucous membranes

    D. Clubbing of fingernails

4. A nurse is caring for a child who is receiving oxygen. The nurse should identify which of the following findings as an indication of oxygen toxicity?

    A. Increased blood pressure

    B. Hyperventilation

    C. Decreased $PaCO_2$

    D. Unconsciousness

5. A nurse is caring for a child who is receiving a bronchodilator medication by nebulized aerosol therapy. Which of the following actions should the nurse take? (Select all that apply.)

    A. Instruct the child that the treatment will last 30 min.

    B. Obtain vital signs prior to the procedure.

    C. Tell the child to take slow deep breaths.

    D. Determine if the child should use a mask.

    E. Attach the device to an air source.

PRACTICE Active Learning Scenario

A nurse is reinforcing teaching with a child about how to use a metered-dose inhaler. What information should the nurse include?

Use the ATI Active Learning Template: Nursing Skill to complete this item.

DESCRIPTION OF SKILL: Outline the steps for using a metered-dose inhaler.

Application Exercises Key

1. A. A DPI is a powder medication and should not be shaken prior to administration.

   B. **CORRECT:** Corticosteroids can cause an oral fungal infection. The client should rinse and expectorate following medication administration.

   C. **CORRECT:** The client should breathe in slowly (about 3 to 5 seconds) to administer the medication into the lungs.

   D. After inhalation of the medication, the client should hold his breath for 5 to 10 seconds and then exhale slowly through pursed lips.

   E. The client should rinse the inhaler as well as the cap and spacer once daily using warm running water.

   Ⓝ *NCLEX® Connection: Pharmacological Therapies, Medication Administration*

2. A. Increasing the oxygen flow rate for a child who has an oxygen saturation of 89% will provide the child with supplemental oxygen; however, there is another action the nurse should take first.

   B. Encouraging the child to take deep breaths will promote lung expansion and better absorption of oxygen in the lungs; however, there is another action the nurse should take first.

   C. **CORRECT:** The first action the nurse should take using the nursing process is to collect data. Ensuring the sensor probe is properly placed to obtain an accurate reading will help the nurse obtain accurate data to determine whether to take further actions.

   D. Placing the child in Fowler's position will promote lung expansion and better absorption of oxygen in the lungs; however, there is another action the nurse should take first.

   Ⓝ *NCLEX® Connection: Physiological Adaptation, Alterations in Body Systems*

3. A. A productive cough is a manifestation of a respiratory infection but is not an indication of acute hypoxemia.

   B. Emesis is a possible manifestation of pneumonia but is not an indication of acute hypoxemia.

   C. **CORRECT:** The nurse should identify pallor of skin and mucous membranes as an indication of acute hypoxemia in an infant.

   D. Clubbing of fingernails is an indication of chronic hypoxemia.

   Ⓝ *NCLEX® Connection: Physiological Adaptation, Basic Pathophysiology*

4. A. Increased blood pressure is not a manifestation of oxygen toxicity.

   B. Hypoventilation is a manifestation of oxygen toxicity.

   C. Increased $PaCO_2$ is a manifestation of oxygen toxicity.

   D. **CORRECT:** Children who exhibit oxygen toxicity progress into an unconscious state rapidly.

   Ⓝ *NCLEX® Connection: Physiological Adaptation, Unexpected Response to Therapies*

5. A. Nebulized medications take approximately 10 to 15 min to deliver.

   B. **CORRECT:** The nurse should obtain baseline vital signs prior to administering a nebulized medication for purposes of comparison with how the client tolerates the medication.

   C. **CORRECT:** The nurse should instruct the child to take slow, deep breaths to inhale the medication deeply into the respiratory tract.

   D. **CORRECT:** The nurse should determine the best method of delivery for nebulized medications. Delivery methods include mask, mouthpiece, or blow-by.

   E. **CORRECT:** Nebulized medications need to have an air source to break the medication into small particles for inhalation.

   Ⓝ *NCLEX® Connection: Pharmacological Therapies, Medication Administration*

PRACTICE Answer

Using the ATI Active Learning Template: Nursing Skill

DESCRIPTION OF SKILL
- Remove the cap from the inhaler
- Shake the inhaler five to six times.
- Attach the spacer. (Encourage the use of a spacer for children to facilitate proper inhalation of the medication.)
- Hold the inhaler with the mouthpiece at the bottom.
- Hold the inhaler with the thumb near the mouthpiece and the index and middle fingers at the top.
  - Open-mouth technique: Hold the inhaler approximately 3 to 4 cm (1.2 to 1.6 in) away from the front of the mouth.
  - Closed-mouth method: Place the inhaler between the lips and instruct the child to form a seal around the inhaler.
- Take a deep breath and then exhale.
- Tilt the head back slightly, and press the inhaler. While pressing the inhaler, begin a slow, deep breath that lasts for 3 to 5 seconds to facilitate delivery to the air passages.
- Hold the breath for approximately 5 to 10 seconds to allow the medication to deposit in the airways.
- If an additional puff is needed, wait 1 min between puffs.
- Take the inhaler out of the mouth and slowly exhale through the nose.
- Resume normal breathing.

Ⓝ *NCLEX® Connection: Pharmacological and Parenteral Therapies, Medication Administration*

UNIT 2 NURSING CARE OF CHILDREN WHO
HAVE SYSTEM DISORDERS
SECTION: RESPIRATORY DISORDERS

CHAPTER 16 *Acute and Infectious Respiratory Illnesses*

Acute and infectious respiratory illnesses prevalent in children include tonsillitis, nasopharyngitis, pharyngitis, croup syndromes, bacterial tracheitis, bronchitis, bronchiolitis, allergic rhinitis, and pneumonia.

Tonsillitis and tonsillectomy

Tonsils are masses of lymph-type tissue found in the pharyngeal area. They filter pathogenic organisms (viral and bacterial), which helps protect the respiratory and gastrointestinal tracts. In addition, they contribute to antibody formation.

Tonsils are highly vascular, which helps them to protect against infection, because foreign materials (viral or bacterial organisms) enter the body through the mouth.

Palatine tonsils are located on both sides of the oropharynx. These are the tonsils removed during a tonsillectomy.

Pharyngeal tonsils located superior to the palatine tonsils, also known as the adenoids, are removed during an adenoidectomy.

Enlarged tonsils
- In some instances, enlarged tonsils can block the nose and throat. This can interfere with breathing, nasal and sinus drainage, sleeping, swallowing, and speaking.
- Enlarged tonsils can also disrupt the function of the Eustachian tube, which can cause otitis media or impede hearing.

Acute tonsillitis occurs when the tonsils become inflamed and reddened. Acute tonsillitis can become chronic.

DATA COLLECTION

RISK FACTORS
- Exposure to a viral or bacterial agent
- Immature immune systems (younger children)

EXPECTED FINDINGS
- Report of sore throat with difficulty swallowing
- History of otitis media and hearing difficulties

PHYSICAL FINDINGS
- Mouth odor
- Mouth breathing
- Snoring
- Nasal qualities in the voice
- Fever
- Persistent cough
- Tonsil inflammation with redness and edema; can meet at midline

LABORATORY TESTS

Throat culture for group A beta-hemolytic streptococci (GABHS)

PATIENT-CENTERED CARE

NURSING CARE

Tonsillitis
- Provide treatment of manifestations for viral tonsillitis (rest, warm fluids, warm salt-water gargles).
- Administer antibiotic therapy for bacterial tonsillitis.
- Encourage soft to liquid diet
- Administer throat lozenges, analgesics, and antipyretics as needed.

MEDICATIONS

Antipyretics/analgesics
- Opioids combined with nonopioids are indicated for routine administration while the child has pain.
- Opioids such as hydrocodone are indicated for the child who has difficulty drinking fluids due to pain.

Antipyretics

Decrease fever and manage pain.

NURSING ACTIONS
- Be aware of allergies.
- Discuss appropriate dosing for acetaminophen and ibuprofen.

Antibiotics

Penicillin or amoxicillin is commonly used for the treatment of tonsillitis caused by GABHS.

NURSING ACTIONS: Be aware of allergies.

CLIENT EDUCATION: Administer antibiotics for the full course of treatment.

THERAPEUTIC PROCEDURES

Tonsillectomy

PREOPERATIVE NURSING ACTION: Maintain NPO status.

POSTOPERATIVE NURSING ACTIONS
- **Positioning**
  - Place in position to facilitate drainage.
  - Elevate head of bed when child is fully awake.
- **Data collection**
  - Check for evidence of bleeding (frequent swallowing, clearing the throat, restlessness, bright red emesis, tachycardia, pallor).
  - Monitor the airway and vital signs.
  - Monitor for difficulty breathing related to oral secretions, edema, or bleeding.
- **Comfort measures**
  - Administer analgesics PO or IV (acetaminophen, hydrocodone).
  - Provide an ice collar.
  - Offer ice chips or sips of water to keep throat moist.
  - Administer pain medication on a regular schedule.
  - Use local anesthetics (tetracaine).
- **Diet**
  - Encourage clear liquids and fluids after return of the gag reflex. Avoid red-colored liquids, citrus juice, and milk-based foods initially.
  - Advance the diet with soft, bland foods.

CLIENT EDUCATION
- Avoid coughing, throat clearing, and nose blowing in order to protect the surgical site.
- Avoid straws as they can damage the surgical site
- Expect some clots or blood-tinged mucus in emesis.
- Notify the provider if bright-red bleeding occurs.
- Rest as much as possible.

CLIENT EDUCATION

- Contact the provider if the child experiences difficulty breathing, lack of oral intake, increase in pain, or indications of infection.
- Ensure that the child does not put objects in the mouth.
- Administer pain medications for discomfort.
- Encourage fluid intake and advancement to a soft diet.
- Avoid foods that are irritating or highly seasoned.
- Limit activity to decrease the potential for bleeding.
- Avoid gargles or vigorous tooth brushing.
- Full recovery usually occurs in approximately 14 days.
- Discuss with the family the manifestations of hemorrhage, dehydration, and infection, and when to notify the provider.

COMPLICATIONS

Hemorrhage

NURSING ACTIONS
- Use a good light source and possibly a tongue depressor to directly observe the throat.
- Check for findings of bleeding (tachycardia, repeated or frequent swallowing and clearing of throat, hemoptysis or bright red emesis, restlessness, pallor). Hypotension is a late indicator of shock.
- Contact the charge nurse and provider immediately if there is any indication of bleeding.

CLIENT EDUCATION: Report indications of bleeding.

Dehydration

NURSING ACTIONS
- Encourage oral fluids (cool water, ice chips).
- Monitor I&O.
- Discuss with the family the manifestations of dehydration.

CLIENT EDUCATION: Encourage oral fluids.

Chronic infection

Chronically infected tonsils with GABHS can pose a potential threat to other parts of the body. Some children who frequently have tonsillitis can develop other diseases (rheumatic fever, kidney infection).

CLIENT EDUCATION: Seek medical attention when the child presents with manifestations of tonsillitis.

Common respiratory illnesses

Disorders can affect both the upper (oronasopharynx, pharynx, larynx, upper part of the trachea) and lower (bronchi, bronchioles, alveoli) respiratory tracts. Infections of the respiratory tract can affect more than one area.

The information in this section applies to a range of common respiratory illnesses.

DATA COLLECTION

RISK FACTORS

Age
- Infants between 3 and 6 months of age are at increased risk for respiratory illnesses due to the decrease of maternal antibodies acquired at birth and the lack of antibody protection.
- Viral infections are more common in toddlers and preschoolers. The incidence of these infections decreases by age 5.
- Certain viral agents can cause serious illness during infancy, but only cause a mild illness in older children.

Anatomy
- A short, narrow airway can become easily obstructed with mucus or edema.
- A short respiratory tract allows infections to travel quickly to the lower airways.
- Infectious agents have easy access to the middle ear through the short and open Eustachian tubes of infants and young children.

Decreased resistance
- Compromised immune system
- Anemia
- Nutritional deficiencies
- Allergies
- Chronic medical conditions (asthma, cystic fibrosis, chronic lung disease, cardiac anomalies)
- Exposure to secondhand smoke
- Daycare attendance

Seasonal variables
- Children who have asthma have a greater incidence of respiratory infections during cold weather.
- Respiratory syncytial virus (RSV) and other common respiratory infections are more common during the winter and spring.
- Infections caused by *Mycoplasma pneumoniae* are more frequent during autumn and early winter.

EXPECTED FINDINGS

- Nursing history that includes recent infections, medications taken, immunization status, and family coping
- Reports of sore throat, decreased activity level, chest pain, fatigue, difficulty breathing, shortness of breath, cough, and decreased appetite

LABORATORY TESTS

Throat culture or rapid antigen testing to rule out GABHS infection

PATIENT-CENTERED CARE

NURSING CARE

- Closely monitor progression of illness and ensuing respiratory distress. Observe for increased heart and respiratory rate, retractions, nasal flaring, and restlessness.
- Check temperature, oxygenation, activity level, and level of comfort.
- Make emergency equipment for intubation readily accessible.
- Position the child to have optimal ventilation without increasing distress that would contribute to increasing respiratory distress.
- Implement isolation precautions as indicated.

CLIENT EDUCATION

- Use a cool-air vaporizer to provide humidity.
- Rest during febrile illness.
- Maintain adequate fluid intake.
  - Infants may be given commercially prepared oral rehydration solutions.
  - Older children may be given sports drinks.
- Administer medications using accurate dosages and appropriate time intervals.
- Develop strategies to decrease the spread of infection.
  - Performing good hand hygiene
  - Covering the nose and mouth with tissues when sneezing and coughing
  - Properly disposing of tissues
  - Not sharing cups, eating utensils, and towels
  - Keeping infected children from contact with children who are well
- Seek further medical attention for the child if manifestations worsen or respiratory distress occurs.

Nasopharyngitis

Also known as the common cold, nasopharyngitis is a self-limiting virus that persists for 4 to 10 days.

DATA COLLECTION

EXPECTED FINDINGS

- Nasal inflammation, coughing, sneezing, dryness and irritation of nasal passages and the pharynx
- Fever, decreased appetite, restlessness

PATIENT-CENTERED CARE

NURSING CARE

Reinforce teaching with parents about home management.
- Give antipyretic for fever.
- Encourage rest.
- Elevate head of bed or crib mattress.
- Suction with bulb syringe.
- Provide vaporized air (cool mist).
- Give decongestants for children older than 6 years.
- Give cough suppressants with caution. (Avoid oversedation.)
- Antihistamines are not recommended.
- Antibiotics are not indicated for the treatment of a viral infection.
- Encourage fluids for hydration.
- Methods to decrease spread of infection include hand hygiene, covering mouth when coughing, and avoiding contact with individuals who have a respiratory infections.

Acute streptococcal pharyngitis

GABHS: Infection of the upper airway (strep throat)

DATA COLLECTION

EXPECTED FINDINGS

- Onset is abrupt and characterized by pharyngitis, headache, fever, and abdominal pain.
- Tonsils and pharynx can be inflamed and covered with white exudate, usually appears by second day of illness.
- Petechiae can be visible on the palate.

LABORATORY TESTS:

Throat culture or rapid antigen testing to determine GABHS infection

PATIENT-CENTERED CARE

NURSING CARE

- Administer antibiotics.
  - Oral penicillin in a dose sufficient to control the acute local manifestations is administered for at least 10 days.
  - Amoxicillin once a day for 10 days is also effective.
  - IM penicillin G benzathine is also appropriate.
  - Oral erythromycin for children allergic to penicillin.
  - Clarithromycin, azithromycin, clindamycin, oral cephalosporins, and amoxicillin with clavulanic acid are also effective to treat GABHS.
  - Instruct to take complete full dose of antibiotics.
- Administer antipyretics for fever.
- Apply cold/warm neck compresses.
- Advise to discard old toothbrush after 24 hr of antibiotics.
- No school or daycare until after 24 hr of antibiotics are taken.

Bronchitis (tracheobronchitis)

- Associated with an upper respiratory infection and inflammation of large airways
- Self-limiting (treatment is focused on relief of manifestations)

DATA COLLECTION

EXPECTED FINDINGS

- Persistent dry, hacking, nonproductive cough that worsens at night as a result of inflammation
- Rhonchi, crackles, fever, nasal congestion
- Resolves in 5 to 10 days

LABORATORY TESTS

Test nasopharyngeal secretions.

PATIENT-CENTERED CARE

NURSING CARE

Instruct parents about home management.
- Give antipyretics for fever.
- Give analgesics for pain or discomfort.
- The use of cough suppressants is limited to promote expectoration of sections. Use them at night to promote rest.
- Provide increased humidity (cool mist vaporizer).

Bronchiolitis

- Mostly caused by RSV
- Primarily affects the bronchi and bronchioles
- Occurs at the bronchiolar level
- Transmitted from exposure to contaminated secretions
- Increased incidence during the winter months

DATA COLLECTION

EXPECTED FINDINGS

INITIALLY: Rhinorrhea, intermittent fever, pharyngitis, coughing, sneezing, wheezing, possible ear or eye infection

WITH ILLNESS PROGRESSION: Increased coughing and sneezing, fever, tachypnea and retractions, refusal to breast- or bottle-feed, copious secretions

INFANT: Lethargy, poor feedings, wheezing, retractions

SEVERE ILLNESS: Tachypnea (greater than 70/min), listlessness, apneic spells, poor air exchange, poor breath sounds, cyanosis

LABORATORY TESTS

Test nasopharyngeal secretions using either rapid immunofluorescent antibody-direct fluorescent antibody staining or enzyme-linked immunosorbent assay techniques for RSV antigen detection.

PATIENT-CENTERED CARE

NURSING CARE

Initiate droplet, contact, and standard precautions for clients receiving acute care.

MANIFESTATION MANAGEMENT

- Provide supplemental oxygen to maintain oxygen saturation equal to or greater than 90%.
- Encourage fluid intake if able to tolerate oral fluids. Otherwise IV fluids until acute phase has passed.
- Maintain airway.
- Chest physiotherapy (CPT) is not recommended.
- Provide nasopharyngeal or nasal suctioning as needed.
- Encourage breastfeeding.
- Provide emotional support to parents and family.
- Avoid exposure to tobacco smoke.

MEDICATIONS

- Corticosteroid use is controversial. Bronchodilators are not recommended.
- Administer inhaled antiviral medications.
- Administer antibiotics if a coexisting bacterial infection is present.

Allergic rhinitis

Caused by seasonal reaction to allergens, most often in the autumn or spring

DATA COLLECTION

EXPECTED FINDINGS

- Watery rhinorrhea; nasal obstruction; itchiness of the nose, eyes, pharynx, and conjunctiva
- Dark circles under the eyes ("allergic shiners") from impaired lymphatic and venous drainage
- Snoring
- Fatigue, malaise, headache, poor performance in school

LABORATORY TESTS

- Nasal smear to determine amount of eosinophils in nasal secretions
- Blood exam for total IgE and elevated eosinophils
- Skin tests
- Various challenge tests

PATIENT-CENTERED CARE

NURSING CARE

Instruct parents about home management.
- Avoid allergens.
- Give nasal corticosteroids (first-line medications used).
- Give antihistamines, beta adrenergic decongestants, mast cell stabilizers, leukotriene modifiers, and ipratropium.

Pneumonia

- Viral pneumonias are more common among children of all ages than bacterial pneumonia, and usually follow a viral upper-respiratory infection.
- Bacterial pneumonia is often caused by *Streptococcus pneumoniae*, Group A streptococci, *Staphylococcus aureus*, *Mycoplasma catarrhalis*, or *Mycoplasma pneumoniae*.

DATA COLLECTION

EXPECTED FINDINGS

- High fever
- Cough that can be productive of white sputum
- Tachypnea with shallow respirations
- Retractions and nasal flaring
- Chest pain
- Dullness with percussion
- Adventitious breath sounds (rhonchi, fine crackles)
- Pale color that progresses to cyanosis
- Irritability, restlessness, lethargy
- Abdominal pain, diarrhea, lack of appetite, vomiting

LABORATORY TESTS

- Radiographic examination to detect presence of infiltrates
- Gram stain and culture of sputum in older children
- Nasopharyngeal specimens
- Blood cultures
- Occasionally lung aspiration and biopsy
- Elevated antistreptolysin titer if streptococcal infection present
- WBC can be within the expected reference range (streptococcal infection) or elevated

PATIENT-CENTERED CARE

NURSING CARE

Viral

- Administer oxygen with cool mist.
- Monitor continuous oximetry.
- Administer antipyretics for fever.
- Monitor I&O.
- Perform CPT and postural drainage.

Bacterial

- Encourage rest.
- Collaborate with the RN to ensure the child receives IV antibiotics.
- Promote increased oral intake.
- Monitor I&O.
- Administer antipyretics for fever.
- CPT and postural drainage can be helpful.
- Collaborate with the RN to ensure the child receives IV fluids.
- Administer oxygen.
- Monitor continuous oximetry.

CLIENT EDUCATION: The pneumococcal conjugate vaccine is used for the prevention of pneumonia.

COMPLICATIONS

Pneumothorax

Accumulation of air in the pleural space with decreased lung expansion

MANIFESTATIONS: Dyspnea, chest pain, back pain, labored respirations, decreased oxygen saturations, tachycardia

NURSING ACTIONS
- Monitor respiratory status.
- Administer oxygen.
- Assist with preparations for chest tube insertion.

Pleural effusion

Accumulation of fluid in the pleural space

MANIFESTATIONS: Dyspnea, chest pain, back pain, labored respirations, decreased oxygen saturations, tachycardia

NURSING ACTIONS
- Monitor vital signs and respiratory status.
- Administer oxygen.
- Administer analgesics for discomfort.
- Assist with preparations for chest tube insertion.

Croup syndromes: Bacterial epiglottitis (acute supraglottitis)

- Medical emergency
- Usually caused by *Haemophilus influenza*

DATA COLLECTION

EXPECTED FINDINGS

- Predictive indicators: Absence of cough, drooling, agitation
- Sitting upright with chin pointing out, mouth opened, and tongue protruding (tripod position)
- Dysphonia (thick, muffled voice; froglike croaking sound)
- Dysphagia (difficulty swallowing)
- Tachycardia and tachypnea
- Inspiratory stridor (noisy inspirations)
- Suprasternal and substernal retractions
- Sore throat, high fever, restlessness

DIAGNOSTIC PROCEDURES

Lateral neck radiograph of the soft tissues

PATIENT-CENTERED CARE

NURSING CARE

- Protect the airway. Have resuscitation equipment and suction equipment at bedside.
- Avoid throat culture or using a tongue blade.
- Assist with preparations for intubation or tracheostomy for severe respiratory distress.
- Provide humidified oxygen.
- Monitor continuous oximetry.
- Administer corticosteroids.
- Collaborate with the RN to ensure the child receives IV fluids and antibiotic therapy. IV antibiotics are initially followed by a 10-day course of oral antibiotics.
- Maintain droplet isolation precautions for first 24 hr after IV antibiotics initiated.
- Provide a calm, supportive environment for the child and parents.

Croup syndromes: Acute laryngotracheobronchitis and acute spasmodic laryngitis

Acute laryngotracheobronchitis (LTB): Causative agents include RSV, influenza A and B, *Mycoplasma pneumonia*, parainfluenza types 1, 2, and 3, and measles.

Acute spasmodic laryngitis
- Self-limiting illness that can result from allergens
- Characterized by paroxysmal attacks of laryngeal obstruction that occur mainly at night

DATA COLLECTION

EXPECTED FINDINGS

Acute laryngotracheobronchitis
- Low-grade fever, restlessness, hoarseness, barking cough, dyspnea, inspiratory stridor, retractions
- INFANTS AND TODDLERS: nasal flaring, intercostal retractions, tachypnea, continuous stridor

Acute spasmodic laryngitis: Croupy, barking cough; restlessness; difficulty breathing; hoarseness; nighttime episodes of laryngeal obstruction

PATIENT-CENTERED CARE

NURSING CARE

- Home care: Advise parents to run hot shower and sit with the child in the steamy environment.
- Administer oxygen if needed.
- Monitor continuous oximetry.
- Administer nebulized racemic epinephrine.
- Administer corticosteroids: oral or IM (dexamethasone), or nebulized (budesonide).
- Encourage oral intake if tolerated.
- Administer IV fluids.
- Provide reassurance and promote rest.
- Monitor for severe respiratory distress. If present, keep the child NPO to prevent aspiration.

Influenza A and B

Mild, moderate, or severe

DATA COLLECTION

EXPECTED FINDINGS
- Sudden onset of fever and chills
- Dry throat and nasal mucosa
- Dry cough and hoarseness
- Flushed face
- Photophobia
- Myalgia
- Fatigue
- GI manifestations (vomiting, diarrhea)

LABORATORY TESTS

- Analyze nasopharyngeal secretions for viral culture or rapid detection testing
- Influenza A and B detected by fluorescent antibody and indirect immunofluorescent antibody staining

PATIENT-CENTERED CARE

NURSING CARE

Instruct parents about home management.

MANIFESTATION TREATMENT
- Promote increased fluid intake.
- Encourage rest.
- Give medications (acetaminophen or ibuprofen for fever).

MEDICATIONS

Amantadine (type A)

- Shortens the length of the illness.
- Administer within 24 to 48 hr of onset of manifestations.

Rimantadine (type A)

- Treats manifestations.
- Give orally two times per day for 7 days for children older than 1 year.

Zanamivir (type A and B)

- Treatment of influenza for children 7 and older or for prophylaxis for children 5 and older.
- Start within 48 hr of manifestations.
- Inhaled two times per day for 5 days.

Oseltamivir (type A and B)

- Decreases manifestations.
- Give orally for 5 days for children older than 1 year.
- Start within 48 hr of manifestations.

Influenza vaccine (prevention)

- Inactivated yearly influenza vaccine is recommended for children 6 months and older.
- Recommendations for the influenza vaccine change periodically. Check the CDC's website (www.cdc.gov) for current recommendations.

Application Exercises

1. A nurse is caring for a child who has bronchiolitis. Which of the following actions should the nurse take? (Select all that apply.)

   A. Administer a bronchodilator.

   B. Initiate chest percussion and postural drainage.

   C. Administer humidified oxygen.

   D. Suction the nasopharynx as needed.

   E. Administer oral penicillin.

2. A nurse is reinforcing teaching with a group of parents about influenza. Which of the following information should the nurse include in the teaching?

   A. "Amantadine will prevent the illness."

   B. "Rimantadine is administered intramuscularly."

   C. "Zanamivir can be given to children 1 year and older."

   D. "Oseltamivir should be given within 48 hours of onset of symptoms."

3. A nurse is collecting data from a child who is in the postoperative period following a tonsillectomy. Which of the following findings indicates postoperative bleeding?

   A. Hgb 11.6 and Hct 37%

   B. Inflamed and reddened throat

   C. Frequent swallowing and clearing of the throat

   D. Blood-tinged mucus

4. A nurse is caring for a child in the postoperative period following a tonsillectomy. Which of the following actions should the nurse take?

   A. Encourage the child to blow her nose gently.

   B. Administer analgesics on a schedule.

   C. Offer orange juice.

   D. Position the child supine.

5. A nurse is collecting data from a child who has epiglottitis. Which of the following findings should the nurse expect? (Select all that apply.)

   A. Hoarseness and difficulty speaking

   B. Difficulty swallowing

   C. Low-grade fever

   D. Drooling

   E. Dry, barking cough

   F. Stridor

PRACTICE Active Learning Scenario

A nurse is reinforcing teaching with a parent of a child who has an infectious respiratory illness. What should the nurse include in the teaching? Use the ATI Active Learning Template: Basic Concept to complete this item.

RELATED CONTENT: Identify at least three strategies to decrease the spread of infection.

Application Exercises Key

1. A. Bronchodilators are not recommended for a client who has bronchiolitis.

   B. Chest percussion and postural drainage are not indicated for a client who has bronchiolitis.

   C. **CORRECT:** The nurse should administer humidified oxygen to provide moisture to the airway.

   D. **CORRECT:** The nurse should suction the nasopharynx to assist the client to clear secretions.

   E. Antibiotics are not indicated for a client who has bronchiolitis unless a coexisting bacterial infection is present.

   NCLEX® Connection: Physiological Adaptation, Alterations in Body Systems

2. A. Amantadine does not prevent influenza, but it can shorten the length of the illness.

   B. Rimantadine is administered orally two times per day for 7 days.

   C. Zanamivir is approved for children older than 5 years of age.

   D. **CORRECT:** The nurse should instruct the parents that oseltamivir decreases the manifestations of influenza in clients who have manifestations for less than 48 hr.

   Ⓝ NCLEX® Connection: Pharmacological Therapies, Expected Actions/Outcomes

3. A. Hgb 11.6 and Hct 37% are within the expected reference range.

   B. Inflamed and reddened throat is an expected finding following a tonsillectomy.

   C. **CORRECT:** Frequent swallowing and clearing of the throat indicates that there is an increased amount of fluid in the back of the throat, which is a finding of postoperative bleeding.

   D. Blood-tinged mucus is an expected finding following a tonsillectomy.

   Ⓝ NCLEX® Connection: Reduction of Risk Potential, Potential for Complications from Surgical Procedures and Health Alterations

4. A. Blowing the nose causes pressure and increases the risk of postoperative bleeding.

   B. **CORRECT:** The nurse should administer analgesics on a schedule to provide and maintain pain relief.

   C. Citrus juices such as orange juice can cause discomfort and should be avoided postoperatively.

   D. The client should be positioned on the abdomen or side-lying following a tonsillectomy.

   Ⓝ NCLEX® Connection: Reduction of Risk Potential, Potential for Complications from Surgical Procedures and Health Alterations

5. A. **CORRECT:** Hoarseness and difficulty speaking are manifestations of epiglottitis.

   B. **CORRECT:** Difficulty swallowing is a manifestation of epiglottitis.

   C. A high fever is a manifestation of epiglottitis.

   D. **CORRECT:** Drooling is a manifestation of epiglottitis.

   E. The absence of a cough is a manifestation of epiglottitis.

   F. **CORRECT:** Inspiratory stridor is a manifestation of epiglottitis.

   Ⓝ NCLEX® Connection: Physiological Adaptation, Basic Pathophysiology

---

PRACTICE Answer

Using the ATI Active Learning Template: Basic Concept

RELATED CONTENT
- Perform appropriate hand hygiene.
- Cover the nose and mouth with tissues when sneezing and coughing.
- Dispose of tissues properly.
- Do not share cups, eating utensils, or towels.
- Keep infected children from contact with children who are well.

Ⓝ NCLEX® Connection: Safety and Infection Control, Standard Precautions/Transmission-Based Precautions/Surgical Asepsis

UNIT 2   NURSING CARE OF CHILDREN WHO
HAVE SYSTEM DISORDERS
SECTION: RESPIRATORY DISORDERS

CHAPTER 17 *Asthma*

Asthma is a chronic inflammatory disorder of the airways that results in intermittent and reversible airflow obstruction of the bronchioles. The obstruction occurs either by inflammation or airway hyper-responsiveness. Asthma diagnoses are categorized based on effects on the child: intermittent, mild persistent, moderate persistent, and severe persistent. (17.1) Q꜀ᴇʙᴘ

DATA COLLECTION

RISK FACTORS

- Family history of asthma
- Family history of allergies
- Sex (male clients affected more than female clients until adolescence, then the incidence is greater among female clients)
- Exposure to smoke
- Low birth weight
- Being overweight

TRIGGERS TO ASTHMA
- Allergens
  - Indoor: Mold, cockroach antigen, dust, dust mites
  - Outdoor: Grasses, pollen, trees, shrubs, molds, spores, air pollution, weeds
  - Irritants: Tobacco smoke, wood smoke, odors, sprays
- Exercise
- Cold air or changes in weather or temperature
- Environmental change (new home or school)
- Infections/colds
- Animal hair or dander: Cats, dogs, rodents, horses
- Medications: Aspirin, nonsteroidal anti-inflammatory drugs, antibiotics, beta blockers

- Strong emotions: Fear, anger, laughing, crying
- Conditions: Gastroesophageal reflux, tracheoesophageal fistula
- Food allergies or additives (sulfites): Nuts, milk
- Endocrine factors: Menses, pregnancy, thyroid disease

EXPECTED FINDINGS

- Chest tightness and discomfort
- History regarding current and previous asthma exacerbations
  - Onset and duration
  - Precipitating factors
  - Changes in medication regimen
  - Medications that relieve manifestations
  - Other medications
  - Self-care methods used to relieve manifestations

PHYSICAL FINDINGS
- Dyspnea
- Hacking, nonproductive cough
- Audible wheezing
- Coarse lung sounds, wheezing throughout possible crackles
- Mucus production
- Restlessness, irritability, shortness of breath
- Anxiety
- Sweating
- Use of accessory muscles; retractions in infants
- Decreased oxygen saturation (low SaO_2)

LABORATORY TESTS

CBC with differential: Elevated WBC, band cells, and eosinophils due to allergic or inflammatory response and possible respiratory infection

DIAGNOSTIC PROCEDURES

Pulmonary function testing: Spirometry
- The most accurate tests for diagnosing asthma and its severity Q꜀ᴇʙᴘ
- Baseline test at time of diagnosis
- Repeat testing after treatment is initiated and child is stabilized
- Test every 1 to 2 years

17.1 Effects of asthma on the child

		Intermittent	Mild persistent	Moderate persistent	Severe persistent
FREQUENCY OF FINDINGS		0 to 2 times/week	More than twice/week, but not daily	Daily	Continually
NIGHTTIME FINDINGS	0- TO 4-YEAR-OLD	None	1 to 2 times/month	3 to 4 times/month	Frequent
	5- TO 11-YEAR-OLD	Two times a month or less	3 to 4 times/month	More than once/week, but not daily	
ACTIVITY LIMITATIONS		None	Minor	Some	Extreme
USE OF A SHORT-ACTING BETA AGONIST		Less than twice/week	More than 2 days/week, but not daily	Daily	Several times/day

---

Peak expiratory flow rates (PEFR)
- Measures the amount of air that can be forcefully exhaled in 1 second
- Each child needs to establish personal best during a 2- to 3-week time frame when asthma manifestations are under control

Bronchoprovocation testing
- Exposure to methacholine, cold air, or histamine determines the reactivity of the client's airway to attempt to identify inhaled allergens.
- Exercise challenge identifies child's respiratory response to increased physical activity.

Skin prick testing: Identifies allergens that trigger asthma

Chest x-ray: Showing hyperexpansion and infiltrates

PATIENT-CENTERED CARE

NURSING CARE

- Monitor airway patency, respiratory rate, symmetry, effort, and use of accessory muscles.
- Auscultate breath sounds in all lung fields.
- Monitor for shortness of breath, dyspnea, and audible wheezing. An absence of wheezing can indicate severe constriction of the alveoli.
- Monitor vital signs and oxygen saturation.
- Check CBC and chest x-ray results, possible ABGs.
- Position the child to maximize ventilation.
- Administer oxygen therapy as prescribed. Keep endotracheal intubation equipment nearby. Qs
- Assist with obtaining and maintaining IV access as prescribed.
- Maintain a calm and reassuring demeanor.
- Encourage appropriate vaccinations and prompt medical attention for infections.
- Administer medications. The provider can prescribe antibiotics if a bacterial infection is confirmed.

MEDICATIONS

Bronchodilators (inhalers)

Short-acting beta₂ agonists (SABA): albuterol, levalbuterol, terbutaline
- Used for acute exacerbations
- Decreases bronchospasm by relaxing the smooth muscle
- Prevention of exercise-induced asthma

Long-acting beta₂ agonists (LABA): formoterol, salmeterol
- Used to prevent exacerbations, especially at night, and reduce use of SABA
- Must be used along with anti-inflammatory therapy
- Cannot be used to treat acute exacerbations

Cholinergic antagonists (anticholinergic medications; atropine, ipratropium) block the parasympathetic nervous system, providing relief of acute bronchospasms.

NURSING ACTIONS
- Watch the child for tremors and tachycardia when taking albuterol.
- Observe the child for dry mouth when taking ipratropium.

CLIENT EDUCATION
- Instruct the child and family in the proper use of metered-dose inhaler or nebulizer.
- Encourage older children who are taking ipratropium to suck on hard candies to help with dry mouth.
- Instruct children to administer prior to exercise or activity.
- Reinforce teaching with the parents about possible adverse effects.

Anti-inflammatory agents

Decrease airway inflammation.

Corticosteroids can be given parenterally (methylprednisolone), orally (prednisone), or by inhalation (fluticasone).
- Oral systemic steroids can be given for short periods (3 or 10 days).
- Inhaled corticosteroids are administered daily as a preventive measure.
- Considered first line of therapy for a child greater than 5 years old.

Leukotriene modifiers (zafirlukast, montelukast)

Mast cell stabilizers (cromolyn)

Monoclonal antibodies (omalizumab) are used to treat moderate to severe persistent allergic asthma uncontrolled by inhaled corticosteroids in children 12 years and older.

Combination medications contain an inhaled corticosteroid and a LABA (fluticasone/salmeterol).

NURSING ACTIONS
- Observe the oral mucosa for infection secondary to use of inhaled medication.
- Monitor weight, blood pressure, electrolytes, glucose, and growth with oral corticosteroid use.

CLIENT EDUCATION
- Encourage the child to drink plenty of fluids to promote hydration.
- Encourage the child to take oral corticosteroids with food.
- Instruct the child to rinse her mouth after the use of a corticosteroid inhaler.
- Instruct the child and family to watch for redness, sores, or white patches in the mouth, and report them to the provider.
- Instruct the family to follow prescription for medication administration (dosage, tapering off medication, length of time to take).

INTERPROFESSIONAL CARE

- Consult respiratory services for inhalers and breathing treatments. Qrc
- Contact nutritional services for weight loss or gain related to medications or diagnosis.
- Consult rehabilitation if the child has prolonged weakness and needs assistance with increasing level of activity.

CLIENT EDUCATION

- Instruct the family and child to identify personal triggering agents.
- Assist the child in avoiding triggering agents.
- Provide the family and child with an asthma action plan.
- Instruct the child how to properly self-administer medications (nebulizers, inhalers, and spacer).
- Reinforce teaching with the child about how to use a peak flow meter.
  - Use at the same time each day.
  - Ensure the marker is zeroed.
  - Stand up straight.
  - Remove gum or food from mouth.
  - Close lips tightly around the mouthpiece. (Ensure the tongue is not occluding.)
  - Blow out as hard and as quickly as possible.
  - Read the number on the meter.
  - Repeat three more times. (Wait at least 30 seconds between attempts.)
  - Record highest number.
- Instruct the family to keep a record of PEFR results. Readings over time show the child's "best" efforts, and to provide a warning of increased airway impairment.
- Reinforce with the family and child how to recognize an asthma exacerbation (decreased PEFR, increased use of SABA, difficulty speaking or eating). Qs
- Reinforce teaching with the family and the child about when to use each of the prescribed medications (rescue medications vs. maintenance medications).
- Reinforce education with the child and family regarding infection prevention techniques.
  - Promote good nutrition.
  - Reinforce importance of good hand hygiene.
  - Reduce allergens in the child's environment.
- Encourage prompt medical attention for infections.
- Stress the importance of keeping immunizations, including seasonal influenza and pneumonia vaccines, up to date.
- Encourage regular exercise as part of asthma therapy.
  - Promotes ventilation and perfusion
  - Maintains cardiac health
  - Enhances skeletal muscle strength
- Children can require medication before exercise.

COMPLICATIONS

Status asthmaticus

A life-threatening episode of airway obstruction that is often unresponsive to common treatment.

MANIFESTATIONS include wheezing, labored breathing, nasal flaring, lack of air movement in lungs, use of accessory muscles, distended neck veins, diaphoresis, and risk for cardiac and respiratory arrest.

NURSING ACTIONS
- Monitor oxygen saturations continuously.
- Place on continuous cardiorespiratory monitoring.
- Position the child sitting upright, standing, or leaning slightly forward.
- Administer humidified oxygen.
- Administer three nebulizer treatments of a beta₂ agonist, 20 to 30 min apart or continuously. Ipratropium bromide can be added to the nebulizer to increase bronchodilation.
- Assist in obtaining IV access.
- Monitor ABGs and serum electrolytes.
- Administer corticosteroid.
- Ensure that emergency intubation supplies are available.
- Heliox (a mixture of helium and oxygen) can be administered via a nonrebreather mask to decrease airway resistance and work of breathing.

Respiratory failure

Persistent hypoxemia related to asthma can lead to respiratory failure.

NURSING ACTIONS
- Monitor oxygenation levels and acid-base balance.
- Assist with preparations for intubation and mechanical ventilation as indicated.

Application Exercises

1. A nurse is collecting data from a child who has asthma. Which of the following findings should the nurse identify as indicating the child's respiratory status is deteriorating? (Select all that apply.)

   A. Oxygen saturation 95%
   B. Wheezing
   C. Retraction of sternal muscles
   D. Agitation
   E. Nasal flaring

2. A nurse is reinforcing teaching with an adolescent about the prescribed use of his asthma medications. Which of the following medications should the nurse instruct the client to use as needed before exercise?

   A. Fluticasone/salmeterol
   B. Montelukast
   C. Prednisone
   D. Albuterol

3. A nurse is contributing to the plan of care for a child who has asthma. Which of the following interventions should the nurse recommend during an asthma exacerbation? (Select all that apply.)

   A. Perform chest percussion.
   B. Place the child in an upright position.
   C. Monitor oxygen saturation.
   D. Administer bronchodilators.
   E. Administer dornase alfa.

4. A nurse is reinforcing teaching with a child who has asthma about how to use a peak flow meter. Which of the following information should the nurse include? (Select all that apply.)

   A. Zero the meter before each use.
   B. Record the average of the attempts.
   C. Perform three attempts.
   D. Deliver a long, slow breath into the meter.
   E. Sit in a chair with feet on the floor.

5. A nurse is discussing risk factors for asthma with a group of parents. Which of the following conditions should the nurse include? (Select all that apply.)

   A. Family history of asthma
   B. Family history of allergies
   C. Exposure to smoke
   D. Low birth weight
   E. Being underweight

PRACTICE Active Learning Scenario

A nurse is reinforcing teaching with a child about asthma triggers. What information should the nurse include? Use the ATI Active Learning Template: System Disorder to complete this item.

CLIENT EDUCATION: List at least eight possible asthma triggers.

Application Exercises Key

1. A. The nurse should expect a child experiencing respiratory difficulty to have an oxygen saturation below the expected reference range.

   B. **CORRECT:** Bronchoconstriction causes wheezing, which is an indicator of deterioration in a child's respiratory status.

   C. **CORRECT:** Increased work of breathing causes retraction of the sternal muscles, which is an indicator of deterioration in a child's respiratory status.

   D. **CORRECT:** Increased work of breathing and decreased oxygenation causes the child to exhibit agitation, which is an indicator of deterioration in a child's respiratory status.

   E. **CORRECT:** Increased work of breathing causes nasal flaring, which is an indicator of deterioration in a child's respiratory status.

   Ⓝ *NCLEX® Connection: Physiological Adaptation, Unexpected Response to Therapies*

2. A. The nurse should instruct the adolescent that fluticasone/salmeterol is a combination of LABA and corticosteroid medications, and to use it for maintenance control of asthma.

   B. The nurse should instruct the adolescent that montelukast affects the immune response to prevent inflammation, and to use it for maintenance control of asthma.

   C. The nurse should instruct the adolescent that prednisone is an anti-inflammatory medication used short-term for exacerbations of asthma.

   D. **CORRECT:** Albuterol is a beta₂ agonist used for bronchodilation. The nurse should instruct the adolescent the medicine is quick-acting, indicated for prevention of exercise-induced asthma, and used to provide immediate relief of bronchoconstriction.

   Ⓝ *NCLEX® Connection: Pharmacological Therapies, Medication Administration*

3. A. The nurse should use chest percussion to promote movement of mucus plugs for a child who has cystic fibrosis.

   B. **CORRECT:** Children who are experiencing an asthma exacerbation have decreased oxygenation. The nurse should place the child an upright position to promote ventilation.

   C. **CORRECT:** Children who are experiencing an asthma exacerbation have decreased oxygenation. The nurse should monitor oxygen saturation to detect changes in the child's condition.

   D. **CORRECT:** Children who are experiencing an asthma exacerbation experience bronchoconstriction. The nurse should administer bronchodilators to promote ventilation.

   E. The nurse should administer dornase alfa to a child who has cystic fibrosis to help with removal of respiratory secretions.

   Ⓝ *NCLEX® Connection: Physiological Adaptation, Alterations in Body Systems*

4. A. **CORRECT:** The nurse should instruct the child to zero the monitor before each use to achieve accurate results.

   B. The nurse should instruct the child to record the highest number reading.

   C. **CORRECT:** The child should perform three attempts to achieve accurate results.

   D. The nurse should instruct the child to breathe hard and fast when using the peak flow meter to measure airflow.

   E. The nurse should instruct the child to stand upright when using a peak flow meter.

   Ⓝ *NCLEX® Connection: Reduction of Risk Potential, Diagnostic Tests*

5. A. **CORRECT:** A familial history of asthma is a risk factor for the development asthma.

   B. **CORRECT:** A familial history of allergies is a risk factor for the development of asthma.

   C. **CORRECT:** Exposure to smoke is a risk factor for the development of asthma.

   D. **CORRECT:** Low birth weight is a risk factor for the development of asthma.

   E. Being overweight is a risk factor for the development of asthma.

   Ⓝ *NCLEX® Connection: Health Promotion and Maintenance, Health Promotion/Disease Prevention*

PRACTICE Answer

Using the ATI Active Learning Template: System Disorder

CLIENT EDUCATION

- Allergens
  - Indoor: mold, cockroach antigen, dust mites
  - Outdoor: grasses, pollen, trees, shrubs, molds, spores, air pollution
- Exercise/activity
- Cold air or changes in weather or temperature
- Tobacco smoke
- Infections/colds
- Animal hair or dander
- Medications
- Strong odors
- Emotions
- Food allergies or additives

Ⓝ *NCLEX® Connection: Physiological Adaptation, Alterations in Body Systems*

UNIT 2 NURSING CARE OF CHILDREN WHO HAVE SYSTEM DISORDERS
SECTION: RESPIRATORY DISORDERS

CHAPTER 18 *Cystic Fibrosis*

Cystic fibrosis is a respiratory disorder that results from inheriting a mutated gene. It is characterized by mucus glands that secrete increase in the quantity of thick, tenacious mucus, which leads to mechanical obstruction of organs (pancreas, lungs, liver, small intestine, reproductive system); an increase in organic and enzymatic constituents in the saliva; an increase in the sodium and chloride content of sweat; and autonomic nervous system abnormalities.

DATA COLLECTION

RISK FACTORS

- Both biological parents carrying the recessive trait for cystic fibrosis
- Caucasian ethnicity

EXPECTED FINDINGS

- Family history of cystic fibrosis
- Medical history of respiratory infections, growth failure
- Meconium ileus at birth manifested as distention of the abdomen, vomiting, and inability to pass stool. Meconium ileus is the earliest indication of cystic fibrosis in the newborn.

RESPIRATORY FINDINGS
- **Early manifestations**
  - Wheezing, rhonchi
  - Dry, nonproductive cough
- **Increased involvement**
  - Dyspnea
  - Paroxysmal cough
  - Obstructive emphysema and atelectasis on chest x-ray
- **Advanced disease**
  - Cyanosis
  - Pneumothorax
  - Barrel-shaped chest
  - Clubbing of fingers and toes
  - Multiple episodes of bronchitis or bronchopneumonia

GASTROINTESTINAL FINDINGS
- Large, frothy, bulky, greasy, foul-smelling stools (steatorrhea)
- Voracious appetite (early), loss of appetite (late)
- Failure to gain weight or weight loss
- Delayed growth patterns
- Prolapsed rectum
- GERD
- Distended abdomen
- Thin arms and legs
- Deficiency of fat-soluble vitamins
- Anemia
- Newborn failure to pass meconium stool within the first 24 hr after birth

INTEGUMENTARY FINDINGS
Sweat, tears, and saliva have an excessively high content of sodium and chloride.

ENDOCRINE AND REPRODUCTIVE SYSTEM FINDINGS
- Viscous cervical mucus
- Decreased or absent sperm
- Delayed puberty in females

LABORATORY TESTS

Blood specimen: Nutritional panel to detect a deficiency of fat-soluble vitamins (A, D, and E)

Sputum culture for detection of infection: *Pseudomonas aeruginosa, Haemophilus influenzae, Burkholderia cepacia, Staphylococcus aureus, Escherichia coli,* or *Klebsiella pneumoniae*

DIAGNOSTIC PROCEDURES

Duodenal analysis: Detects pancreatic enzymes

DNA testing: To isolate the mutation

Pulmonary function tests (PFTs)

Chest x-ray: Can indicate diffuse atelectasis and obstructive emphysema

Abdominal x-ray: Detects meconium ileus

Stool analysis
- For presence of fat and enzymes
- 72 hr sample with documented food intake

Sweat chloride test
- The child must be well hydrated to ensure accurate test results.
- A device that uses an electrical current stimulates sweat production. Q EBP
- Test involves collection of sweat from two different sites for an adequate sample.
- Expected reference range is chloride content less than 40 mEq/L and sodium content less than 70 mEq/L.

> **Diagnostic confirmation of cystic fibrosis:** Chloride greater than 40 mEq/L for infants younger than 3 months of age and greater than 60 mEq/L for all others; sodium greater than 90 mEq/L

PATIENT-CENTERED CARE

NURSING CARE

- Monitor newborn feeding and stool patterns.
- Check lung sounds and respiratory status.
- Vital signs with oxygen saturation.
- Assist in obtaining IV access. The provider might prescribe a peripherally inserted central catheter to allow for home IV antibiotic therapy.
- Obtain sputum for culture and sensitivity.
- Provide support to the child and family.
- Provide good oral hygiene.

Pulmonary management

- Assist in providing airway clearance therapy (ACT) to promote expectoration of pulmonary secretions. ACT is usually prescribed twice a day in the morning and evening. Avoid ACT immediately before or after meals. Several methods of ACT are available.
  - Chest physiotherapy (CPT) with postural drainage as prescribed (manual or mechanical percussion).
  - Positive expiratory therapy (PEP) uses a device, such as a flutter mucus clearance device, to encourage the client to breathe with forceful exhalations.
  - Active-cycle-of-breathing techniques, such as huffing or forced expiration with thoracic expansion, are encouraged.
  - Autogenic drainage uses an electronic chest vibrator or handheld percussor along with breathing techniques.
  - High-frequency chest compression uses a mechanical vest-like chest device combined with nebulization therapy.
- Administer aerosol therapy (bronchodilator, human deoxyribonuclease), often recommended prior to ACT.
- Administer IV or aerosolized antibiotics.
- Administer nebulized hypertonic saline for airway hydration and the clearance of mucus.
- Encourage physical aerobic exercise.
- Provide oxygen as prescribed. (Monitor for carbon dioxide retention.)

Gastrointestinal management

- Provide a well-balanced diet high in protein and calories with unrestricted fats.
- Give three meals a day with snacks.
- Encourage oral fluid intake.
- Administer pancreatic enzymes with meals or within 30 min of eating a meal or snack.
- Administer vitamin supplements (multivitamin; vitamins A, D, E, K).
- Administer laxatives or stool softeners for constipation. Polyethylene-glycol electrolyte solution is administered orally or via nasogastric tube.
- Administer histamine-receptor antagonist and motility medications for GERD.
- Administer possible formula supplements in addition to breastfeeding.
- Monitor stools and for the presence of abdominal distention.
- Administer supplemental feedings through an NG tube or gastrostomy tube if unable to maintain weight.
- Guide rectal prolapse back into place with a lubricated, gloved finger.
- Assist with a referral to a dietitian.

Endocrine management

- Cystic fibrosis-related diabetes (CFRD) necessitates monitoring of blood glucose levels.
- Administer insulin. Oral glycemic medications are not effective for CFRD.
- Monitor HbA1c levels.
- Identify the need to check for bone density for child older than 8 years to detect osteoporosis.

MEDICATIONS

Respiratory medications

Short-acting beta₂ agonists, such as albuterol; cholinergic antagonists (anticholinergics), such as ipratropium bromide; fluticasone propionate/salmeterol
- NURSING ACTIONS
  - Monitor for tremors and tachycardia when the child is taking albuterol.
  - Observe for dry mouth when the child is taking ipratropium.
- CLIENT EDUCATION
  - Instruct the child and family about how to properly use an MDI, PEP, or nebulizer.
  - Instruct the child to rinse her mouth after fluticasone propionate/salmeterol.

Ibuprofen
- NURSING ACTIONS: Monitor for adverse effects (conjunctivitis, epistaxis).
- CLIENT EDUCATION: Administer high-dose ibuprofen as prescribed. Long-term use slows the progression of pulmonary damage through suppression of the inflammatory response.

Dornase alfa decreases the viscosity of mucus and improves lung function
- NURSING ACTIONS
  - Monitor sputum thickness and ability of the client to expectorate.
  - Monitor for improvement in PFTs.
  - Monitor for adverse effects such as hoarseness, pharyngitis, rash, chest pain
- CLIENT EDUCATION
  - Instruct the child how to use a nebulizer.
  - Instruct the child to administer once or twice a day.

Antibiotics

- Administer through IV or aerosol.
- Specific to treat pulmonary infection. Common medications include tobramycin, ticarcillin, and gentamicin. Q EBP

NURSING ACTIONS
- Check for allergies.
- High doses can be prescribed. Schedule the collection of blood specimens before and after some IV antibiotics to maintain therapeutic levels.

Pancreatic enzymes

Pancrelipase treats pancreatic insufficiency associated with cystic fibrosis.

NURSING ACTIONS

- Monitor stools for adequate dosing (one to two stools per day).
- Administer capsules with all meals and snacks.
- Client can swallow or sprinkle capsules on food.
- Increase dosage of enzymes when eating high-fat foods.

Vitamins

Daily multivitamin and vitamins A, E, D, and K

INTERPROFESSIONAL CARE

- Respiratory and physical therapy, social services, pulmonologist, pharmacist, pediatrician, infectious disease specialists, and dietitians can be involved in the care of the child who has cystic fibrosis.
- Transplantation of heart, lung, pancreas, and liver can be a consideration for clients who have advanced disease.

CLIENT EDUCATION

- Ensure that the family has information regarding access to medical equipment and medications.
- Reinforce teaching about equipment and medications prior to discharge.
- Instruct the family about ways to provide CPT and breathing exercises.

- Discuss the importance of oral hygiene.
- Promote regular provider visits.
- Emphasize the need for up-to-date immunizations and a yearly influenza vaccine.
- Discuss diet and ways to increase calorie intake.
- Identify indications of infection and when to call the provider.
- Reinforce teaching with parents about ways to manage chronic illness in children.
- Promote regular physical activity and frequent position changes.
- Encourage the family to participate in a support group and use community resources. Provide information on respite care.
- Assist the family in accessing information provided by the Cystic Fibrosis Foundation.
- Identify specific needs based on the client's developmental level. For example, older adolescents are at a higher risk for depression due to the emotional and physical effects of cystic fibrosis.
- Provide home palliative care for the child or adolescent in the terminal stages of CF.

COMPLICATIONS

RESPIRATORY: Respiratory infections, respiratory colonizations, bronchial cysts, emphysema, pneumothorax, nasal polyps

GASTROINTESTINAL: Meconium ileus, prolapse of the rectum, intestinal obstruction, GERD

ENDOCRINE: Diabetes mellitus

Application Exercises

1. A nurse is reviewing the diagnostic findings for a preschool-age child who is suspected of having cystic fibrosis. Which of the following findings should the nurse identify as an indication of cystic fibrosis?

   A. Sweat chloride content 85 mEq/L

   B. Increased serum levels of fat-soluble vitamins

   C. 72-hr stool analysis sample indicating hard, packed stools

   D. Chest x-ray negative for atelectasis

2. A nurse is assisting with the admission of a child who has cystic fibrosis. For which of the following medications should the nurse anticipate receiving a prescription? (Select all that apply.)

   A. Tobramycin

   B. Loperamide

   C. Fat-soluble vitamins

   D. Albuterol

   E. Dornase alfa

3. A nurse is collecting data from a child who has cystic fibrosis. Which of the following findings should the nurse expect? (Select all that apply.)

   A. Wheezing

   B. Clubbing of fingers and toes

   C. Barrel-shaped chest

   D. Thin, watery mucus

   E. Rapid growth spurts

4. A nurse is reinforcing discharge teaching with the parents of a child who has cystic fibrosis. Which of the following instructions should the nurse include?

   A. Provide a low-calorie, low-protein diet.

   B. Administer pancreatic enzymes with meals and snacks.

   C. Implement a fluid restriction during times of infection.

   D. Restrict physical activity.

Application Exercises Key

1. A. **CORRECT:** Children who have cystic fibrosis excrete an excessive amount of sodium and chloride in their sweat. A sweat chloride content of 85 mEq/L is above the expected reference range and is an indication of cystic fibrosis.

   B. Children who have cystic fibrosis are expected to have decreased serum levels of fat-soluble vitamins.

   C. Children who have cystic fibrosis are expected to have large, bulky, frothy, greasy, foul-smelling stools (steatorrhea).

   D. Children who have cystic fibrosis are expected to have obstructive emphysema and atelectasis on chest x-ray.

   Ⓝ *NCLEX® Connection: Reduction of Risk Potential, Diagnostic Tests*

2. A. **CORRECT:** Children who have cystic fibrosis have frequent pulmonary infections. Administering antibiotics is an expected part of the plan of care.

   B. Children who have cystic fibrosis have constipation and are expected to take a laxative or stool softener as part of the plan of care. Loperamide is an antidiarrheal medication.

   C. **CORRECT:** Children who have cystic fibrosis have difficulty absorbing fat. Supplementation of the fat-soluble vitamins is an expected part of the plan of care.

   D. **CORRECT:** Children who have cystic fibrosis have mucus plugs. Administering a bronchodilator is an expected part of the plan of care.

   E. **CORRECT:** Children who have cystic fibrosis have mucus plugs. Administering dornase alfa, which decreases the viscosity of the mucus, is an expected part of the plan of care.

   Ⓝ *NCLEX® Connection: Pharmacological Therapies, Expected Actions/Outcomes*

3. A. **CORRECT:** Wheezing is an expected finding of cystic fibrosis.

   B. **CORRECT:** Clubbing is an expected finding of cystic fibrosis.

   C. **CORRECT:** A barrel-shaped chest is an expected finding of cystic fibrosis.

   D. Thick, viscous mucus is an expected finding of cystic fibrosis.

   E. Delayed growth is an expected finding of cystic fibrosis.

   Ⓝ *NCLEX® Connection: Physiological Adaptation, Basic Pathophysiology*

4. A. Children who have cystic fibrosis should eat a high-calorie, high-protein diet to allow for proper growth.

   B. **CORRECT:** Children who have cystic fibrosis have pancreatic insufficiency. The nurse should provide instruction about administering pancreatic enzymes with meals or within 30 min of a meal or snack.

   C. Children who have cystic fibrosis should increase fluids to assist in thinning thick mucus.

   D. Children who have cystic fibrosis should engage in daily aerobic activity to assist with lung expansion and to stimulate mucus expectoration.

   Ⓝ *NCLEX® Connection: Physiological Adaptation, Alterations in Body Systems*

NCLEX® Connections

When reviewing the following chapters, keep in mind the relevant topics and tasks of the NCLEX outline, in particular:

Pharmacological Therapies

EXPECTED ACTIONS/OUTCOMES: Reinforce education to the client regarding medications.

MEDICATION ADMINISTRATION: Administer a subcutaneous, intradermal, or intramuscular medication.

Reduction of Risk Potential

DIAGNOSTIC TESTS: Perform diagnostic testing (blood glucose, oxygen saturation, testing for occult blood).

POTENTIAL FOR COMPLICATIONS OF DIAGNOSTIC TESTS/ TREATMENTS/PROCEDURES: Implement measures to prevent complication of the client's condition or procedure (circulatory complication, seizure, aspiration, potential neurological disorder).

Physiological Adaptation

ALTERATIONS IN BODY SYSTEMS
Provide care to correct client alteration in body system.

Reinforce education to the client regarding care and condition.

BASIC PATHOPHYSIOLOGY
Identify signs and symptoms related to an acute or chronic illness.

Consider general principles of client disease process when providing care (injury and repair, immunity, cellular structure).

UNIT 2   NURSING CARE OF CHILDREN WHO
HAVE SYSTEM DISORDERS
SECTION: CARDIOVASCULAR AND HEMATOLOGIC DISORDERS

CHAPTER 19 # Cardiovascular Disorders

Heart disease can be congenital or acquired. Anatomic abnormalities present at birth can lead to congenital heart disease (CHD). These abnormalities result primarily in heart failure and hypoxemia. Heart failure occurs when the heart is unable to pump adequate blood to meet the metabolic and physical demands of the body.

Due to changing lifestyles and socioeconomic conditions, the incidence of hyperlipidemia is on the rise in children. The result is obesity in childhood and leads to heart disease during adulthood.

Congenital heart disease

Anatomic defects of the heart prevent normal blood flow to the pulmonary and/or systemic system. Defects are categorized by blood flow patterns in the heart, and are a major cause of death in neonates and infants.
- Increased pulmonary blood flow: atrial septal defect (ASD), ventricular septal defect (VSD), and patent ductus arteriosus (PDA)
- Decreased pulmonary blood flow: Tetralogy of Fallot, tricuspid atresia
- Obstruction to blood flow: Coarctation of the aorta, pulmonary stenosis, aortic stenosis
- Mixed blood flow: Transposition of the great arteries, truncus arteriosus, hypoplastic left heart syndrome

DATA COLLECTION

RISK FACTORS

MATERNAL FACTORS
- Infection
- Alcohol or substance use during pregnancy
- Poorly controlled diabetes mellitus or other chronic condition

GENETIC FACTORS
- History of congenital heart disease in other family members
- Syndromes such as trisomy 21 (Down syndrome)
- Presence of other congenital or chromosomal abnormalities

EXPECTED FINDINGS

Defects that increase pulmonary blood flow

Defects with increased pulmonary blood flow allow blood to shift from the high-pressure left side of the heart to the right, lower pressure side of the heart.
- Increased pulmonary blood volume on the right side of the heart increases pulmonary blood flow.
- These defects cause manifestations of heart failure.

Ventricular septal defect (19.1)
A hole in the septum between the right and left ventricle that results in increased pulmonary blood flow (left-to-right shunt)
- Most common congenital defect
- Loud, harsh murmur auscultated at the left sternal border
- A vibration (thrill) might be palpable in this area
- Heart failure
- Many VSDs close spontaneously

Atrial septal defect
A hole in the septum between the right and left atria that results in increased pulmonary blood flow (left-to-right shunt)
- Loud, harsh murmur with a fixed split second heart sound
- Heart failure
- Asymptomatic (possibly)

Patent ductus arteriosus
A condition in which the normal fetal circulation conduit between the pulmonary artery and the aorta fails to close and results in increased pulmonary blood flow (left-to-right shunt)
- Murmur (machine hum)
- Wide pulse pressure
- Bounding pulses
- Asymptomatic (possibly)
- Heart failure

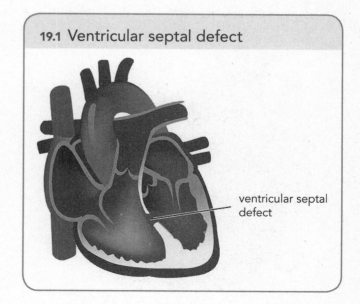

19.1 Ventricular septal defect

ventricular septal defect

Obstructive defects

Obstructive defects include those where blood flow exiting the heart meets an area of narrowing (stenosis), which causes obstruction of blood flow.
- The pressure that occurs before the defect is increased (ventricle) and the pressure that occurs after the defect is decreased. This results in a decrease in cardiac output.
- These children can present with manifestations of heart failure.

Pulmonary stenosis (19.2)
A narrowing of the pulmonary valve or pulmonary artery that results in obstruction of blood flow from the ventricles
- Systolic ejection murmur
- Asymptomatic (possibly)
- Cyanosis varies with defect, worse with severe narrowing
- Cardiomegaly
- Heart failure

Aortic stenosis
A narrowing of the aortic valve causes decreased cardiac output and left ventricular hypertrophy.
- INFANTS: Faint pulses, hypotension, tachycardia, poor feeding tolerance
- CHILDREN: Intolerance to exercise, dizziness, chest pain, possible ejection murmur

Coarctation of the aorta (19.3)
A narrowing of the lumen of the aorta, usually at or near the ductus arteriosus, that results in obstruction of blood flow from the ventricle
- Elevated blood pressure in the arms
- Bounding pulses in the upper extremities
- Decreased blood pressure in the lower extremities
- Cool skin of lower extremities
- Weak or absent femoral pulses
- Heart failure in infants
- Dizziness, headaches, fainting, or nosebleeds in older children

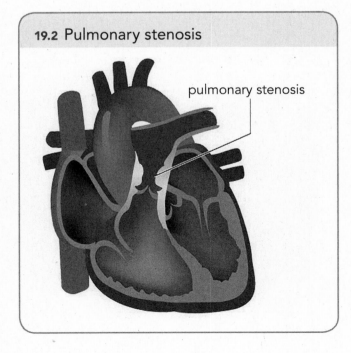

19.2 Pulmonary stenosis

pulmonary stenosis

Defects that decrease pulmonary blood flow

- Defects that decrease pulmonary blood flow have an obstruction of pulmonary blood flow and an anatomic defect (ASD or VSD) between the right and left sides of the heart.
- In these defects, there is a right to left shift allowing deoxygenated blood to enter the systemic circulation.
- Hypercyanotic (blue, "Tet") spells manifest as acute cyanosis and hyperpnea.

Tricuspid atresia
A complete closure of the tricuspid valve that results in mixed blood flow. An atrial septal opening needs to be present to allow blood to enter the left atrium.
- Infants: Cyanosis, dyspnea, tachycardia
- Older children: Hypoxemia, clubbing of fingers

Tetralogy of Fallot (19.4)
Four defects that result in mixed blood flow: Pulmonary stenosis, ventricular septal defect, overriding aorta, right ventricular hypertrophy
- Cyanosis at birth: progressive cyanosis over the first year of life
- Systolic murmur
- Episodes of acute cyanosis and hypoxia (Tet spells), especially while crying or after feeding Qs

Mixed defects

Transposition of the great arteries
A condition in which the aorta is connected to the right ventricle instead of the left, and the pulmonary artery is connected to the left ventricle instead of the right. A septal defect or a PDA must exist in order to oxygenate the blood.
- Murmur depending on presence of associated defects
- Low to severe cyanosis depending on the size of the associated defect
- Cardiomegaly
- Heart failure

Truncus arteriosus
Failure of septum formation, resulting in a single vessel that comes off of the ventricles
- Heart failure
- Murmur
- Variable cyanosis
- Delayed growth
- Lethargy
- Fatigue
- Poor feeding habits

Hypoplastic left heart syndrome
Left side of the heart is underdeveloped. ASD or patent foramen ovale allows for oxygenation of the blood.
- Mild cyanosis
- Heart failure
- Lethargy
- Cold hands and feet
- Once PDA closes, progression of cyanosis and decreased cardiac output result in eventual cardiac collapse.

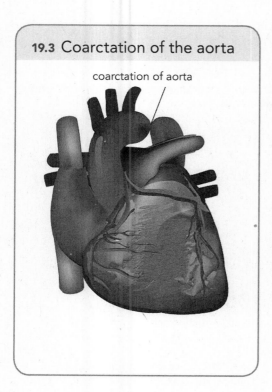

19.3 Coarctation of the aorta

coarctation of aorta

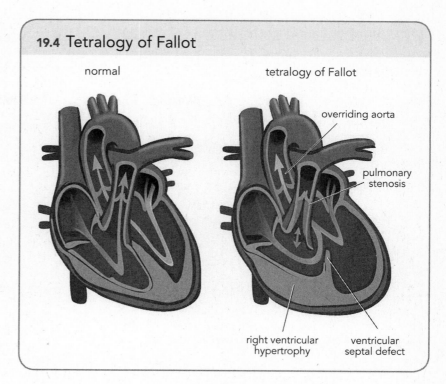

19.4 Tetralogy of Fallot

normal

tetralogy of Fallot

overriding aorta

pulmonary stenosis

right ventricular hypertrophy

ventricular septal defect

PATIENT-CENTERED CARE

THERAPEUTIC PROCEDURES

Ventricular septal defect

NONSURGICAL PROCEDURE: Closure during cardiac catheterization

SURGICAL PROCEDURES
- Pulmonary artery banding (palliative care)
- Complete repair with polyethylene terephthalate patch (procedure of choice)

Atrial septal defect

NONSURGICAL PROCEDURE: Closure during cardiac catheterization

SURGICAL PROCEDURE: Patch closure

Patent ductus arteriosus

NONSURGICAL PROCEDURES
- Administration of a prostaglandin inhibitor (indomethacin)
- Insertion of polyethylene terephthalate coated coils to occlude PDA during cardiac catheterization

SURGICAL PROCEDURE: Thoracoscopic repair

Pulmonary stenosis

NONSURGICAL PROCEDURE: Balloon angioplasty with cardiac catheterization

SURGICAL PROCEDURES
- INFANTS: Brock procedure
- CHILDREN: pulmonary valvotomy

Aortic stenosis

NONSURGICAL PROCEDURE: Balloon dilation with cardiac catheterization

SURGICAL PROCEDURES
- Norwood procedure
- Aortic valvotomy using a human donor valve (homograft)

Coarctation of the aorta

NONSURGICAL PROCEDURES
- Infants and children: Balloon angioplasty
- Adolescents: Placement of stents

SURGICAL PROCEDURE: Repair of defect recommended for infants less than 6 months of age

Tricuspid atresia

SURGICAL PROCEDURES: Surgery in 3 stages: shunt placement, Glenn procedure, modified Fontan procedure

Tetralogy of Fallot

SURGICAL PROCEDURES
- Shunt placement until able to undergo primary repair
- Complete repair within the first year of life

Transposition of the great arteries

SURGICAL PROCEDURE: Surgery to switch the arteries within the first 2 weeks of life

Truncus arteriosus

SURGICAL PROCEDURE: Surgical repair within the first month of life

Hypoplastic left heart syndrome

SURGICAL PROCEDURES: Surgery in three stages starting shortly after birth: Norwood procedure, Glenn shunt, and Fontan procedure

Pulmonary artery hypertension

Pulmonary hypertension (PAH) is high blood pressure in the arteries of the lungs that is a progressive and eventually fatal disease. There is no cure for PAH.

DATA COLLECTION

RISK FACTORS

Although anyone can develop PAH, there can be a genetic link in children who have family members who have PAH.

EXPECTED FINDINGS

- Dyspnea with exercise
- Chest pain
- Syncope

DIAGNOSTIC PROCEDURES

- Chest x-ray
- Electrocardiogram (ECG)
- Echocardiography
- Cardiac catheterization

PATIENT-CENTERED CARE

NURSING CARE

- Advise parents to avoid high altitude areas because of hypoxia.
- Reinforce teaching to parents about supplemental oxygen therapy.
- Support clients and family regarding diagnosis and treatment options.
- Reinforce teaching to parents about importance of adhering to the medication schedule.
- Reinforce teaching to parents that the prostacyclin infusion cannot be interrupted for any reason.
- Assist in preparing the child and family for possible lung transplantation.

Infective (bacterial) endocarditis

- Infective endocarditis is an infection of the inner lining of the heart and the valves.
- Causative organisms include *Streptococcus viridans* and *Staphylococcus aureus*.

DATA COLLECTION

RISK FACTORS

- Congenital or acquired heart disease
- Indwelling catheters
- Previous heart surgery

EXPECTED FINDINGS

- Fever, malaise, new murmur or change in existing murmur, myalgias, arthralgias, headache, diaphoresis, weight loss
- Neonates: Feeding problems, respiratory distress, tachycardia, heart failure, septicemia
- Splenomegaly

LABORATORY TESTS

- CBC: anemia, increased WBC
- Erythrocyte sedimentation rate (ESR) elevated
- Urinalysis: microscopic hematuria
- Positive blood cultures

DIAGNOSTIC PROCEDURES

- ECG might show AV block
- Echocardiogram shows vegetation on valves
- Chest x-ray shows cardiomegaly
- CT
- MRI

PATIENT CENTERED CARE

NURSING CARE

- Ensure administration of antibiotics parenterally for an extended length of time (2 to 8 weeks) usually via a peripherally inserted central catheter.
- Reinforce teaching to the family of high-risk children about the need for prophylactic antibiotics prior to dental and surgical procedures.
- Inform the family's regular dentist of existing cardiac problems in high-risk children to ensure preventative treatment. Qᴛᴄ
- Maintain a high level of oral care.
- Reinforce teaching to families regarding expected manifestations of infection.
- Advise families of follow-up appointments.
- Reinforce teaching to the family about manifestations of endocarditis (low-grade fever, malaise, decreased appetite with weight loss).

MEDICATIONS

High-dose anti-infectives are given for 2 to 8 weeks IV.

CLIENT EDUCATION Qpcc

- Follow the American Heart Association's recommendations for infective endocarditis prophylaxis. Only high-risk clients should receive prophylactic antibiotic therapy.
- High-risk clients should receive prophylactic antibiotic therapy prior to dental procedures, surgical procedures that involve the respiratory tract, and procedures on infected skin or musculoskeletal tissue.
- The high-risk group requiring prophylaxis treatment includes children who have artificial heart valves; previous diagnosis of infective endocarditis; unrepaired cyanotic congenital heart disease; repaired congenital heart disease using prosthetic material or device during the first 6 months of the procedure; and residual defects after congenital heart disease repair.

COMPLICATIONS

- Heart failure
- Myocardial infarction
- Embolism

Cardiomyopathy

Cardiomyopathy refers to abnormalities of the myocardium that interfere with its ability to contract effectively.

DATA COLLECTION

RISK FACTORS

Genetic factors, infection, deficiency states, metabolic conditions, collagen diseases, drug toxicity, dysrhythmias

EXPECTED FINDINGS

- Tachycardia and dysrhythmias
- Dyspnea
- Hepatosplenomegaly
- Fatigue and poor growth

DIAGNOSTIC PROCEDURES

- Chest x-ray
- ECG
- Echocardiogram
- Cardiac catheterization

COMPLICATIONS

- Infection
- Embolic complications

Shock

Cardiogenic shock results from impaired cardiac function that leads to a decrease in cardiac output.

Anaphylactic shock results from a hypersensitivity to a foreign substance that leads to massive vasodilation and capillary leak and can occur in response to an allergy to latex or medications, insect stings, or blood transfusions.

DATA COLLECTION

RISK FACTORS

- Cardiogenic shock can be seen in children following cardiac surgery and with acute dysrhythmias, congestive heart failure, trauma, or cardiomyopathy.
- Anaphylaxis can be seen in children who have allergies, asthma, or a family history of anaphylaxis.

EXPECTED FINDINGS

- Dyspnea
- Breath sounds with crackles
- Grunting
- Hypotension
- Tachycardia
- Weak peripheral pulses

MANIFESTATIONS OF HEART FAILURE

- **Impaired myocardial function:** Sweating, tachycardia, fatigue, pallor, cool extremities with weak pulses, hypotension, gallop rhythm, cardiomegaly
- **Pulmonary congestion:** Tachypnea, dyspnea, retractions, nasal flaring, grunting, wheezing, cyanosis, cough, orthopnea, exercise intolerance
- **Systemic venous congestion:** Hepatomegaly, peripheral edema, ascites, neck vein distention, periorbital edema, weight gain

MANIFESTATIONS OF HYPOXEMIA: Cyanosis, poor weight gain, tachypnea, dyspnea, clubbing, polycythemia **(19.5)**

MANIFESTATIONS OF ANAPHYLAXIS: Urticaria, periorbital or perioral angioedema, stridor, bronchospasm

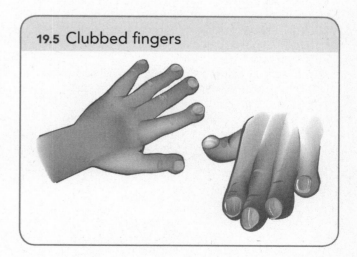

19.5 Clubbed fingers

LABORATORY TESTS

- ABGs including pH
- Hemoglobin, hematocrit, and serum electrolytes

DIAGNOSTIC PROCEDURES

ECG monitoring

To identify cardiac dysrhythmias

NURSING ACTIONS
- Assist with the application of electrodes.
- Assist with maintaining the child in a quiet position.

CLIENT EDUCATION: The test will not be painful.

Radiography (chest x-ray)

To determine heart size and blood flow

NURSING ACTIONS: Assist with positioning the child.

Echocardiography

To determine cardiac defects and heart function

NURSING ACTIONS: Assist with positioning the child.

Cardiac catheterization

An invasive test used for diagnosing, repairing some defects, and evaluating dysrhythmias. A radiopaque catheter is peripherally inserted and threaded into the heart with the use of fluoroscopy. A contrast medium (can be iodine-based) is injected, and images of the blood vessels and heart are taken as the medium is diluted and circulated throughout the body.

PREPROCEDURE NURSING ACTIONS
- Collect data from parents and child. Evidence of infection, such as a severe diaper rash, can necessitate canceling the procedure if femoral access is required.
- Check for allergies to iodine and shellfish.
- Witness signing of informed consent for procedure.
- Reinforce age-appropriate teaching.
- Reinforce how long the procedure will take, how the child will feel, and what care will be required after the procedure.
- Provide for NPO status 4 to 6 hr prior to the procedure. (If the procedure is performed as outpatient, be sure the child and family are given instructions in advance.)
- Obtain baseline vital signs, including oxygen saturation.
- Locate and mark the dorsalis pedis and posterior tibial pulses on both extremities.
- Ensure administration of pre-sedation based on the child's age, height, weight, condition, and type of procedure being performed.

POSTPROCEDURE NURSING ACTIONS
- Provide for continuous cardiac monitoring and oxygen saturation to check for bradycardia, dysrhythmias, hypotension, and hypoxemia.
- Check heart and respiratory rate for 1 full minute.
- Palpate pulses for equality and symmetry.
- Observe temperature and color of affected extremity. A cool extremity with skin that blanches can indicate arterial obstruction.
- Observe insertion site (femoral or antecubital area) for bleeding or hematoma.
- Maintain clean pressure dressing.
- Prevent bleeding by maintaining the affected extremity in a straight position for 4 to 8 hr.
- Monitor I&O for adequate urine output, hypovolemia, or dehydration.
- Monitor for hypoglycemia. IV fluids with dextrose can be necessary.
- Encourage oral intake, starting with clear liquids.
- Encourage the child to void to promote excretion of the contrast medium.

CLIENT EDUCATION
- Fluid intake will help with the removal of the dye from the body.
- Monitor the site for infection.

PATIENT-CENTERED CARE

NURSING CARE

- Remain calm when providing care.
- Keep the child well-hydrated.
- Conserve the child's energy by providing frequent rest periods; clustering care; providing small, frequent meals; bathing PRN; and keeping crying to a minimum in cyanotic children.
- Perform daily weight and I&O to monitor fluid status and nutritional status.
- Monitor heart rate, blood pressure, serum electrolytes, and kidney function to check for complications.
- Provide support and resources for parents to promote developmental growth in the child.
- Monitor family coping and provide support.
- Administer medications.
- Maintain fluid and electrolyte balance.
  - Administer potassium supplements if prescribed. These might not be indicated if the child is concurrently taking an ACE inhibitor.
  - Maintain sodium and fluid restrictions if prescribed.
  - Monitor administration of IV fluids.

- Decrease workload of the heart.
  - Maintain bed rest.
  - Position the infant in a car seat or hold at a 45° angle. Keep safety restraints low and loose on the abdomen.
  - Allow the child to sleep with several pillows and encourage a semi-Fowler's or Fowler's position while awake. Q℗
- Provide adequate nutrition.
  - Plan to feed the infant using a feeding schedule of every 3 hr. Feeding just after waking ensures the infant is well-rested.
  - Use a soft preemie nipple or a regular nipple with a slit to provide an enlarged opening.
  - Hold the infant in a semi-upright position.
  - Allow the infant to rest during feedings, taking approximately 30 min to complete the feeding.
  - Gavage feed the infant if he is unable to consume enough formula or breast milk.
  - Increase caloric density of formula gradually from 20 kcal/oz to 30 kcal/oz.
  - Encourage mothers who are breastfeeding to alternate feedings with high-density formula or fortified breast milk.
- Increase tissue oxygenation.
  - Provide cool, humidified oxygen via an oxygen hood (or tent), mask, or nasal cannula.
  - Suction the airway as indicated.
  - Monitor oxygen saturation every 2 to 4 hr.

MEDICATIONS

Digoxin

Improves myocardial contractility

NURSING ACTIONS
- Monitor pulse and withhold the medication as prescribed. Generally, if an infant's pulse is less than 90/min, the medication should be withheld. In children, the medication should be withheld if the pulse is less than 70/min.
- Monitor for toxicity as evidenced by bradycardia, dysrhythmias, nausea, vomiting, or anorexia.
- Monitor serum digoxin levels. Therapeutic serum digoxin levels range from 0.5 to 2 ng/mL.

Captopril or enalapril

Angiotensin-converting enzyme (ACE) inhibitors reduce afterload by causing vasodilation, resulting in decreased pulmonary and systemic vascular resistance.

NURSING ACTIONS
- Monitor blood pressure before and after medication administration.
- Monitor for evidence of hyperkalemia.

CLIENT EDUCATION: Monitor blood pressure frequently.

Metoprolol or carvedilol

Beta blockers decrease heart rate and blood pressure, and promote vasodilation.

NURSING ACTIONS
- Monitor blood pressure and pulse prior to administration.
- Monitor for adverse effects (dizziness, hypotension, headache).

Furosemide or chlorothiazide

Potassium-wasting diuretics rid the body of excess fluid and sodium.

NURSING ACTIONS
- Encourage a diet high in potassium.
- Monitor I&O.
- Monitor for adverse effects (hypokalemia, nausea, vomiting, dizziness).
- Monitor weight daily.

INTERPROFESSIONAL CARE

Dietitians should be consulted to assist the family with appropriate food choices.

CLIENT EDUCATION Q℗

Cardiac catheterization

- Monitor for possible complications (bleeding, infection, thrombosis).
- Limit activity for 24 hr.
- Consume fluids.

Digoxin administration

- Measure heart rate prior to medication administration. Notify provider if heart rate is lower than specified rate.
- Administer digoxin every 12 hr.
- Direct oral elixir toward the side and back of mouth when administering. Q℗
- Give water following administration to prevent tooth decay if the child has teeth.
- If a dose is missed, do not give an extra dose or increase the next dose.
- If the child vomits, do not re-administer the dose.
- Observe for indications of digoxin toxicity (decreased heart rate, decreased appetite, nausea, vomiting). Notify the provider if these occur.
- Keep the medication in a locked cabinet.

Diuretic administration

- Mix the oral elixir in a small amount of juice to disguise the bitter taste and prevent intestinal irritation.
- Observe for adverse effects of diuretics, (nausea, vomiting, diarrhea).
- Observe for manifestations of serum potassium level imbalances (muscle weakness, irritability, excessive drowsiness, increased or decreased heart rate).
- Encourage the child to eat foods high in potassium (bran cereals, potatoes, tomatoes, bananas, melons, oranges, orange juice).
- Monitor daily weight.
- Report evidence of worsening heart failure, such as increased sweating and decreased urinary output (fewer wet diapers or less frequent toileting).

COMPLICATIONS

Cardiac catheterization (potential)

- Nausea, vomiting
- Low-grade fever
- Loss of pulse in the catheterized extremity
- Transient dysrhythmias
- Acute hemorrhage from entry site

NURSING ACTIONS
- Apply direct continuous pressure at 2.5 cm (1 in) above the catheter entry site to localize pressure over the location of the vessel puncture.
- Position the child flat to reduce the gravitational effect on the rate of bleeding.
- Notify the provider immediately.
- Ensure possible administration of replacement fluids and/or medication to control emesis.

CLIENT EDUCATION
- Monitor for infection.
- Monitor for bleeding.

Hypoxemia

A hypercyanotic spell can result in severe hypoxemia, which leads to cerebral hypoxemia, and should be treated as an emergency.

NURSING ACTIONS: Immediately place the child in the knee-chest position, attempt to calm the child, and call for help.

Heart failure requiring transplant

Cardiomyopathy and congenital heart disease are causes of heart failure.

NURSING ACTIONS
- Maintain pharmacological support (oxygen, diuretics, digoxin, afterload reducers such as ACE inhibitors).
- Provide family and child support.
- Inform the child and family about infection control precautions.

CLIENT EDUCATION: Adhere to the medication regimen.

Rheumatic fever

Rheumatic fever is an inflammatory disease that occurs as a reaction to group A beta-hemolytic streptococcus (GABHS) infection of the throat.

DATA COLLECTION

RISK FACTORS

Rheumatic fever usually occurs within 2 to 6 weeks following an untreated or partially treated upper respiratory infection (strep throat) with GABHS and is most common in children 5 to 14 years old.

EXPECTED FINDINGS

- Recent upper respiratory infection
- Fever
- Tachycardia, cardiomegaly, prolonged PR interval, new or changed heart murmur, muffled heart sounds, pericardial friction rub, and report of chest pain, which can indicate carditis.
- Nontender, subcutaneous nodules over bony prominence
- Large joints (knees, elbows, ankles, wrists, shoulders) with painful swelling, indicating polyarthritis Qpcc
  - Findings can be present for a few days and then disappear without treatment, frequently returning in another joint.
- Pink, nonpruritic macular rash on the trunk and inner surfaces of extremities that appears and disappears rapidly, indicating erythema marginatum
- CNS involvement (chorea) including involuntary, purposeless muscle movements; muscle weakness; involuntary facial movements; difficulty performing fine motor activities; labile emotions; and random, uncoordinated movements of the extremities
- Irritability, poor concentration, and behavioral problems

LABORATORY TESTS

Throat culture for GABHS

Serum antistreptolysin-O titer: Elevated or rising titer, most reliable diagnostic test

C-reactive protein (CRP): Elevated in response to an inflammatory reaction

Erythrocyte sedimentation rate: Elevated in response to an inflammatory reaction

DIAGNOSTIC PROCEDURES

Cardiac function

- ECG to reveal the presence of conduction disturbances and to evaluate the function of the heart and valves.
- Echocardiography to document pericardial effusions.

NURSING ACTIONS: Position the child correctly for the procedure.

CLIENT EDUCATION: Decrease movement during the procedure.

Jones criteria

The diagnosis of rheumatic fever is made on the basis of modified Jones criteria. The child should demonstrate the presence of two major criteria or the presence of one major and two minor criteria following an acute infection with GABHS infection.

MAJOR CRITERIA
- Carditis
- Subcutaneous nodules
- Polyarthritis
- Rash (erythema marginatum)
- Chorea

MINOR CRITERIA
- Fever
- Arthralgia

PATIENT-CENTERED CARE

NURSING CARE

- Encourage bed rest during the acute illness.
- Administer antibiotic.
- Encourage nutritionally balanced meals.
- Check for chorea.
- Provide information and reassurance related to the development of chorea and its self-limiting nature.

MEDICATIONS

Antibiotic prophylaxis

Follow the prophylactic treatment regimen, which can include one of the following.
- Two daily oral doses of 200,000 units of penicillin
- Monthly IM injection of 1.2 million units of penicillin G
- Daily oral dose of 1 g sulfadiazine

The length of treatment varies according to residual heart disease, ranging from 5 years to indefinitely.

NURSING ACTIONS
- Monitor for an allergic response (anaphylaxis, hives, rashes).
- Monitor for nausea, vomiting, or diarrhea.

CLIENT EDUCATION: Adhere to medication regimen.

CLIENT EDUCATION Qᴘᴄᴄ

- Rest during the acute phase.
- Consume well-balanced meals.
- Seek medical care if infection recurrence is suspected.

COMPLICATIONS

Carditis and heart disease

Dyslipidemia

Dyslipidemia refers to disorders of lipid metabolism that can result in abnormalities in the lipid profile. Cholesterol is part of the lipoprotein complex in blood.

Triglycerides come from two sources: Naturally made in the body from carbohydrates, and the end product of fat ingestion.

Total cholesterol: The sum of all forms of cholesterol.

High density lipoprotein (HDL) cholesterol: "Good" cholesterol, having low level of cholesterol and triglycerides and high level of protein.

Low density lipoprotein (LDL) cholesterol: "Bad" cholesterol, having a high level of cholesterol, low level of triglycerides, and moderate levels of protein.

DATA COLLECTION

RISK FACTORS

- Genetic
- Obesity
- Lack of exercise
- History of health condition: diabetes, kidney disease, hypothyroidism
- Congenital heart disease and transplant patients
- Cancer survivors
- History of Kawasaki disease with coronary artery aneurysms
- Chronic inflammatory diseases
- Medications: birth control pills, diuretics, beta blockers

LABORATORY TESTS

Lipid profile: fasting for 12 hr prior to test

Fasting blood glucose

PATIENT-CENTERED CARE

NURSING CARE

- Assist in screening clients who are at risk.
- Ask parents, child about febrile illness 3 weeks prior to screening. (Illness will alter results.)

CLIENT EDUCATION Qᴘᴄᴄ

- Keep a diet history for review by the dietitian.
- Diet to lower cholesterol includes low fat, whole grains, fruit, and vegetables.
- Use of olive oil and canola oil.
- Adhere to an exercise program (60 min/day of aerobic exercise 5 days/week).

MEDICATION

Cholestyramine and colestipol

- These bile acid resin binders are used in clients who do not respond to conventional treatment.
- Used in children 10 years and older who have LDL 190 mg/dL or higher, or 160 mg/dL in clients who have risk factors.

NURSING ACTIONS

- Mix powdered medication in 4 to 6 oz water or juice, then administer immediately.
- Monitor for adverse effects (constipation, abdominal pain, flatulence, nausea, abdominal bloating).
- Monitor laboratory findings (liver function tests, CBC, creatinine kinase, fasting lipid profile) at 4- and 8-week intervals and with any dosage change.
- Reinforce teaching to the child and family how to administer medications.

CLIENT EDUCATION: Discontinue medication if the child exhibits dark urine or muscle aches, and notify the provider.

INTERPROFESSIONAL CARE

Dietary counseling

COMPLICATIONS

Atherosclerosis and coronary heart disease

NURSING ACTIONS

- Identify clients who are at risk and promote early screening.
- Reinforce teaching about healthy eating to families and clients.

Kawasaki disease

Acute systemic vasculitis that is self-limiting and can resolve or can cause cardiac complications within 8 weeks.

DATA COLLECTION

RISK FACTORS

Etiology unknown

EXPECTED FINDINGS

Acute phase

Onset of high fever that is unresponsive to antipyretics, with development of other manifestations

- Fever greater than 38.9° C (102° F) lasting 5 days to 2 weeks and unresponsive to antipyretics
- Irritability
- Red eyes without drainage
- Bright red, chapped lips

- Strawberry tongue with white coating or red bumps on the posterior aspect
- Red oral mucous membranes with inflammation including the pharynx
- Swelling of hand and feet with red palms and soles
- Nonblistering rash
- Bilateral joint pain
- Enlarged lymph nodes
- Desquamation of the perineum
- Cervical lymphadenopathy.
- Cardiac manifestations: myocarditis, decreased left ventricular function, pericardial effusion, mitral regurgitation

Subacute phase

Resolution of fever and gradual subsiding of other manifestations
- Irritability
- Peeling skin around the nails, on the palms and soles
- Temporary arthritis

Convalescent

No manifestations except altered laboratory findings. Resolution in about 6 to 8 weeks from onset.

LABORATORY TESTS

CBC, CRP, ESR, serum albumin

DIAGNOSTIC PROCEDURES

Chest x-ray

Echocardiogram and/or ECG to indicate myocarditis, pericarditis, arthritis, meningitis, inflammation

PATIENT-CENTERED CARE

NURSING CARE

- Monitor vital signs and cardiac status. Maintain cardiac monitoring.
- Monitor for heart failure (decreased urine output, gallop heart rhythm, tachycardia, respiratory distress).
- Monitor I&O.
- Obtain daily weight.
- Ensure IV fluids are administered to prevent dehydration.
- Offer clear liquids and soft foods.
- Ensure IV gamma globulin is administered according to facility policy.
- Administer aspirin.
- Provide care to promote comfort due to findings.
  - Perform oral hygiene.
  - Apply cool cloths to skin.
  - Apply skin lotions to maintain hydration.
  - Provide for a calm, quiet environment.
  - Promote rest by clustering care.
- Reinforce teaching to the family about disease progression.

MEDICATION

Gamma globulin

NURSING ACTIONS
- Ensure administration via IV infusion.
- High dosage: 2 g/kg over 8 to 12 hr.
- Ideally, administer within the first 7 days of illness.
- Repeat for clients who remain febrile.
- Monitor vital signs.
- Monitor for allergic reaction.

Aspirin (inflammation and anti-platelet therapy)

- High dose: 80 to 100 mg/kg/day divided every 6 hr.
- Once afebrile: 3 to 5 mg/kg/day to continue until platelet count returns to expected range which can be approximately 6 to 8 weeks.
- If coronary abnormalities develop, low-dose aspirin therapy can be prescribed indefinitely.

CLIENT EDUCATION Qpcc

- Maintain follow-up appointments.
- Irritability can last 2 months.
- Arthritic manifestations can last several weeks.
- Skin manifestations are painless, but the skin could be tender.

- Use passive range-of-motion exercises in the bathtub.
- Avoid live immunizations for 11 months.
- Notify the provider of any fever.

CARE AFTER DISCHARGE
- Avoid smoking.
- Maintain a heart healthy diet.
- Screen for heart disease as child ages.
  - Serum cholesterol testing
  - Blood pressure monitoring
  - Periodic imaging of the heart

COMPLICATIONS

Coronary artery dilation or aneurysm formation

- Most common in the subacute phase
- Echocardiogram to monitor for changes
- Administer anticoagulation medications (enoxaparin)

> **PRACTICE** Active Learning Scenario
>
> A nurse is discussing care of a child who has Kawasaki disease with a newly hired nurse. What should the nurse include in the discussion? Use the ATI Active Learning Template: System Disorder to complete this item.
>
> **EXPECTED FINDINGS:** Identify for the acute, subacute, and convalescent phase.
>
> **NURSING CARE:** List seven nursing actions for this client.

Application Exercises

1. A nurse is collecting data from an infant who has coarctation of the aorta. Which of the following manifestations should the nurse expect? (Select all that apply.)

   A. Weak femoral pulses

   B. Cool skin of lower extremities

   C. Severe cyanosis

   D. Clubbing of the fingers

   E. Elevated blood pressure in the arms

2. A nurse is collecting data from an infant who has infective endocarditis. Which of the following manifestations should the nurse expect? (Select all that apply.)

   A. Bradycardia

   B. Increased WBC

   C. Elevated erythrocyte sedimentation rate

   D. Increased appetite

   E. Heart murmur

3. A nurse is reinforcing teaching to the parent of a 9-month-old who has a prescription for digoxin. Which of the following instructions should the nurse include?

   A. "Do not offer your baby fluids after giving the medication."

   B. "Stop the medication and call your provider if your baby is sleeping poorly."

   C. "Give the correct dose of medication at regularly scheduled times."

   D. "If your baby vomits a dose, you should repeat the dose to ensure that he gets the correct amount."

4. A nurse is caring for a 2-year-old child who has a heart defect and is scheduled for cardiac catheterization. Which of the following actions should the nurse take?

   A. Place on NPO status for 12 hr prior to the procedure.

   B. Check for iodine or shellfish allergies prior to the procedure.

   C. Elevate the affected extremity following the procedure.

   D. Limit fluid intake following the procedure.

5. A nurse is caring for a child who is suspected of having rheumatic fever. Which of the following findings should the nurse expect? (Select all that apply.)

   A. Nonpruritic macular rash

   B. Continuous joint pain of the digits

   C. Fever

   D. Decreased erythrocyte sedimentation rate

   E. Elevated C-reactive protein

Application Exercises Key

1. A. **CORRECT:** Narrowing of the lumen of the aorta results in obstruction of blood flow from the ventricle, resulting in weak or absent femoral pulse and bounding pulses in the arms.

   B. **CORRECT:** Narrowing of the lumen of the aorta results in obstruction of blood flow from the ventricle, resulting in cool skin of the lower extremities.

   C. A client who has coarctation of the aorta exhibits adequate oxygenation of blood. Severe cyanosis is not present.

   D. Clubbing of the fingers is a manifestation of chronic hypoxemia and will not be observed in an infant who has coarctation of the aorta.

   E. **CORRECT:** Narrowing of the aorta causes increased blood pressure in the upper extremities and lower blood pressure in the lower extremities.

   Ⓝ *NCLEX® Connection: Physiological Adaptation, Basic Pathophysiology*

2. A. An infant who has infective endocarditis will exhibit tachycardia and fever due to infection with *Streptococcus viridans* or *Staphylococcus aureus*.

   B. **CORRECT:** An infant who has infective endocarditis has an increased WBC due to the presence of a bacterial infection.

   C. **CORRECT:** An infant who has infective endocarditis has an elevated ESR due to the presence of inflammation caused by bacterial infection.

   D. An infant who has infective endocarditis has feeding difficulties and weight loss due to malaise, fever, and discomfort due to myalgia.

   E. **CORRECT:** An infant who has infective endocarditis often exhibits a new heart murmur or a change in a previously existing heart murmur caused by damage to heart valves by bacterial infection.

   Ⓝ *NCLEX® Connection: Physiological Adaptation, Basic Pathophysiology*

3. A. Digoxin can be given without regard to food or fluids. For an infant whose teeth have erupted, giving water following administration of the elixir helps to prevent tooth decay.

   B. Digoxin slows the heart rate by increasing contractility of the heart. The parent should be instructed to notify the provider if an infant is eating poorly or if her heart rate has decreased below a level specified by the provider (often 90/minute for an infant and 70/minute for an older child).

   C. **CORRECT:** The correct amount of digoxin should be administered at regularly scheduled times to maintain therapeutic blood levels.

   D. It is not recommended to repeat digoxin following vomiting because it is impossible to determine how much medication was lost.

   Ⓝ *NCLEX® Connection: Pharmacological Therapies, Medication Administration*

4. A. The child should remain NPO 4 to 6 hr prior to the procedure.

   B. **CORRECT:** Iodine-based dyes can be used in this procedure, so the child is monitored for allergies to iodine or shellfish which could lead to anaphylaxis.

   C. The affected extremity should be maintained in a straight position following the procedure.

   D. Fluids should be encouraged after the procedure to maintain adequate urine output and promote excretion of the dye.

   Ⓝ *NCLEX® Connection: Reduction of Risk Potential, Potential for Complications from Surgical Procedures and Health Alterations*

5. A. **CORRECT:** Rheumatic fever is caused by Group A beta-hemolytic streptococcus. A nonpruritic, macular rash on the trunk and inner aspects of extremities, called erythema marginatum is a manifestation.

   B. A client who has rheumatic fever exhibits migratory joint pain of the large joints.

   C. **CORRECT:** Fever is a common manifestation of rheumatic fever.

   D. Rheumatic fever is caused by Group A beta-hemolytic streptococcus, which results in an elevated erythrocyte sedimentation rate.

   E. **CORRECT:** Rheumatic fever is caused by Group A beta-hemolytic streptococcus. An increase in C-reactive protein is a manifestation.

   Ⓝ *NCLEX® Connection: Physiological Adaptation, Basic Pathophysiology*

PRACTICE Answer

Using the ATI Active Learning Template: System Disorder

EXPECTED FINDINGS

- Acute phase: onset of high fever that is unresponsive to antipyretics, with development of other manifestations
  - Fever greater than 38.9° C (102° F) lasting 5 days to 2 weeks and unresponsive to antipyretics
  - Irritability
  - Red eyes without drainage
  - Bright red, chapped lips
  - Strawberry tongue with white coating or red bumps on the posterior aspect
  - Red oral mucous membranes
  - Swelling of hands and feet with red palms and soles
  - Nonblistering rash
  - Bilateral joint pain
  - Enlarged lymph nodes
- Subacute phase: resolution of the fever and gradual subsiding of other manifestations
  - Irritability
  - Peeling skin around the nails, on the palms and soles
- Convalescent phase: No manifestations except altered laboratory findings. Resolution in about 6 to 8 weeks from onset.

NURSING CARE

- Monitor vital signs, ECG, and cardiac status.
- Collect data for heart failure (decreased urine output, gallop heart rhythm, tachycardia, respiratory distress).
- Monitor I&O. Obtain daily weight.
- Administer IV fluids. Offer clear liquids and soft foods.
- Ensure IV administration of gamma globulin according to facility policy.
- Administer aspirin.
- Provide care to include oral hygiene, cool cloths to extremities, and application of skin lotion.
- Provide a quiet environment to promote rest. Cluster nursing care.

Ⓝ *NCLEX® Connection: Physiological Adaptation, Unexpected Response to Therapies*

CHAPTER 20 *Hematologic Disorders*

Blood disorders that can affect children include epistaxis, iron deficiency anemia, sickle cell anemia, and hemophilia.

Epistaxis

- Short, isolated occurrences of epistaxis (nosebleeds) are common in childhood.
- Although epistaxis is rarely an emergency, it causes anxiety for the child and caregivers.

DATA COLLECTION

RISK FACTORS

- Trauma (picking, rubbing the nose) can cause mucous membranes in the nose, which are vascular and fragile, to tear and bleed.
- Low humidity, allergic rhinitis, upper respiratory infection, blunt injury, or a foreign body in the nose can precipitate a nosebleed.
- Medications that affect clotting factors can increase bleeding.
- Epistaxis can be the result of underlying diseases (von Willebrand disease, hemophilia, idiopathic thrombocytopenia purpura, leukemia).

EXPECTED FINDINGS

- History of bleeding gums or blood in body fluids or stool
- History of trauma, illness, allergies, or placing foreign bodies in the nose

PHYSICAL FINDINGS
- Active bleeding from nose
- Restlessness and agitation

PATIENT-CENTERED CARE

NURSING CARE

- Maintain a calm demeanor with the child and family.
- Have the child sit up with the head tilted slightly forward to prevent aspiration of blood. Qs
- Apply pressure to the lower nose with the thumb and forefinger for at least 10 min.
- If needed, pack cotton or tissue into the side of the nose that is bleeding.
- Encourage the child to breathe through her mouth while her nose is bleeding.
- Apply ice across the bridge of the nose if bleeding continues.

CLIENT EDUCATION

- For recurrences, sit up and slightly forward so blood does not flow down the throat and cause coughing.
- Bleeding usually stops within 10 min.

COMPLICATIONS

Hemorrhage

NURSING ACTIONS: Provide support to the child during cauterization or packing.

CLIENT EDUCATION
- Seek medical care if bleeding lasts longer than 30 min.
- Repeated episodes require further evaluation for bleeding disorders.

Iron deficiency anemia

- Iron deficiency anemia is the most common anemia in the U.S.
- Adolescents are at risk due to poor diet, rapid growth, menses, strenuous activities, and obesity.
- The production of hemoglobin (Hgb) requires iron. Iron deficiency will result in decreased Hgb levels.
- Iron deficiency anemia usually results from an inadequate dietary supply of iron, and is the most preventable mineral disturbance.

DATA COLLECTION

RISK FACTORS

- Premature birth resulting in decreased iron stores
- Excessive intake of cows' milk in toddlers
  - Milk is not a good source of iron.
  - Milk takes the place of iron-rich solid foods.
- Malabsorption disorders
- Poor dietary intake of iron
- Increased iron requirements (blood loss)

EXPECTED FINDINGS

- Tachycardia
- Pallor
- Brittle, spoon-shaped fingernails
- Fatigue, irritability, and muscle weakness
- Systolic heart murmur

LABORATORY TESTS

CBC: Decreased RBC count, Hgb, and Hct

Hgb levels: Vary with age

RBC indices: Decreased, indicating microcytic/
hypochromic RBCs
- **Mean corpuscular volume:** Average size of RBC
- **Mean corpuscular Hgb:** Average weight of RBC
- **Mean corpuscular hemoglobin concentration:**
  Amount of Hgb relative to size of cell

Reticulocyte count: Can be decreased (indicates bone
marrow production of RBCs)

Total iron binding capacity: Elevated

PATIENT-CENTERED CARE

NURSING CARE

- Provide iron supplements for preterm and
  low-birth-weight infants by the age of 2 months. **Q**EBP
- Provide iron supplements to full-term infants by the age
  of 4 to 6 months.
- Recommend iron-fortified formula for infants when
  solids are introduced.
- Modify the infant's diet to include high iron,
  and vitamin C.
- Monitor formula intake in infants.
  - Limit formula intake to 32 oz (960 mL) per day.
  - Encourage intake of iron-rich foods.
  - Provide iron-fortified cereal when solid foods
    are introduced
  - Allow frequent rest periods.
- Provide information regarding appropriate iron
  administration.

MEDICATIONS

Iron supplements

NURSING ACTIONS
- Give 1 hr before or 2 hr after milk or antacid to prevent
  decreased absorption.
- Gastrointestinal (GI) upset (diarrhea, constipation,
  nausea) is common at the start of therapy. These will
  decrease over time.
- If tolerated, administer iron supplements on an empty
  stomach. Give with meals and start with reduced dose
  and gradually increase if GI distress occurs.

- Give with vitamin C (ascorbic acid) to increase
  absorption.
- Use a straw with liquid preparation to prevent
  staining of teeth.
- Use a Z-track into deep muscle for parenteral injections.
  Do not massage after injection.
- Expect to administer a small test dose before a full dose
  of parenteral iron due to a high risk for anaphylaxis.
- Monitor for an allergic reaction for at least 30 min
  following iron injection.

CLIENT EDUCATION
- Expect stools to turn a tarry green color if dose
  is adequate.
- Brush teeth after oral dose to minimize or
  prevent staining.
- Store iron supplements in the original container and out
  of reach of children. **Q**s

CLIENT EDUCATION

- Diarrhea, constipation, or nausea can occur at the
  start of therapy, but these adverse effects are usually
  self-limiting.
- Increase fiber and fluids if constipation develops.
- To prevent overdose, store no more than 1 month's
  supply in a child-proof bottle out of reach of children.
- Allow the child to rest.
- The length of treatment will be determined by the
  child's response to the treatment. If Hgb levels are not
  increased after 1 month of therapy, further evaluation
  is warranted. Return for follow-up laboratory tests to
  determine the effectiveness of treatment.

Dietary sources of iron
- **INFANTS:** Iron-fortified cereals and formula
- **OLDER CHILDREN:** Dried beans and lentils; peanut
  butter; green, leafy vegetables; iron-fortified breads and
  flour; poultry; red meat

COMPLICATIONS

Developmental delay

NURSING ACTIONS
- Monitor level of functioning.
- Improve nutritional intake.
- Recommend referral to appropriate developmental
  services. **Q**PCC
- Provide support to the family.

Sickle cell anemia

SICKLE CELL DISEASE (SCD) is a group of diseases in which abnormal sickle hemoglobin S (HbS) replaces normal adult hemoglobin (Hgb A).

- **Sickle cell anemia (SCA)** is the homozygous and most common form of SCD.
  - Manifestations and complications of SCA are the result of RBC sickling, which leads to increased blood viscosity, obstruction of blood flow, and tissue hypoxia. Manifestations of SCA are not usually apparent until later in infancy due to the presence of fetal Hgb.
  - Tissue hypoxia causes tissue ischemia, which results in pain.
  - Increased destruction of RBCs occurs.
- **Sickle cell crisis** is the exacerbation of SCA.

DATA COLLECTION

RISK FACTORS

- SCD is an autosomal recessive genetic disorder.
- In the U.S., SCA primarily affects people of African, Indian, Mediterranean, and Middle Eastern descent.
- Children who have the sickle cell trait are usually asymptomatic, but can pass the trait to their offspring.

EXPECTED FINDINGS

- Family history of sickle cell anemia or sickle cell trait
- Reports of pain
- Shortness of breath, fatigue
- Pallor, pale mucous membranes
- Jaundice
- Hands and feet cool to touch
- Dizziness
- Headache

Vaso-occlusive crisis (painful episode)

Usually lasts from minutes to days and is caused by acute ischemia

Acute
- Severe pain, usually in bones, joints, and abdomen
- Swollen joints, hands, and feet
- Abdominal pain
- Hematuria
- Obstructive jaundice
- Low-grade fever
- Visual disturbances

Chronic
- Increased risk of respiratory infections and osteomyelitis
- Retinal detachment and blindness
- Systolic murmurs
- Kidney failure and enuresis
- Liver cirrhosis; hepatomegaly
- Seizures
- Skeletal deformities; shoulder or hip avascular necrosis

Sequestration

- Excessive pooling of blood primarily in the spleen (splenomegaly) and sometimes the liver (hepatomegaly)
- Reduced circulating blood volume results in hypovolemia and can progress to shock.
- Hypovolemic shock: irritability, tachycardia, pallor, decreased urinary output, tachypnea, cool extremities, thready pulse, hypotension

Aplastic crisis

- Extreme anemia as a result of decreased RBC production
- Typically triggered by an infection with a virus

Hyperhemolytic crisis

Increased rate of RBC destruction leading to anemia, jaundice, and/or reticulocytosis

LABORATORY TESTS

Screening for SCA in newborns is mandatory in most states.

CBC to detect anemia.

Sickle-turbidity screening tool detects the presence of HbS but will not differentiate the trait from the disease.

Hemoglobin electrophoresis separates the various forms of Hgb and is the definitive diagnosis of sickle cell anemia.

Sickle-cell crisis

Hgb: decreased

WBC count: elevated

Bilirubin and reticulocyte levels: elevated

Peripheral blood smear reveals sickled cells

DIAGNOSTIC PROCEDURES

Transcranial Doppler (TCD) test
- Used to assess intracranial vascular flow and detect the risk for cerebrovascular accident (CVA). **Qs**
- A TCD is performed annually on children ages 2 to 16 years who have SCD.

PATIENT-CENTERED CARE

NURSING CARE

- Promote rest to decrease oxygen consumption.
- Administer oxygen if hypoxia is present.
- Maintain fluid and electrolyte balance.
  - Monitor I&O.
  - Give oral fluids.
  - Ensure administration of IV fluids with electrolyte replacement.
- Ensure administration of blood products, usually packed RBCs, and exchange transfusions per facility protocol. Observe for manifestations of hypervolemia and transfusion reaction.
- Treat and prevent infection.
  - Administer antibiotics.
  - Perform frequent hand hygiene.
  - Give oral prophylactic penicillin. Qᴇʙᴘ
  - Administer pneumococcal conjugate vaccine, meningococcal vaccine, and *Haemophilus influenzae* type B vaccine.
- Monitor and report laboratory results
- Allogeneic hematopoietic stem cell transplant (permanent cure for clients unresponsive to therapy).
- Chelation therapy decreases iron overload.
- Provide emotional support, and refer to social services if appropriate.
- Reinforce teaching to child and family about manifestations of crisis and infection.
- Give specific directions regarding fluid intake requirements, such as how many ounces of fluid should be consumed daily.
- Provide information about genetic counseling. Qᴘᴄᴄ

Pain management

- Use an interprofessional approach. Qᴛᴄ
- Treat mild to moderate pain with acetaminophen or ibuprofen. Manage severe pain with opioid analgesics.
- Apply comfort measures, such as warm packs to painful joints.
- Schedule administration of analgesics to prevent pain.

MEDICATIONS

Opioids

Codeine, morphine sulfate, oxycodone, hydromorphone, and methadone provide analgesia for pain management

NURSING ACTIONS
- Administer orally (immediate- or sustained-release) if possible.
- Administer on a regular schedule to maintain control, or prevent pain if possible.
- Use patient-controlled analgesia if appropriate.

CLIENT EDUCATION
- Avoid activities that require mental alertness. Qs
- Analgesics can be necessary in high doses, and addiction is rare.

CLIENT EDUCATION

- Promote rest and provide adequate nutrition for the child.
- Practice good hand hygiene and avoid individuals who have colds/infections/viruses.
- Maintain up-to-date immunizations.
- Wear a medical identification wristband or medical identification tags.

COMPLICATIONS

Cerebrovascular accident

NURSING ACTIONS: Monitor and report manifestations.
- Seizures
- Abnormal behavior
- Weakness of or inability to move an extremity
- Slurred speech
- Visual changes
- Vomiting
- Severe headache

CLIENT EDUCATION: Blood transfusions are usually performed every 3 to 4 weeks to prevent a repeat CVA.

Acute chest syndrome

Can be life-threatening

NURSING ACTIONS: Monitor and report manifestations.
- Chest, back, or abdominal pain
- Fever of 38.5° C (101.3° F) or higher
- Cough
- Tachypnea
- Dyspnea
- Wheezing
- Retractions
- Decreased oxygen saturations

Hemophilia

Hemophilia is a group of bleeding disorders characterized by difficulty controlling bleeding.

- Bleeding time is extended due to lack of a factor required for blood to clot. Bleeding is internal or external.
- Bleeding tendencies are sometimes recognized during infancy following circumcision, but might not become apparent until the infant becomes more active and prone to injuries during the toddler years.
- Hemophilia varies in severity based on the percentage of clotting factor a child's body contains. For example, a child who has mild hemophilia can have up to 49% of the normal factor VIII in his body, while a child who has severe hemophilia has very little factor VIII.
- Both hemophilia A and B are X-linked recessive disorders.

Hemophilia A

- Deficiency of factor VIII
- Referred to as classic hemophilia
- Accounts for 80% of cases

Hemophilia B

- Deficiency of factor IX
- Referred to as Christmas disease

DATA COLLECTION

EXPECTED FINDINGS

- Episodes of bleeding, excessive bleeding
- Reports of joint pain and stiffness
- Impaired mobility, easy bruising
- Activity intolerance

PHYSICAL FINDINGS

- Active bleeding (bleeding gums, epistaxis, hematuria, tarry stools)
- Hematomas and/or bruising, even with minor injuries
- Hemarthrosis as evidenced by joint pain, stiffness, warmth, swelling, redness, loss of range of motion, and deformities
- Headache, slurred speech, and decreased level of consciousness

LABORATORY TESTS

- Prolonged partial thromboplastin time (aPTT)
- Factor-specific assays to determine deficiency
- Platelets and prothrombin time within expected reference ranges
- Whole blood clotting time within expected range or prolonged

DIAGNOSTIC PROCEDURES

DNA testing: Detects classic hemophilia trait in females

PATIENT-CENTERED CARE

NURSING CARE

Management of bleeding in the hospital

- Administer injections via the subcutaneous route instead of IM whenever possible. Qs
- Avoid unnecessary skin punctures.
- Use surgical aseptic technique.
- Venipunctures are preferred over finger or heel sticks for blood sampling.
- Monitor urine, stool, and nasogastric fluid for occult blood.
- Do not administer products that contain aspirin.
- Acetaminophen is an acceptable substitute for aspirin.
- Control localized bleeding.
  - Ensure administration of factor replacement.
  - Observe for adverse effects (headache, flushing, low sodium, alterations in heart rate and blood pressure).
  - Encourage the child to rest and immobilize the affected joints.
  - Elevate and apply ice to the affected joints.
- Reinforce teaching about manifestations of internal bleeding and hemarthrosis.

MEDICATIONS

1-deamino-8-d-arginine vasopressin (DDAVP)

DDAVP is a synthetic form of vasopressin that increases plasma factor VIII (antihemophilic factor).

- Effective for mild, but not severe, hemophilia
- Not effective for hemophilia B, which involves a factor IX deficiency

NURSING ACTIONS: Can be given prior to dental or surgical procedures

Factor VIII, products that contain factor VIII, pooled plasma, and recombinant products

Used to prevent and treat hemorrhage

NURSING ACTIONS: Administered by IV infusion.

CLIENT EDUCATION

- Treatment can require numerous doses.
- Periodic administration has proven effective for preventing bleeding complications.

Corticosteroids

Used to treat hematuria, acute episodes of hemarthrosis, and chronic synovitis

NURSING ACTIONS: Monitor for infection and bleeding.

CLIENT EDUCATION: Maintain good hand hygiene and avoid individuals who have colds/infection/viruses.

Nonsteroidal anti-inflammatory agents

Used to treat chronic synovitis

NURSING ACTIONS: Monitor for infection.

CLIENT EDUCATION
- Administer cautiously due to potential inhibition of platelet function.
- Take the medication with food.

INTERPROFESSIONAL CARE

An interprofessional approach includes the pediatrician, hematologist, orthopedist, nurse, nurse practitioner, physical therapist, and social worker.

CLIENT EDUCATION

- To prevent bleeding at home: Qs
  - Make the environment as safe as possible to prevent injury.
  - Set activity restrictions to avoid injury. Acceptable activities include low-contact sports (bowling, fishing, swimming, golf). While participating in these activities, wear protective equipment.
  - Encourage the use of soft-bristled toothbrushes.
- Practice regular exercise and physical therapy after active bleeding is controlled.
- Maintain up-to-date immunizations.
- Wear medical identification.
- Control bleeding episodes using the RICE (rest, ice, compression, elevation) method.
- Participate in a support group such as the National Hemophilia Foundation.

COMPLICATIONS

Uncontrolled bleeding

Intracranial hemorrhage, airway obstruction from bleeding in mouth, neck, or chest

NURSING ACTIONS
- Monitor vital signs for evidence of impending shock.
- Take measures to control bleeding.
- Ensure administration of appropriate factor replacement during bleeding episodes to treat excessive bleeding or hemarthrosis.
- Ensure administration of a blood transfusion.
- Identify manifestations that can indicate presence of an intracranial bleed.
- Provide prophylaxis treatment. Regimens include infusion of factor VIII concentrate:
  - Prior to joint bleed
  - Three times a week or every other day after the first joint bleed.

CLIENT EDUCATION: Report manifestations of bleeding.

Joint deformity

- Most often elbows, knees, and ankles
- Repeated episodes of hemarthrosis (bleeding into joint spaces) lead to impaired range of motion, pain, tenderness, and swelling, which can develop into joint deformities.

NURSING ACTIONS
- Take appropriate measures to rest, immobilize, elevate, and apply ice to the affected joints during active bleeding.
- Encourage active range of motion after active bleeding is controlled.
- Encourage maintenance of ideal weight to minimize stress on joints.
- Encourage maintenance of regular exercise and physical therapy.

Application Exercises

1. A nurse is reinforcing teaching about the management of epistaxis with a school-age child. Which of the following positions should the nurse instruct the child to take when experiencing a nosebleed?

   A. Sit up and lean forward.

   B. Sit up and tilt the head up.

   C. Lie in a supine position.

   D. Lie in a prone position.

2. A nurse is reinforcing teaching about epistaxis with the parent of a school-age child. Which of the following should the nurse include as actions to take when managing an episode of epistaxis? (Select all that apply.)

   A. Press the nares together for at least 10 min.

   B. Breathe through the nose until bleeding stops.

   C. Pack cotton or tissue into the naris that is bleeding.

   D. Apply a small ice pack across the bridge of the nose.

   E. Insert petroleum into the naris after the bleeding stops.

3. A nurse is reinforcing teaching with the parent of a child who has a new prescription for liquid oral iron supplements. Which of the following statements by the parent indicates an understanding of the teaching?

   A. "I should take my child to the emergency department if his stools become dark."

   B. "My child should avoid eating citrus fruits while taking the supplements."

   C. "I should give the iron with milk to help prevent an upset stomach."

   D. "My child should take the supplement through a straw."

4. A nurse is preparing to administer iron dextran IM to a school-age child who has iron deficiency anemia. Which of the following actions by the nurse is appropriate?

   A. Administer the dose in the deltoid muscle.

   B. Use the Z-track method when administering the dose.

   C. Monitor the child for flu-like manifestations after the injection.

   D. Massage the injection site for 1 min after administering the dose.

5. A nurse is caring for an infant whose screening test reveals that he might have sickle cell disease. Which of the following tests should be performed to distinguish if the infant has the trait or the disease?

   A. Sickle solubility test

   B. Hemoglobin electrophoresis

   C. Complete blood count

   D. Transcranial Doppler

PRACTICE Active Learning Scenario

A nurse is caring for a child who has a new diagnosis of hemophilia A. Use the ATI Active Learning Template: System Disorder to complete this item.

EXPECTED FINDINGS: List two data collection findings associated with hemophilia.

CLIENT EDUCATION: List three concepts to include in the teaching with the family and child.

Application Exercises Key

1. A. **CORRECT:** The nurse should instruct the child to sit up and lean to prevent aspiration when experiencing a nosebleed.

   B. Sitting up and tilting the head up could cause aspiration of blood.

   C. Lying in a supine position could cause aspiration of blood.

   D. Lying in a prone position could cause aspiration of blood.

   Ⓝ *NCLEX® Connection: Physiological Adaptation, Alterations in Body Systems*

2. A. **CORRECT:** Pressing the nares together for at least 10 min is an appropriate action to take when managing an episode of epistaxis.

   B. The child should breathe through the mouth until the bleeding stops.

   C. **CORRECT:** Packing cotton or tissue into the naris that is bleeding is an appropriate action when managing an episode of epistaxis.

   D. **CORRECT:** Applying a ice pack across the bridge of the nose is an appropriate action when managing an episode of epistaxis.

   E. Inserting petroleum into the naris after the bleeding stops is not an appropriate action when managing an episode of epistaxis.

   Ⓝ *NCLEX® Connection: Physiological Adaptation, Alterations in Body Systems*

3. A. The child's stools will become a tarry-green color if the iron supplement dose is adequate.

   B. Vitamin C increases absorption of the iron and should be encouraged while taking the supplement.

   C. Milk prevents absorption of the iron. The supplement should be given 1 hr before or 2 hr after consuming milk.

   D. **CORRECT:** The child should take the supplement through a straw to prevent or minimize staining of the teeth.

   Ⓝ *NCLEX® Connection: Pharmacological Therapies, Medication Administration*

4. A. The nurse should administer the dose into a large muscle mass.

   B. **CORRECT:** The nurse should use the Z-track method when administering an IM dose to prevent staining of the skin at the injection site.

   C. The nurse should monitor carefully for an allergic reaction following the injection because parenteral iron can cause anaphylaxis.

   D. To reduce irritation and skin staining, the nurse should not massage the injection site after administering the dose.

   Ⓝ *NCLEX® Connection: Pharmacological Therapies, Medication Administration*

5. A. The sickle solubility test is a screening tool that detects the presence of abnormal hemoglobin, but it does not distinguish between the trait and the disease.

   B. **CORRECT:** The hemoglobin electrophoresis test should be performed to distinguish if the infant has the trait or the disease.

   C. A complete blood count tests for anemia. It indicates the average size of the red blood cells, and the amount of hemoglobin in the red blood cells. It will not distinguish between sickle cell disease and sickle cell trait.

   D. The transcranial Doppler is performed to assess intracranial vascular flow and detect the risk for cerebrovascular accident. It will not distinguish between sickle cell disease and sickle cell trait.

   Ⓝ *NCLEX® Connection: Reduction of Risk Potential, Diagnostic Tests*

PRACTICE Answer

Using the ATI Active Learning Template: System Disorder

EXPECTED FINDINGS
- Active bleeding (possibly from the gums, epistaxis, hematuria, and/or gastrointestinal tract).
- Hematomas and bruising occur easily even with minor injuries.
- Joint pain and stiffness, warmth, swelling, redness, loss of range of motion of the joints.
- Cerebral bleeding can cause headaches, slurred speech, and decreased level of consciousness.

CLIENT EDUCATION
- Prevent bleeding at home.
- Provide a safe home and a play environment that is free of clutter.
- Place padding on corners of furniture.
- Set activity restrictions to avoid injury. Wear protective equipment during activities.
- Use soft-bristled toothbrushes or disposable oral sponges.
- Practice regular exercise and physical therapy when not actively bleeding.
- Remain up to date on recommended immunizations.
- Wear medical identification.
- Report manifestations of internal bleeding and hemarthrosis
- Use the RICE (rest, ice, compression, elevation) method to control active bleeding.

Ⓝ *NCLEX® Connection: Physiological Adaptation, Alterations in Body Systems*

NCLEX® Connections

When reviewing the following chapters, keep in mind the relevant topics and tasks of the NCLEX outline, in particular:

Reduction of Risk Potential

DIAGNOSTIC TESTS: Perform diagnostic testing (blood glucose, oxygen saturation, testing for occult blood).

POTENTIAL FOR COMPLICATIONS OF DIAGNOSTIC TESTS/TREATMENTS/PROCEDURES: Identify the client's response to diagnostic tests/treatments/procedures.

Physiological Adaptation

ALTERATIONS IN BODY SYSTEMS
Perform care for the client after surgical procedure.

Reinforce education to the client regarding care and condition.

BASIC PATHOPHYSIOLOGY
Identify signs and symptoms related to an acute or chronic illness.

Consider general principles of the client's disease process when providing care (injury and repair, immunity, cellular structure).

FLUID AND ELECTROLYTE IMBALANCES
Identify signs and symptoms of the client's fluid and/or electrolyte imbalances.

Provide interventions to restore the client's fluid and/or electrolyte balances.

CHAPTER 21 *Acute Infectious Gastrointestinal Disorders*

Diarrhea can be mild to severe, and acute or chronic. It can result in mild to severe dehydration.

Acute diarrhea is a sudden increase in frequency and change in consistency of stool. It is usually secondary to an infectious agent in the gastrointestinal (GI) tract, upper respiratory infection, urinary tract infection, antibiotic use, or laxative use. Self-resolution occurs in less than 14 days if dehydration does not occur. Acute infectious diarrhea is caused by a variety of viral, bacterial, or parasitic pathogens.

Chronic diarrhea is an increase in frequency and change of consistency of stools for more than 14 days. It is caused by chronic conditions such as malabsorption syndrome, food allergies, or inflammatory bowel disease. Chronic nonspecific diarrhea has no identified cause.

Dehydration is a body fluid disturbance when the output exceeds intake. It results from causes such as fluid losses through the skin, or respiratory, urinary, or GI tract.

DATA COLLECTION

RISK FACTORS

- Lack of normal elimination pattern
- Lack of clean water, poor hygiene
- Crowded living environments, poor sanitation
- Nutritional deficiency

EXPECTED FINDINGS

- Reports of fatigue, malaise, change in behavior, change in stool pattern, poor appetite, weight loss, and pain.
- Monitor for manifestations of dehydration.

Rotavirus

Viral infection
- Most common cause of diarrhea in children younger than 5 years
- Affects children of all ages

MANIFESTATIONS
- Fever
- Onset of foul-smelling, watery stools
- Diarrhea for 5 to 7 days
- Vomiting for approximately 2 days

TRANSMISSION: Fecal-oral

INCUBATION PERIOD: 48 hr

Norwalk-like organisms: Caliciviruses

Viral infection

MANIFESTATIONS
- Abdominal cramps, nausea, vomiting
- Malaise, watery diarrhea
- Lasts 2 to 3 days

TRANSMISSION: Contaminated water

INCUBATION PERIOD: 12 to 48 hr

Yersinia enterocolitis

Bacterial infection

MANIFESTATIONS
- Mucoid, possibly bloody diarrhea
- Abdominal pain, fever, and vomiting

TRANSMISSION: Pets and food

INCUBATION PERIOD: 1 to 3 weeks

Escherichia coli

Bacterial infection

MANIFESTATIONS
- Watery diarrhea for 1 to 2 days, followed by abdominal cramping and bloody diarrhea
- Can lead to hemolytic uremic syndrome

TRANSMISSION: Depends on strain of *E. coli* (foodborne, contact with cattle, person-to-person)

INCUBATION PERIOD: 3 to 4 days

Salmonella nontyphoidal groups

Bacterial infection

MANIFESTATIONS
- Mild to severe nausea, vomiting, abdominal cramping, bloody diarrhea, and fever (can be afebrile in infants)
- Diarrhea can last 2 to 3 weeks
- Possible headache, confusion, drowsiness, seizures Qs
- Can lead to meningitis or septicemia

TRANSMISSION: Person to person; undercooked meats and poultry; household pets

INCUBATION PERIOD: 6 to 72 hr

Clostridium difficile

Bacterial infection

MANIFESTATIONS
- Mild, watery diarrhea for a few days
- Possibly less severe findings in children than adults
- Possible leukocytosis, hypoalbuminemia, and high fever
- Possible pseudomembranous colitis

TRANSMISSION: Contact with colonized spores, commonly in health care settings

INCUBATION PERIOD: Nonspecified

Clostridium botulinum

Bacterial infection

MANIFESTATIONS
- Findings depend on strain
- Abdominal pain, cramping, and diarrhea
- Possible respiratory or central nervous system problems

TRANSMISSION: Contaminated food products

INCUBATION PERIOD: 12 to 26 hr

Shigella groups: Shigellosis

Bacterial infection

MANIFESTATIONS
- Sick appearance
- Fever, fatigue, and anorexia
- Cramping abdomen followed by watery or bloody diarrhea lasting 5 to 10 days

TRANSMISSION: Contaminated food or water

INCUBATION PERIOD: 1 to 7 days

Staphylococcus

Bacterial infection

MANIFESTATIONS: Diarrhea, nausea, and vomiting

TRANSMISSION: Inadequately cooked or refrigerated food

INCUBATION PERIOD: 1 to 8 hr

Enterobius vermicularis (pinworm)

Helminthic infection

Ingested or inhaled eggs hatch in the upper intestine, and mature. After mating, worms migrate out of the intestine and lay eggs. Eggs can survive for 2 to 3 weeks on surfaces.

MANIFESTATIONS: Perianal itching, enuresis, sleeplessness, restlessness, and irritability due to itching

TRANSMISSION: Fecal-oral

Giardia intestinalis: Parasitic pathogen

The nonmotile stage of protozoa can survive in the environment for months.

MANIFESTATIONS
- **Children 5 years old or younger**
  - Diarrhea
  - Vomiting
  - Anorexia
- **Older children**
  - Abdominal cramps
  - Intermittent loose, malodorous, pale, greasy stools

TRANSMISSION: Person to person, food, animals

LABORATORY TESTS

- CBC with differential determines anemia and infection.
- Hct, Hgb, BUN, creatinine, and urine-specific gravity levels are usually elevated with dehydration. QEBP
- Stool test for occult blood.
- Perform a urinalysis.
- Check serum electrolytes

DIAGNOSTIC PROCEDURES

Tape test

Performed to check for *Enterobius vermicularis*.

CLIENT EDUCATION
- Place transparent tape over the child's anus at night. Remove the tape the following morning prior to the child toileting or bathing. If possible, apply the tape after the child has gone to sleep and remove it before the child awakens.
- Bring the specimen to the laboratory for microscopic evaluation.
- Use good hand hygiene during this procedure.

Infectious gastroenteritis

Rotavirus: Enzyme immunoassay (stool sample)

E. coli: Sorbitol-MacConkey agar (stool sample)

Salmonella: Gram-stained stool culture

C. difficile: Stool culture

C. botulinum: Blood and stool culture

Staphylococcus: Identification of organism in stool, blood, food, or aspirate

G. intestinalis: Enzyme immunoassay (stool sample)

Shigellosis: Blood and stool culture

Caliciviruses: Enzyme immunoassay (stool sample)

Yersinia enterocolitis: Identification of organism in stool or other body fluids

PATIENT-CENTERED CARE

NURSING CARE

- Obtain baseline height and weight.
- Obtain daily weights at the same time each day.
- Avoid taking a rectal temperature.
- Check and monitor I&O (urine and stool).
- Monitor administration of IV fluids as ordered.
- Administer antibiotic (Shigella, C. difficile, G. intestinalis) Q EBP
- Avoid antibiotics (C. botulinum, E. coli, Salmonella).
- Avoid antimotility agents (E. coli, Salmonella, Shigella).
- Instruct prevention measures, including immunization for rotavirus.

Oral rehydration therapy

- Start replacement with an oral replacement solution (ORS) of 75 to 90 sodium mEq/L at 40 to 50 mL/kg over 4 hr. Q EBP
- Determine the need for further rehydration after initial replacement.
- Initiate maintenance therapy with ORS of 40 to 60 sodium mEq/L and limit to 150 mL/kg/day.
  - Give ORS alternately with appropriate intake.
  - Give infants water, breast milk, or lactose-free formula if supplementary fluid is needed.
  - Older children may resume their regular diets for additional intake.
- Replace each diarrheal stool with 10 mL/kg of ORS for ongoing diarrhea.

MEDICATIONS

Metronidazole, tinidazole

Indicated for C. difficile and G. intestinalis

NURSING ACTIONS: Monitor for allergies and GI upset.

CLIENT EDUCATION: Take the medication as prescribed and report any GI disturbances.

Mebendazole, albendazole, pyrantel pamoate

Indicated for Enterobius vermicularis

NURSING ACTIONS
- Administer in a single dose that can need to be repeated in 2 weeks.
- Administer mebendazole for children older than 2 years of age.

CLIENT EDUCATION: The entire family should be treated at the same time.

CLIENT EDUCATION

- Inform the child's school or day care of the infection/infestation. The child should stay home during the incubation period.
- Provide frequent skin care to prevent skin breakdown.
- Avoid the spread of infectious diseases. Q PCC
  - Change bed linens and underwear daily for several days.
  - Cleanse toys and child care areas thoroughly to prevent further spread or reinfestation.
  - Keep toys separate and avoid shaking linens to prevent the spread of disease.
  - Shower frequently.
  - Avoid undercooked or under-refrigerated food.
  - Perform proper hand hygiene after toileting and after changing diapers.
  - Do not share dishes and utensils. Wash them in hot, soapy water or in the dishwasher.
  - Clip nails and discourage nail biting and thumb sucking.
  - Clean toilet areas.
- Use commercially prepared ORS when the child experiences diarrhea.

Foods and fluids to avoid
- Fruit juices, carbonated sodas, and gelatin, which all have high carbohydrate content, low electrolyte content, and a high osmolality
- Caffeine, due to its mild diuretic effect
- Chicken or beef broth, which have too much sodium and not enough carbohydrates
- Bananas, rice, applesauce, and toast (BRAT diet, which has low nutritional value, high carbohydrate content, and low electrolytes)

COMPLICATIONS

Dehydration

TYPES OF DEHYDRATION

Isotonic
- Water and sodium are lost in nearly equal amounts.
- Major loss of fluid from extracellular fluid leads to a reduced volume of circulating fluid.
- Hypovolemic shock can result.
- Serum sodium is within the expected reference range (130 to 150 mEq/L).

Hypotonic
- Electrolyte loss is greater than water loss.
- Water changes from extracellular fluid to intracellular fluid.
- Physical manifestations are more severe with smaller fluid loss.
- Shock is likely.
- Serum sodium is less than 130 mEq/L.

Hypertonic
- Water loss is greater than electrolyte loss.
- Fluid shifts from intracellular to extracellular.
- Shock is less likely.
- Neurologic changes (change in level of consciousness, irritability, hyperreflexia, seizures) can occur.
- Serum sodium concentration is greater than 150 mEq/L

LEVELS OF DEHYDRATION

Mild
- WEIGHT LOSS
  - 3% to 5% in infants
  - 3% to 4% in children
- MANIFESTATIONS
  - Slightly dry buccal mucous membranes
  - Anterior fontanel, unchanged; pulse and blood pressure within expected reference ranges
  - Capillary refill greater than 2 seconds
  - Slight increase in thirst

Moderate
- WEIGHT LOSS
  - 6% to 9% in infants
  - 6% to 8% in children
- MANIFESTATIONS
  - Capillary refill between 2 and 4 seconds
  - Possible thirst and irritability
  - Pulse slightly increased possible orthostatic hypotension
  - Dry buccal mucous membranes
  - Decreased ability to produce tears and sluggish skin turgor
  - Possible sunken anterior fontanel on infants

Severe
- WEIGHT LOSS: 10% or more for infants or children
- MANIFESTATIONS
  - Capillary refill greater than 4 seconds
  - Rapid thready pulse
  - Orthostatic hypotension can progress to shock
  - Extreme thirst
  - Very dry mucous membranes and tented skin
  - Hyperpnea
  - Sunken eyeballs and inability to produce tears
  - Mottled skin or cyanosis
  - Sunken anterior fontanel
  - Lethargy
  - Oliguria or anuria

NURSING ACTIONS
- Oral rehydration is attempted first for mild and moderate cases of dehydration.
  - **Mild:** 50 mL/kg oral rehydration fluid within 4 hr
  - **Moderate:** 100 mL/kg oral rehydration fluid within 4 hr
  - **Replacement of diarrhea losses** with 10 mL/kg each stool
- Administer parenteral fluid therapy.
  - Initiated when a child is unable to drink enough oral fluids to correct fluid losses, and those who have severe dehydration or continued vomiting. Qs
  - Isotonic solution 20 mL/kg IV bolus with possible repeat for isotonic and hypotonic dehydration. Sodium bicarbonate may be added for severe dehydration if acidosis present.
  - Rapid fluid replacement is contraindicated in hypertonic dehydration because of the risk of cerebral edema.
  - Monitor administration of maintenance IV fluids.
  - Avoid potassium replacement until kidney function is verified.
- Check capillary refill.
- Monitor vital signs.
- Monitor weight.
- Maintain accurate I&O.

CLIENT EDUCATION
- Encourage oral fluids.
- Resume normal diet as soon as possible.
- Monitor how many times the child voids.

Application Exercises

1. A nurse is caring for a child who has had watery diarrhea for the past 3 days. Which of the following is an appropriate action for the nurse to take?

   A. Offer chicken broth.

   B. Initiate oral rehydration therapy.

   C. Start hypertonic IV solution.

   D. Keep the child NPO until the diarrhea subsides.

2. A nurse is caring for a child who is suspected to have *Enterobius vermicularis*. Which of the following actions should the nurse take?

   A. Perform a tape test.

   B. Collect stool specimen for culture.

   C. Test the stool for occult blood.

   D. Ensure IV fluids are initiated.

3. A nurse is collecting data from a preschooler who has a rotavirus infection. Which of the following are expected manifestations? (Select all that apply.)

   A. Fever

   B. Vomiting

   C. Watery stools

   D. Bloody stools

   E. Confusion

4. A nurse is reinforcing teaching to the parents of a toddler who has salmonella. Which of the following information should the nurse include in the teaching? (Select all that apply.)

   A. Incubation period is nonspecific.

   B. It is a bacterial infection.

   C. Bloody diarrhea is common.

   D. Transmission can be from house pets.

   E. Antibiotics are used for treatment.

5. A nurse is reinforcing teaching with a group of parents about *E. coli*. Which of the following information should the nurse include in the teaching? (Select all that apply.)

   A. Severe abdominal cramping occurs.

   B. Bloody diarrhea is the first manifestation.

   C. It can lead to hemolytic uremic syndrome.

   D. It is a foodborne pathogen.

   E. Antibiotics are given for treatment.

PRACTICE Active Learning Template

A nurse is reinforcing teaching with the parent of a child who has an acute gastrointestinal infection. What information should the nurse include in the teaching? Use the ATI Active Learning Template: System Disorder to complete this item.

CLIENT EDUCATION: Describe at least 10 points to review regarding care after discharge.

Application Exercises Key

1. A. Chicken broth is avoided for children who have diarrhea due to its increased sodium and inadequate carbohydrates.

   B. **CORRECT:** Oral rehydration therapy is recommended to replace lost electrolytes for children who have diarrhea.

   C. Isotonic IV solutions are recommended for children who experience severe dehydration.

   D. Children who experience diarrhea are at risk for dehydration. Keeping them NPO is contraindicated.

   ⓝ *NCLEX® Connection: Physiological Adaptation, Fluid and Electrolyte Imbalances*

2. A. **CORRECT:** A tape test is used when diagnosing *Enterobius vermicularis*.

   B. Stool cultures are obtained to diagnose salmonella or *C. difficile*.

   C. A manifestation of *E. coli* is bloody stools.

   D. IV fluids are initiated for children who are dehydrated.

   ⓝ *NCLEX® Connection: Reduction of Risk Potential, Diagnostic Tests*

3. A. **CORRECT:** Fever is a manifestation of rotavirus infection.

   B. **CORRECT:** Vomiting for approximately 2 days is a manifestation of rotavirus infection.

   C. **CORRECT:** Foul-smelling, watery stools are a manifestation of rotavirus infection.

   D. Bloody stools are a manifestation of *E. coli*.

   E. Confusion and other neurologic manifestations can occur as complications of salmonella infection.

   ⓝ *NCLEX® Connection: Physiological Adaptation, Basic Pathophysiology*

4. A. The incubation period of salmonella is 6 to 72 hr.

   B. **CORRECT:** Salmonella is classified as a bacterial infection.

   C. **CORRECT:** Salmonella manifestations include bloody diarrhea, nausea, vomiting, and abdominal cramping.

   D. **CORRECT:** Salmonella can be transmitted to children from household pets such as cats, dogs, hamsters, and turtles.

   E. Salmonella is a bacterial infection. However, antibiotics are not prescribed unless complications occur.

   ⓝ *NCLEX® Connection: Physiological Adaptation, Alterations in Body Systems*

5. A. **CORRECT:** Severe abdominal cramping is a manifestation of *E. coli*.

   B. Manifestations begin with watery diarrhea lasting 1 to 2 days and then advancing to bloody diarrhea.

   C. **CORRECT:** *E. coli* can lead to hemolytic uremic syndrome.

   D. **CORRECT:** *E. coli* is a foodborne pathogen.

   E. Antibiotics can worsen an *E. coli* infection. They are not recommended.

   ⓝ *NCLEX® Connection: Physiological Adaptation, Alterations in Body Systems*

PRACTICE Answer

Using the ATI Active Learning Template: System Disorder

CLIENT EDUCATION

- Inform the child's school or day care center of the infection/infestation.
- Use commercially prepared oral rehydration therapy when the child experiences diarrhea. Foods and fluids to avoid include the following.
  ○ Fruit juices, carbonated sodas, and gelatin, which have high carbohydrate content, low electrolyte content, and high osmolality
  ○ Caffeine, due to its mild diuretic effect
  ○ Chicken or beef broth, which have high sodium content and inadequate carbohydrates
  ○ Bananas, rice, applesauce, and toast (BRAT diet) due to low nutritional value, high carbohydrate content, and low electrolytes
- Use prevention measures, including immunization for rotavirus.
- Provide frequent skin care to prevent skin breakdown.
- Avoid the spread of infectious diseases.
- Change bed linens and underwear daily for several days.
- Cleanse toys and child care areas thoroughly to prevent further spread or reinfestation.
- Keep toys separate, and avoid shaking linens to prevent the spread of disease.
- Shower frequently.
- Avoid undercooked or under-refrigerated food.
- Perform proper hand hygiene after toileting and after changing diapers.
- Do not share dishes and utensils. Wash them in hot, soapy water or in the dishwasher.
- Clip nails, and discourage nail-biting and thumb-sucking.
- Clean toilet areas.

ⓝ *NCLEX® Connection: Physiological Adaptation, Illness Management*

CHAPTER 22 Gastrointestinal Structural and Inflammatory Disorders

Gastrointestinal structural disorders include cleft lip and palate, gastroesophageal reflux disease, hypertrophic pyloric stenosis, Hirschsprung's disease, and intussusception. Inflammatory disorders include appendicitis and Meckel's diverticulum.

Cleft lip and palate

- Cleft lip (CL) results from the incomplete fusion of the oral cavity during intrauterine life. Cleft palate (CP) results from the incomplete fusion of the palates during intrauterine life.
- Although a CL and CP can occur together, either defect can appear alone. The defects can be unilateral (one-sided) or bilateral (two-sided).

DATA COLLECTION

RISK FACTORS

- Other syndromes
- Maternal and environmental factors
- Family history of cleft lip or palate
- Exposure to alcohol, cigarette smoke, anticonvulsants, retinoids, or steroids during pregnancy
- Folate deficiency during pregnancy

EXPECTED FINDINGS

PHYSICAL FINDINGS

- Cleft lip is an externally visible separation from the upper lip toward the nose.
- Cleft palate is a visible or palpable opening of the palate connecting the mouth and the nasal cavity.

PATIENT-CENTERED CARE

NURSING CARE

- Support and encourage parents in the general care of their child.
- Promote parent-infant bonding. Qpcc
- Promote healthy self-esteem throughout the child's development.

THERAPEUTIC PROCEDURES

Cleft lip
- Repair is typically done between 2 and 3 months of age.
- Revisions are usually required in severe defects.

Cleft palate
- Repair is typically done between 6 and 12 months of age.
- Most require a second surgery.

PREOPERATIVE NURSING ACTIONS
- Inspect the lip and palate, using a gloved finger to palpate the palate.
- Check the infant's ability to suck.
- Obtain baseline weight.
- Observe interaction between the family and infant.
- Determine family coping and support.
- Inform parents of appropriate support groups.
- Consult with social services to provide needed services (financial, insurance) for the family and infant.
- Instruct parents about proper feeding and care.
- Monitor the child's ability to feed.
- Initiate strategies for successful feeding.
  - **For isolated cleft lip**
    - Encourage breast feeding.
    - Use a wide-based nipple for bottle feeding.
    - Squeeze the infant's cheeks together during feeding to decrease the gap.
  - **For cleft palate with or without cleft lip**
    - Position the infant upright while cradling the head during feeding.
    - Use a specialized nipple and bottle with a one-way flow valve.
    - Burp the infant frequently.
    - Syringe feeding can be necessary for the infant who is unsuccessful with other methods.

22.1 Cleft palate

incomplete cleft palate

unilateral complete lip and palate

bilateral complete lip and palate

POSTOPERATIVE NURSING ACTIONS

- Perform standard postoperative care (monitoring vital signs and oxygen saturation; providing pain management using an age-appropriate tool). Q_{EBP}
- Keep the infant pain-free to decrease crying and stress on repair.
- Administer analgesics.
- Monitor operative sites for indications of crusting, bleeding, and infection.
- Avoid having the infant suck on a nipple or pacifier.
- Avoid spoons, forks, and other objects the infant might bring to her mouth that could damage the incision site.
- Monitor I&O and weigh daily.
- Observe the family's interaction with the infant.
- Collect data regarding family coping and support.
- Reinforce teaching to parents on the postoperative diet and feeding techniques.
- **For cleft lip**
  - Monitor the integrity of the postoperative protective device to ensure proper positioning.
  - Position the infant on her back and upright, or on her side during the immediate postoperative period to maintain the integrity of the repair.
  - Apply elbow restraints to keep the infant from injuring the repair site.
  - Restraints should be removed periodically to check skin, allow limb movement, and provide for comfort.
  - Use normal saline, water, or diluted hydrogen peroxide to clean the incision site. Apply antibiotic ointment if prescribed.
  - Gently aspirate secretions of mouth and nasopharynx to prevent respiratory complications.
- **For cleft palate**
  - Change the infant's position frequently to facilitate drainage and breathing.
  - Place the infant in a side-lying position to facilitate drainage of secretions and prevent aspiration. Q_S
  - Ensure maintenance of IV fluids until the infant is able to eat and drink.
  - Provide a clear liquid diet for first 24 hr.
  - Avoid placing a straw, tongue depressor, hard pacifier, rigid utensils, hard-tipped sippy cups, or suction catheters in the infant's mouth after cleft palate repair.
  - Elbow restraints can be used to prevent the infant from injuring the repair.
  - Closely observe for manifestations of airway obstruction, hemorrhage, and laryngeal spasm.
  - Use a face mask to deliver oxygen.

CLIENT EDUCATION

- Infant can require elbow restraints until lip and palate are healed.
- Practice proper care of operative site.

INTERPROFESSIONAL CARE

Care of the child who has CL and CP requires care from members of various disciplines (plastic surgeon, orthodontist, otolaryngologist, speech-language pathologist, pediatrician, nurse, audiologist, social worker, psychologist). Q_{TC}

COMPLICATIONS

Ear infections, hearing loss

Related to altered structure and recurrent otitis media

NURSING ACTIONS

- Feed the infant in an upright position.
- Monitor temperature.
- Inform the parents that the provider might insert pressure-equalizing tubes to facilitate fluid drainage from the ears and prevent middle ear effusion and otitis media.
- Reinforce teaching to parents about manifestations of ear infections.
- Encourage early intervention.

Speech and language impairment

More common with cleft palate than cleft lip

NURSING ACTIONS

- Recommend referral to state/national support groups and interprofessional team members as appropriate.
- Provide information to parents about a speech therapist for care.

Dental problems

Teeth might not erupt normally. Orthodontia is usually necessary later in life.

CLIENT EDUCATION

- Promote healthy dental hygiene.
- Seek early dental care.

Gastrointestinal reflux disease

- Gastroesophageal reflux (GER) occurs when gastric contents reflux back up into the esophagus, making esophageal mucosa vulnerable to injury from gastric acid and resulting in gastroesophageal reflux disease (GERD).
- GERD is tissue damage from GER.
- GER is self-limiting and usually resolves by 1 year of age.

DATA COLLECTION

RISK FACTORS

GER: Prematurity, bronchopulmonary dysplasia, neurological impairments, asthma, cystic fibrosis, cerebral palsy, scoliosis

GERD: Neurologic impairments, hiatal hernia, morbid obesity

EXPECTED FINDINGS

INFANTS
- Spitting up or forceful vomiting, irritability, excessive crying, blood in vomitus, arching of back, stiffening
- Respiratory problems
- Failure to thrive
- Apnea

CHILDREN: Heartburn, abdominal pain, difficulty swallowing, chronic cough, noncardiac chest pain

DIAGNOSTIC PROCEDURES

- Upper GI endoscopy to detect GI structural abnormalities
- 24-hr intraesophageal pH study to measure the amount of gastric acid reflux into the esophagus
- Endoscopy with biopsy to detect esophagitis and strictures
- Scintigraphy to identify the cause of gastric content aspiration

PATIENT-CENTERED CARE

NURSING CARE

GER
- Depends on the severity of the findings.
- Offer small, frequent meals.
- Thicken formula or breast milk with 1 tsp to 1 tbsp rice cereal per 1 oz formula.
- Avoid foods that cause reflux (caffeine, citrus, peppermint, spicy or fried foods).
- Assist with weight control.
- Position the child upright or with the head elevated after meals.
- Avoid feeding right before bedtime.
- Position infants prone with extreme caution; supine is still the recommended position for sleep Qs

GERD: Initiate interventions for GER, plus administering a proton pump inhibitor (omeprazole, esomeprazole, pantoprazole, rabeprazole) or an H_2–receptor antagonist (ranitidine, cimetidine, famotidine).

THERAPEUTIC PROCEDURES

Nissen fundoplication
- Laparoscopic surgical procedure that wraps the fundus of the stomach around the distal esophagus to decrease reflux
- Used for clients who have severe cases of GERD

COMPLICATIONS

Recurrent pneumonia, weight loss, failure to thrive

Repeated reflux of stomach contents can lead to erosion of the esophagus or pneumonia if stomach contents are aspirated.

NURSING ACTIONS
- Assist with evaluation of the treatment plan.
- Monitor for manifestations of pneumonia and failure to thrive.
- Reinforce the plan of care with the family.
- Reinforce teaching to the parents about manifestations of pneumonia.

Hypertrophic pyloric stenosis

- Hypertrophic pyloric stenosis is the thickening of the pyloric sphincter, which creates an obstruction.
- Usually occurs the first few weeks of life.

DATA COLLECTION

RISK FACTORS

Genetic predisposition

EXPECTED FINDINGS

- Vomiting that often occurs following a feeding but can occur up to several hours following a feeding and becomes projectile as obstruction worsens
- Nonbilious vomitus that can be blood-tinged
- Constant hunger
- Olive-shaped mass in the right upper quadrant of the abdomen and possible peristaltic wave that moves from left to right when lying supine Qebp
- Failure to gain weight and findings of dehydration (dry and/or pale skin, cool lips, dry mucous membranes, decreased skin turgor, diminished urinary output, concentrated urine, thirst, rapid pulse, sunken eyes)

LABORATORY TESTS

Serum electrolytes

DIAGNOSTIC PROCEDURES

Ultrasound reveals an elongated, mass surrounding an elongated pyloric canal.

PATIENT-CENTERED CARE

NURSING CARE

Prepare the child for surgery.

THERAPEUTIC PROCEDURES

Pyloromyotomy

Performed by laparoscope

PREOPERATIVE NURSING ACTIONS
- Monitor administration of IV fluids for correction of dehydration and electrolyte imbalances
- Insert a nasogastric (NG) tube for decompression.
- Maintain NPO status.
- Monitor I&O.
- Obtain daily weights.

POSTOPERATIVE NURSING ACTIONS

- Obtain routine postoperative vital signs.
- Ensure provision of IV fluids.
- Monitor daily weights and I&O.
- Administer analgesics for pain.
- Check for manifestations of infection.
- Start clear liquids 4 to 6 hr after surgery. Advance to breast milk or formula as tolerated 24 hr after surgery.
- Document tolerance to feedings.

Hirschsprung's disease

Hirschsprung's disease (congenital aganglionic megacolon) is a structural anomaly of the GI tract caused by lack of ganglionic cells in segments of the colon resulting in decreased motility and mechanical obstruction.

DATA COLLECTION

RISK FACTORS

Family history of Hirschsprung's disease

EXPECTED FINDINGS

Newborn
- Failure to pass meconium within 24 to 48 hr after birth
- Episodes of vomiting bile
- Refusal to eat
- Abdominal distention

Infant
- Failure to thrive
- Constipation
- Vomiting
- Episodes of diarrhea and vomiting

Child
- Undernourished, anemic appearance
- Abdominal distention
- Visible peristalsis
- Palpable fecal mass
- Constipation
- Foul-smelling, ribbonlike stool

LABORATORY TESTS

- Serum electrolytes
- CBC

DIAGNOSTIC PROCEDURES

Rectal biopsy to confirm the absence of ganglion cells

PATIENT-CENTERED CARE

NURSING CARE

- Prepare family and client for surgery.
- Assist family with improving nutritional status until surgery.
  - High-protein, high-calorie, low-fiber diet Q EBP
  - Total parenteral nutrition in some cases

THERAPEUTIC PROCEDURES

- Surgical removal of the aganglionic section of the bowel.
- Temporary colostomy can be required.

PREOPERATIVE NURSING ACTIONS
- Assist in preparing the child and family for surgery using developmentally appropriate techniques.
- Administer electrolyte and fluid replacement.
- Monitor for enterocolitis.
- Bowel prep with saline enemas and oral antibiotics.

POSTOPERATIVE NURSING ACTIONS
- Monitor respiratory status and maintain airway.
- Provide supplemental oxygen.
- Obtain vital signs.
- Administer analgesics for pain.
- Check surgical site for bleeding or other abnormalities.
- Provide Foley catheter care.
- Check bowel sounds and bowel function.
- Provide ostomy care if appropriate.
- Recommend appropriate referrals.
- Reinforce teaching to the family about ostomy care if indicated. Q PCC
- Reinforce teaching to the family about incisional care and how to monitor for infection.
- Ensure that family knows the manifestations of dehydration.

COMPLICATIONS

Enterocolitis (inflammation of the bowel)

Treatment focuses on resolving inflammation, preventing bowel perforation, maintaining hydration, initiating antibiotic therapy, and performing surgery for colostomy if there is extensive bowel involvement.

NURSING ACTIONS
- Monitor vital signs.
- Check abdominal girth.
  - Measure girth with a paper tape at the level of the umbilicus or at the widest point of the abdomen.
  - Mark the area with a pen to ensure continuity of future measurements.
- Monitor for manifestations of sepsis, peritonitis, or shock caused by enterocolitis.
- Monitor and manage fluid, electrolyte, and blood product replacement.
- Administer antibiotics.

Anal stricture and incontinence

- Bowel-retaining therapy
- Can require further procedures, such as dilatation

Intussusception

- Proximal segment of the bowel telescopes into a more distal segment, resulting in lymphatic and venous obstruction causing edema in the area. With progression, ischemia and increased mucus into the intestine will occur.
- Common in infants and children ages 3 months to 6 years.

DATA COLLECTION

EXPECTED FINDINGS

- Sudden episodic abdominal pain
- Screaming with drawing knees to chest during episodes of pain
- Abdominal mass (sausage-shaped)
- Stools mixed with blood and mucus that resemble the consistency of red currant jelly
- Vomiting
- Fever
- Tender, distended abdomen

DIAGNOSTIC PROCEDURES

Ultrasound

PATIENT-CENTERED CARE

NURSING CARE

- Stabilize the child prior to the procedure.
  - IV fluids to correct and prevent dehydration
  - Nasogastric (NG) tube for decompression
- Reinforce teaching to the family and child about the nonsurgical procedure.

THERAPEUTIC PROCEDURES

Air enema

- With or without contrast
- Performed by a radiologist

COMPLICATIONS

Reoccurring intussusception

Surgery is required for reoccurring cases.

Appendicitis

- Inflammation of the vermiform appendix caused from an obstruction of the lumen of the appendix.
- Average client age is 10 years.

DATA COLLECTION

EXPECTED FINDINGS

- Abdominal pain beginning around the umbilicus and then localizing to the right lower quadrant (McBurney's point)
- Rigid abdomen
- Decreased or absent bowel sounds
- Fever
- Diarrhea or constipation
- Lethargy
- Tachycardia
- Rapid, shallow breathing
- Anorexia
- Possible vomiting

LABORATORY TESTS

- CBC
- Urinalysis

DIAGNOSTIC PROCEDURES

Computed tomography scan shows an enlarged diameter of appendix, as well as thickening of the appendiceal wall.

PATIENT-CENTERED CARE

NURSING CARE

- Assist with preparation of the child and family for surgery using developmentally appropriate techniques.
- Avoid applying heat to the abdomen.
- Avoid enemas or laxatives.

THERAPEUTIC PROCEDURES

Removal of the nonruptured appendix

Laparoscopic surgery

PREOPERATIVE NURSING ACTIONS

- Monitor IV fluid replacement.
- Ensure administration of IV antibiotic.

POSTOPERATIVE NURSING ACTIONS

- Monitor respiratory status and maintain airway.
- Provide supplemental oxygen.
- Obtain vital signs.
- Ensure administration of analgesics for pain.
- Monitor surgical site for bleeding or any other abnormalities.
- Check bowel sounds and bowel function.

Removal of the ruptured appendix

Laparoscopic or open surgery

PREOPERATIVE NURSING ACTIONS
- Administer electrolyte and fluid replacement.
- Place NG tube for decompression.
- Monitor administration of IV antibiotics.

POSTOPERATIVE NURSING ACTIONS
- Monitor respiratory status, and maintain airway.
- Provide supplemental oxygen.
- Obtain vital signs.
- Administer analgesics for pain.
- Monitor surgical site for bleeding or other abnormalities.
- Check bowel sounds and bowel function.
- Ensure administration of IV fluids and antibiotics.
- Maintain NPO status.
- Maintain NG tube to low continuous suction.
- Provide wound care for open surgical sites with wound irrigations with antibacterial solution or saline-soaked gauze.
- Provide drain care.
- Monitor for peritonitis. Qs
  - Fever
  - Sudden increase in pain
  - Irritability
  - Rigid abdomen
  - Abdominal distention
  - Tachycardia
  - Rapid, shallow breathing
  - Pallor
  - Chills
- Reinforce teaching to the family about incision care.
- Reinforce teaching to the family about manifestations of infection.

COMPLICATIONS

Peritonitis (inflammation in the peritoneal cavity)

NURSING ACTIONS
- Monitor for peritonitis.
- Provide pain management.
  - Monitor for pain using a developmentally appropriate tool.
  - Administer analgesics.
- Monitor IV fluid therapy.
- Ensure administration of IV antibiotics for infection.
- Manage NG tube suction.
- Assist with preoperative and postoperative nursing care.
- Provide surgical wound care with wound irrigation and dressings if delayed wound closure is necessary.
- Provide psychosocial support for the child and family.
- Reinforce teaching to the child and parents about preoperative care, such as the need to maintain NPO status and the need for pain medication.
- Reinforce teaching about early ambulation, advancement of diet, wound care, and monitoring for infection.

Meckel's diverticulum

Meckel's diverticulum is a complication resulting from failure of the omphalomesenteric duct to fuse during embryonic development.

DATA COLLECTION

EXPECTED FINDINGS
- Rectal bleeding, usually painless
- Abdominal pain
- Bloody, mucus stools

LABORATORY TESTS

CBC and metabolic panel

DIAGNOSTIC EVALUATION

RADIONUCLEOTIDE SCAN: Meckel's scan is the most effective diagnostic test

PATIENT-CENTERED CARE

NURSING CARE

Prepare the child and family for surgery using developmentally appropriate techniques.

THERAPEUTIC PROCEDURES

Surgical removal of the diverticulum

PREOPERATIVE NURSING ACTIONS
- Provide blood transfusions to correct hypovolemia.
- Ensure administration of IV fluid and electrolyte replacement.
- Provide oxygen.
- Ensure administration of IV antibiotics.
- Maintain bed rest.
- Closely monitor blood loss in stools.

POSTOPERATIVE NURSING ACTIONS
- Monitor respiratory status and maintain airway.
- Provide supplemental oxygen.
- Obtain vital signs.
- Administer analgesics for pain.
- Check surgical site for bleeding or any other abnormalities.
- Monitor bowel sounds and bowel function.
- Ensure administration of IV fluids and antibiotics.
- Maintain NPO status.
- Maintain NG tube to low continuous suction.
- Instruct the family about manifestations of infection.

COMPLICATIONS

GI hemorrhage and bowel obstruction (for untreated Meckel's diverticulum)

Application Exercises

1. A nurse is collecting data from an infant who has hypertrophic pyloric stenosis. Which of the following manifestations should the nurse expect? (Select all that apply.)

    A. Projectile vomiting

    B. Dry mucus membranes

    C. Currant jelly stools

    D. Sausage-shaped abdominal mass

    E. Constant hunger

2. A nurse is caring for a child who has Hirschsprung's disease. Which of the following actions should the nurse take?

    A. Encourage a high-fiber, low-protein, low-calorie diet.

    B. Prepare the family for surgery.

    C. Place an NG tube for decompression.

    D. Initiate bed rest.

3. A nurse is caring for an infant who is postoperative following cleft lip and palate repair. Which of the following actions should the nurse take?

    A. Keep the infant NPO for the first 24 hr following surgery.

    B. Place elbow restraints on the infant.

    C. Offer the infant a pacifier containing sucrose.

    D. Inspect the incision site inside the mouth with a tongue blade.

4. A nurse is collecting data from a child who has Meckel's diverticulum. Which of the following manifestations should the nurse expect? (Select all that apply.)

    A. Abdominal pain

    B. Fever

    C. Mucus, bloody stools

    D. Vomiting

    E. Rapid, shallow breathing

5. A nurse is reinforcing teaching with the parents of an infant about gastrointestinal reflux disease. Which of the following interventions should the nurse include in the instructions? (Select all that apply.)

    A. Offer frequent feedings.

    B. Thicken formula with rice cereal.

    C. Use a bottle with a one-way valve.

    D. Position the infant upright after feedings.

    E. Use a wide-based nipple for feedings.

PRACTICE Active Learning Scenario

A nurse is caring for a child who is postoperative following an open appendectomy for a perforated appendix. Use the ATI Active Learning Template: System Disorder to complete this item.

NURSING CARE: List postoperative nursing interventions.

Application Exercises Key

1. A. **CORRECT:** A client who has a pyloric stricture has thickening of the pyloric sphincter, resulting in projectile vomiting.

   B. **CORRECT:** A client who has pyloric stricture is unable to consume adequate food and fluid, resulting in dehydration. Dry mucous membranes is a manifestation of hypertrophic pyloric stenosis.

   C. A client who has intussusception has bloody mucus stools, resulting in currant jelly stools.

   D. A client who has intussusception has telescoping intestine, resulting in a sausage-shaped abdominal mass.

   E. **CORRECT:** A client who has pyloric stricture is unable to consume adequate food and fluid, resulting in constant hunger.

   Ⓝ *NCLEX® Connection: Physiological Adaptation, Basic Pathophysiology*

2. A. A client who has Hirschsprung's disease is encouraged to eat a low-fiber, high-protein, high-calorie diet.

   B. **CORRECT:** A client who has Hirschsprung's disease requires surgery to remove the affected segment of the intestine. Preparing the family for surgery is an appropriate action for the nurse to take.

   C. A client who has Hirschsprung's disease is managed with a special diet or might receive parenteral nutrition. Placing an NG tube for decompression is not an appropriate action for the nurse to take.

   D. A client who has Meckel's diverticulum is placed on bed rest to prevent further bleeding.

   Ⓝ *NCLEX® Connection: Physiological Adaptation, Alterations in Body Systems*

3. A. The infant should be given clear liquids for the first 24 hr following surgery.

   B. **CORRECT:** The nurse should place elbow restraints on the infant to prevent damage to the incision site.

   C. Objects in the mouth, including pacifiers, could injure the surgical site and should be avoided.

   D. Objects in the mouth could injure the surgical site and should be avoided.

   Ⓝ *NCLEX® Connection: Reduction of Risk Potential, Potential for Complications from Surgical Procedures and Health Alterations*

4. A. **CORRECT:** Abdominal pain is a manifestation of Meckel's diverticulum.

   B. Fever is a manifestation of appendicitis.

   C. **CORRECT:** Mucus and bloody stools are a manifestation of Meckel's diverticulum.

   D. Vomiting is a manifestation of appendicitis.

   E. Rapid, shallow breathing is a manifestation of peritonitis and appendicitis.

   Ⓝ *NCLEX® Connection: Physiological Adaptation, Basic Pathophysiology*

5. A. **CORRECT:** Frequent feeding helps decrease the amount of vomiting.

   B. **CORRECT:** Thickened formula helps decrease the amount of vomiting and promote weight gain.

   C. A bottle with a one-way valve is used for an infant who has cleft lip and palate.

   D. **CORRECT:** Positioning the infant in an upright position following feedings will help decrease the number of vomiting episodes. It is still recommended that these infants be positioned supine for sleep.

   E. A wide-based nipple is used for an infant who has cleft lip and palate.

   Ⓝ *NCLEX® Connection: Basic Care and Comfort, Nutrition and Oral Hydration*

PRACTICE Answer

Using the ATI Active Learning Template: System Disorder

NURSING CARE
- Collect data regarding respiratory status.
- Maintain airway.
- Provide supplemental oxygen.
- Obtain vital signs.
- Ensure administration of analgesics for pain.
- Monitor surgical site for bleeding or any other abnormalities.
- Check bowel sounds and bowel function.
- Provide IV fluids and antibiotics.
- Maintain NPO status.
- Maintain NG tube to low continuous suction.
- Provide wound care for open surgical sites with antibacterial solution or saline.
- Provide drain care.
- Monitor for manifestations of for peritonitis.

Ⓝ *NCLEX® Connection: Physiological Adaptation, Alterations in Body Systems*

NCLEX® Connections

When reviewing the following chapters, keep in mind the relevant topics and tasks of the NCLEX outline, in particular:

Basic Care and Comfort

ELIMINATION: Identify the client at risk for impaired elimination (medication, hydration status).

Pharmacological Therapies

DOSAGE CALCULATIONS: Perform calculations needed for medication administration.

EXPECTED ACTIONS/OUTCOMES: Reinforce education to the client regarding medications.

Reduction of Risk Potential

LABORATORY VALUES: Notify the primary health care provider about the client's laboratory test results.

Physiological Adaptation

ALTERATIONS IN BODY SYSTEMS
Provide care to correct client alteration in body system.

Reinforce education to the client regarding care and condition.

BASIC PATHOPHYSIOLOGY
Identify signs and symptoms related to an acute or chronic illness.

Consider general principles of the client's disease process when providing care (injury and repair, immunity, cellular structure).

Apply knowledge of pathophysiology to monitoring client for alterations in body systems.

UNIT 2 NURSING CARE OF CHILDREN WHO HAVE SYSTEM DISORDERS
SECTION: GENITOURINARY AND REPRODUCTIVE DISORDERS

CHAPTER 23 *Enuresis and Urinary Tract Infections*

Enuresis is uncontrolled or unintentional urination that occurs after a child is beyond an age at which bladder control is achieved. A urinary tract infection (UTI) is an infection in any portion of the urinary tract.

Enuresis

Enuresis is uncontrolled or unintentional urination that occurs at least twice a week for at least 3 consecutive months. The child must be at least 5 years of age. Rule out organic causes related to genitourinary dysfunction prior to diagnosis of enuresis.

Primary enuresis: A child who has never been free of bed-wetting for any extended periods of time

Secondary enuresis: A child who started bed-wetting after development of urinary control

DATA COLLECTION

RISK FACTORS

Enuresis has no clear etiology, but it might be related to the following.
- Family history of enuresis
- Disorders associated with bladder dysfunction
- Male sex
- Emotional factors
- Stressful home or family situation

EXPECTED FINDINGS

- Report of day- or night-time enuresis from parent
- Urinary urgency with restlessness and discomfort is primarily associated with daytime enuresis. The child can also have urinary frequency.
- History of alterations in toilet training, voiding behaviors, and bowel movement patterns Qpcc
- History of chronic or acute illness (UTI, diabetes mellitus, sickle cell disease, neurologic deficits)
- History of family disruptions or other emotional stressors
- Family history of enuresis
- Increased fluid intake, especially in the evening
- Possible decreased functional bladder capacity.

Expected capacity = child's age in years + 2 ounces.

PATIENT-CENTERED CARE

NURSING CARE

- Evaluate the child's self-esteem.
- Evaluate the child's and family's coping strategies and available support systems.
- Reinforce teaching on how to perform bladder stretching and Kegel exercises.
- Inform the child and family regarding the management of enuresis.
  - Have the child empty his bladder prior to bedtime.
  - Encourage fluids during the day and restrict fluids in the evening.
  - Avoid caffeinated drinks.
  - Allow the child to wear regular sleepwear and avoid diapers.
  - Use positive reinforcement. Avoid punishing, scolding, or teasing the child following an incident.
  - Assist the child in keeping a calendar of wet and dry days.
  - Make environmental changes to assist the child to get to the bathroom (avoiding the top bunk bed, use of a night light, clear path from bed to bathroom).
  - Avoid holding urine during the day.
  - Have the child change the bed linens and clothing following an incident.
  - Avoid constipation (increase fiber in diet, encourage regular bowel movements).
  - Wake the child up during the night to void.
  - Administer prescribed medications.
  - Offer support to the child and the family.
  - Use conditioning therapy (child awakens by buzzer or bell in order to get up to urinate).

MEDICATIONS

Antidiuretic hormone

Desmopressin reduces the volume of urine.

NURSING ACTIONS
- Can be prescribed either oral or nasal.
- Monitor I&O.

CLIENT EDUCATION
- Restrict the child's fluid intake after the evening meal. Qebp
- Administer the medication at bedtime.
- Store nasal preparation in the refrigerator.
- Possible adverse reactions include headache, nausea, and nasal irritation.

Tricyclic antidepressants

Imipramine inhibits urination.

NURSING ACTIONS
- Monitor children for an increase in suicidality.
- Monitor for therapeutic effectiveness.
- Length of treatment is 6 to 8 weeks. Then, plan gradual withdrawal.
- Administer with food.
- Risk for relapse of manifestations when medication is discontinued.

CLIENT EDUCATION
- Administer the medication 1 hr before bedtime.
- Possible adverse effects include blurred vision, hypotension, and dry mouth.
- Avoid sun exposure.
- Avoid using with over-the-counter medications without consulting with the provider.

Anticholinergics

Oxybutynin chloride reduces bladder contractions.

NURSING ACTIONS: Monitor for effectiveness of therapy.

CLIENT EDUCATION: Possible adverse reactions include drowsiness, dry mouth, constipation, and nausea.

COMPLICATIONS

Emotional problems

Low self-esteem, altered body image, social isolation, fears

NURSING ACTIONS
- Support the child and family by listening to concerns and correcting misperceptions.
- Involve the child when reinforcing teaching about management of enuresis.
- Assist with referrals to appropriate resources (support groups, counseling) as necessary. Q͏ᴛᴄ
- Assist the child and family to understand the emotional aspects of the disorder.

CLIENT EDUCATION: Early interventions can alleviate long-term emotional issues.

Urinary tract infections

Bacteriuria: bacteria in the urine

Recurrent UTI: multiple occurrences of bacteriuria

Persistent UTI: unresolved bacteriuria with antibiotic therapy

Febrile UTI: bacteriuria with fever

Cystitis: inflammation of the bladder

Urethritis: inflammation of the urethra

Pyelonephritis: inflammation of the upper urinary tract and kidneys

Urosepsis: systemic bacterial illness related to urinary bacteria accompanied by febrile UTI

DATA COLLECTION

RISK FACTORS

- Urinary stasis
- Urinary tract anomalies
- Reflux within the urinary tract system
- Constipation
- Onset of toilet training
- Uncircumcised males
- Females (urethra in close proximity to rectum)
- Synthetic, tight underwear and wet bathing suits
- Sexual activity
- Catheter use
- Inadequate hygiene

EXPECTED FINDINGS

INFANTS
- Increase in irritability Q͏ᴘᴄᴄ
- Screaming with urination
- Poor feeding, vomiting, or failure to gain weight
- Increase in thirst
- Frequent urination
- Straining with urination
- Foul-smelling urine
- Fever
- Diaper rash
- Dehydration
- Seizure
- Jaundice
- Tachypnea
- Pallor

CHILDREN
- Abdominal or back pain
- Pain with urination
- Poor appetite
- Vomiting
- Slowed growth
- Increase in thirst
- Fever
- Foul-smelling urine
- Enuresis, frequent urination
- Costovertebral angle pain
- Swelling of the face
- Seizures
- Pallor
- Fatigue
- Blood in the urine
- Edema
- Hypertension
- Tetany

LABORATORY TESTS

Urinalysis, urine culture and sensitivity

- Sterile catheterization is indicated for obtaining urine for urinalysis and culture in children younger than 2 years old.
- Obtain a clean-catch urine sample from children who are able to cooperate.

NURSING ACTIONS
- To prevent a falsely low bacterial count, avoid having the child drink a large amount of oral fluids prior to obtaining a urine specimen.
- Obtain the urine specimen prior to starting antibiotic therapy.
- Send the specimen for culture to the laboratory without delay.
- Review findings indicative of UTI.
  - Urine culture: Positive for infecting organisms (*Escherichia coli*, proteus, pseudomonas, klebsiella, haemophilus, *Staphylococcus aureus*)
  - Urinalysis
    - pH: weak acid or neutral alkaline
    - Protein: positive
    - Glucose: positive
    - Ketones: positive
    - Leukocytes: positive
    - Nitrites: positive
- Educate the child and family about the procedure for invasive urinary catheterization or clean-voided specimen.

DIAGNOSTIC PROCEDURES

Locate the primary infection site or anatomic defects.
- Percutaneous kidney tap
- Bladder washouts
- Ultrasonography
- Voiding cystourethrogram
- Intravenous pyelogram (IVP)
- Dimercaptosuccinic acid scan

NURSING ACTIONS
- Educate the child and family about the procedure for the diagnostic test prescribed.
- Ask about an allergy to iodine or shellfish if a contrast medium is used.
- Assist with sedation of infants and young children if required. Assist an older child to remain quiet during the examinations.
- Maintain the child on NPO status after midnight in preparation for a cystoscopy and IVP. IVP requires bowel preparation.
- Prepare the child for catheterization if necessary.
- Monitor the child after the procedure, according to facility protocol.

PATIENT-CENTERED CARE

NURSING CARE

- Encourage frequent voiding and complete emptying of the bladder.
- Encourage fluids.
- Monitor urine output.
- Prepare the child for diagnostic tests.
- Administer a mild analgesic (acetaminophen) for pain management.

MEDICATIONS

Antibiotics based on findings of urine culture and sensitivity testing (penicillins, sulfonamide, cephalosporins, nitrofurantoin)

NURSING ACTIONS: Monitor for potential allergic response.

CLIENT EDUCATION: Have the child complete all prescribed antibiotics, even if manifestations are no longer present.

CLIENT EDUCATION

- Watch for manifestations of recurrence of UTIs (dysuria, frequency, urgency).
- To prevent recurrence:
  - Females should wipe the perineal area from front to back.
  - Parents of male infants who are uncircumcised should wash the penis with soap and water. If the foreskin has separated from the tip of the penis, which typically occurs by 3 years of age, then it can be gently pulled back and cleaned. The provider should inform the parents when this is safe.
  - Change the infant's diapers frequently
  - Keep underwear dry.
  - Suggest the use of cotton underwear.
  - Maintain adequate hydration.
  - Avoid bubble baths due to perineal irritation, which increases the risk for UTIs.
  - Void frequently.
  - Complete emptying of bladder using double voiding.
  - Avoid constipation and straining with bowel movements.
  - Adolescents who are sexually active should void immediately after intercourse.

COMPLICATIONS

Progressive kidney injury

Urosepsis
NURSING ACTIONS
- Monitor for findings of UTIs.
- Reinforce teaching about prevention, early identification, and treatment of UTIs.

Application Exercises

1. A nurse is reinforcing teaching with the a parent of a child who has a urinary tract infection (UTI). Which of the following should the nurse include? (Select all that apply.)

   A. Wear nylon underpants.

   B. Avoid bubble baths.

   C. Empty the bladder completely with each void.

   D. Report recurrence of urinary frequency.

   E. Wipe perineal area back to front.

2. A nurse is contributing to the plan of care for a child who has a urinary tract infection. Which of the following should the nurse recommend?

   A. Administer an antidiuretic.

   B. Restrict fluids.

   C. Evaluate the child's self-esteem.

   D. Encourage frequent voiding.

3. A nurse is caring for a child who has enuresis. The nurse should monitor for which of the following as a complication of enuresis?

   A. Urinary tract infections

   B. Altered body image

   C. Urosepsis

   D. Progressive kidney disease

4. A nurse is collecting data from an infant who has a suspected urinary tract infection. Which of the following findings should the nurse expect? (Select all that apply.)

   A. Increase in hunger

   B. Irritability

   C. Decrease in urination

   D. Vomiting

   E. Fever

5. A nurse is collecting data from a child who has a urinary tract infection. Which of the following findings should the nurse expect? (Select all that apply.)

   A. Night sweats

   B. Swelling of the face

   C. Pallor

   D. Blood in the urine

   E. Fatigue

PRACTICE Active Learning Scenario

A nurse is reviewing the plan of care for a child who has enuresis with the child's family. What should the nurse include in the review? Use the ATI Active Learning Template: System Disorder to complete this item

ALTERATION IN HEALTH (DIAGNOSIS)

CLIENT EDUCATION: List at least 10 points to review.

Application Exercises Key

1. A. The nurse should discuss the use of cotton underwear to decrease the risk of future UTIs.

   B. **CORRECT:** The nurse should discuss avoiding bubble baths to decrease perineal irritation, which increases the risk for UTIs.

   C. **CORRECT:** The nurse should discuss the need to completely empty the bladder with each void to decrease the risk of bacterial growth and UTIs.

   D. **CORRECT:** The nurse should inform the parent to report recurrence of manifestations of UTIs to promote early treatment.

   E. The nurse should discuss the importance of wiping the perineal area from front to back to reduce the introduction of micro-organisms into the urinary tract, which is a cause of UTIs.

   Ⓝ *NCLEX® Connection: Physiological Adaptation, Alterations in Body Systems*

2. A. An antidiuretic is not indicated for a child who has a urinary tract infection.

   B. The nurse should encourage fluids for a child who has a urinary tract infection.

   C. The nurse should evaluate self-esteem in children who have enuresis.

   D. **CORRECT:** The nurse should encourage frequent voiding. This assists in flushing the bacteria through the urinary system.

   Ⓝ *NCLEX® Connection: Physiological Adaptation, Alterations in Body Systems*

3. A. Urinary tract infections can occur in children. However, they are not a complication of enuresis.

   B. **CORRECT:** The nurse should monitor the child for an altered body image or other emotional problems that can result from enuresis.

   C. Urosepsis is a complication of urinary tract infections.

   D. Progressive kidney disease is a complication of urinary tract infections.

   Ⓝ *NCLEX® Connection: Reduction of Risk Potential, Potential for Alterations in Body Systems*

4. A. An increase in thirst is an expected finding in an infant who has a urinary tract infection. Poor feeding and failure to gain weight are manifestations of a UTI in an infant.

   B. **CORRECT:** Irritability is an expected finding in an infant who has a urinary tract infection.

   C. Frequent urination is an expected finding in an infant who has a urinary tract infection.

   D. **CORRECT:** Vomiting is an expected finding in an infant who has a urinary tract infection.

   E. **CORRECT:** Fever is an expected finding in an infant who has a urinary tract infection.

   Ⓝ *NCLEX® Connection: Physiological Adaptation, Basic Pathophysiology*

5. A. Night sweats are not an expected finding in a child who has a urinary tract infection.

   B. **CORRECT:** Swelling of the face is an expected finding in child who has a urinary tract infection.

   C. **CORRECT:** Pallor is an expected finding in child who has a urinary tract infection.

   D. **CORRECT:** Bloody urine is an expected finding in child who has a urinary tract infection.

   E. **CORRECT:** Fatigue is an expected finding in child who has a urinary tract infection.

   Ⓝ *NCLEX® Connection: Physiological Adaptation, Basic Pathophysiology*

PRACTICE Answer

Using the ATI Active Learning Template: System Disorder

ALTERATION IN HEALTH (DIAGNOSIS): Enuresis is uncontrolled or unintentional urination that occurs after a child is an age at which bladder control is usually achieved. The uncontrolled or unintentional urination occurs at least twice a week for at least 3 consecutive months, and the child must be at least 5 years of age.

CLIENT EDUCATION
- Have the child empty his bladder prior to bedtime.
- Encourage fluids during the day, and restrict fluids in the evening.
- Avoid caffeinated drinks.
- Allow the child to wear regular sleep wear and avoid diapers.
- Use positive reinforcement. Avoid punishing, scolding, or teasing the child following an incident.
- Assist the child in keeping a calendar of wet and dry days.
- Make environmental changes to assist the child to get to the bathroom, such as avoiding the top bunk bed, providing a night light, and clearing a path from the bed to the bathroom.
- Avoid holding urine during the day.
- Have the child change bed linens and clothing following an incident.
- Avoid constipation. Increase fiber in the diet, and encourage regular bowel movements.
- Wake the child during the night to void.
- Administer all medications as prescribed.
- Reinforce teaching on how to perform bladder stretching and Kegel exercises.
- Use conditioning therapy (child awakens by buzzer or bell in order to get up to urinate).

Ⓝ *NCLEX® Connection: Physiological Adaptation, Alterations in Body Systems*

UNIT 2 NURSING CARE OF CHILDREN WHO
HAVE SYSTEM DISORDERS
SECTION: GENITOURINARY AND REPRODUCTIVE DISORDERS

CHAPTER 24 # Structural Disorders of the Genitourinary Tract and Reproductive System

Various structural disorders can be evident at birth and can affect normal genitourinary and reproductive function. Children become aware of and are very interested in the genital area, normality of genital function, and sex differences between 3 and 6 years of age. Due to this, repair of structural defects is recommended between 6 and 15 months of age to minimize impact on body image and promote healthy development.

DATA COLLECTION

RISK FACTORS

Can have a genetic link

EXPECTED FINDINGS

OBSTRUCTIVE DEFECTS: Obstructive uropathy
- Hydronephrosis can be present if the ureteropelvic junction becomes obstructed and the renal pelvis and calyces become dilated.
- Partial obstructions can go undetected.
- Oligohydramnios can be a prenatal indicator of impaired kidney function.
- Inability to concentrate urine
- Urinary tract infections

PATIENT-CENTERED CARE

NURSING CARE

Nursing care should focus on education and support of the family and child.
- Evaluate the family's perception of the child's defect, family support, and coping.
- Assist parents to identify ways to help the child maintain a positive self-image.
- Promote healthy growth and development.
- Assist child with maintaining self-image.

DEFECTS OF THE GENITOURINARY TRACT

Obstructive uropathy

Structural or functional obstruction in the urinary system. More common in males than females.

THERAPEUTIC PROCEDURE: Surgical procedures that divert the flow of urine to bypass the obstruction, including surgical repair with insertion of percutaneous nephrostomy or cutaneous ureterostomy tubes

Chordee

Ventral curvature of the penis

THERAPEUTIC PROCEDURE: Surgical release of the fibrous band

Bladder exstrophy

- Eversion of the posterior bladder through the anterior bladder wall and lower abdominal wall
- Exposed bladder, urethra, and ureteral orifices through the suprapubic area
- Possible epispadias

THERAPEUTIC PROCEDURE: Single-stage or staged closure repair
- Cover the exposed bladder with sterile, nonadherent (plastic wrap or thin film) dressing.
- Assist in preparing the child for surgery. Recommended during the first 2 days of life.

Hypospadias

- Urethral opening located just below the glans penis, behind the glans penis, or on the ventral surface of the penile shaft
- Meatus opening below the glans penis
- Meatus opening along the ventral surface of the penis, scrotum, or perineum
- Possible chordee present

THERAPEUTIC PROCEDURE: Surgical repair recommended between 6 and 12 months of age

Epispadias

MALE
- Widened pubic symphysis
- Urethra opened on dorsal surface of the penis
- Possible exstrophy of the bladder

FEMALE
- Wide urethra
- Bifid clitoris
- Possible exstrophy of the bladder

THERAPEUTIC PROCEDURES
- Surgery performed during the first year of life.
- Traditionally male circumcision not performed; newer surgical techniques do not require an intact foreskin.

Phimosis

- Narrowing of the preputial opening of the foreskin
- Inability to retract foreskin of penis

THERAPEUTIC PROCEDURE

- Normal finding in infants and young boys and usually disappears as the child grows.
- Proper hygiene for phimotic foreskin is external cleansing during routine bathing; the foreskin should not be forcibly retracted.

Cryptorchidism

- One or both testes undescended
- Inability to palpate testes within the scrotum

THERAPEUTIC PROCEDURE

- Surgical orchiopexy
- Surgery performed between 6 and 24 months of age

Hydrocele

- Fluid in the scrotum
- Enlarged scrotal sac
- Diagnosed by ultrasound or transillumination

THERAPEUTIC PROCEDURE

- Can resolve spontaneously
- Surgical repair if not resolved in 1 year

Varicocele

- Elongation, dilation, and tortuosity of the veins of the spermatic cord superior to the testicle
- Possible discomfort during sexual stimulation
- Palpable worm-like mass above the testicle

THERAPEUTIC PROCEDURE: Varicocelectomy

Testicular torsion

- Testis hangs free from its vascular structures.
- Pain is either acute or insidious in onset and radiates to the groin area.

THERAPEUTIC PROCEDURE: Immediate surgery

Ambiguous genitalia

- Genitalia of the newborn that is not clearly defined as male or female.
- DNA analysis confirms the newborn's sex.
- Laparoscopy is performed if it is necessary to identify if internal structures such as ovaries are present.
- Surgical correction depends on the genitalia present and the sex of the newborn. The provider and parents discuss whether reconstructive surgery is indicated while the child is a newborn or whether to wait until the child is older and can provide input into the decision-making process.
- Avoid referring to the newborn by a specific sex until DNA analysis is complete.
- Promote bonding between the parents and newborn.
- Reinforce explanations with the parents, and provide a supportive and caring environment.

THERAPEUTIC PROCEDURES

Structural defects are treated with surgical intervention. The goal of most structural defect repairs is to preserve or create normal urinary and sexual function. Early intervention minimizes emotional trauma.

PREOPERATIVE NURSING ACTIONS

- Provide education to the child and family related to the procedure and expectations for postoperative care.
- Provide emotional support to the child and family.
- Encourage parents to express concerns and fears related to the surgical procedure and outcomes.
- If NPO status is necessary, explain the parameters to the family and child.
- Explain procedures at the appropriate level for the child and parents.
- Use age-appropriate interventions to allay fears and anxiety.
- Help the child understand that surgery is not a punishment, and it will not mutilate the body.

POSTOPERATIVE NURSING ACTIONS

- Assess pain using an appropriate pain assessment tool.
- Administer pain medication. An antispasmodic, such as oxybutynin, can be prescribed to treat painful bladder spasms.
- Monitor I&O.
- Monitor urinary catheters, drains, tubes, or stents.
- Provide wound and dressing care.
- Monitor for indications of infection (redness, warmth, drainage, edema at surgical site).
- Monitor for fever, lethargy, and foul-smelling urine.
- Do not provide tub baths for at least 1 week or as prescribed.
- Limit activity as prescribed.

CLIENT EDUCATION: Practice measures to prevent infection (good hand hygiene; care of wounds, drains, urinary catheters, and drainage bags).

COMPLICATIONS

Infection

NURSING ACTION: Observe for indications of infection (fever, skin inflammation, foul urine odor, cloudy urine, urinary frequency).

CLIENT EDUCATION

- Monitor for infection.
- Report any indications of infection immediately.

Emotional problems

Poor self-esteem, altered body image, social isolation, fears

NURSING ACTIONS

- Support the child and family by listening to concerns and correcting misperceptions.
- Use play therapy for toddlers and preschoolers.
- Encourage peer-to-peer social networking for older children.
- Educate the child and family regarding support groups. Qpcc

Application Exercises

1. A nurse is caring for an infant who has a hydrocele. Which of the following actions should the nurse take?

    A. Prepare the child for surgery.

    B. Explain to the parents that the issue can self-resolve.

    C. Retract the foreskin and cleanse several times daily.

    D. Refer the family for genetic counseling.

2. A nurse is collecting data from a male infant who has an epispadias. Which of the following findings should the nurse expect?

    A. Urethral opening on the dorsal surface of the penis

    B. Exposed bladder through the suprapubic area

    C. Ventral curvature of the penis

    D. Foreskin that does not retract

3. A nurse is caring for a newborn who has ambiguous genitalia. Which of the following actions should the nurse take?

    A. Prepare the child for DNA analysis.

    B. Refer to a specific sex when talking about the newborn.

    C. Gather supplies for an immediate circumcision.

    D. Advise the parents to avoid rooming-in until reconstructive surgery is complete.

4. A nurse is reviewing the medical record of an infant who has obstructive uropathy. Which of the following findings should the nurse expect?

    A. Female sex

    B. Urinary tract infection

    C. Dilute urine

    D. Prenatal excess of amniotic fluid

PRACTICE Active Learning Scenario

A nurse is discussing structural disorders of the genitourinary tract and reproductive system with a newly licensed nurse. What should the nurse include in the discussion? Use the ATI Active Learning Template: Basic Concept to complete this item.

RELATED CONTENT: Describe six structural disorders of the genitourinary tract and reproductive system.

Application Exercises Key

1. A. Hydroceles are surgically repaired if they have not resolved spontaneously in 1 year.

   B. **CORRECT:** Hydrocele is fluid in the scrotum and resolves spontaneously in the majority of cases.

   C. Cleansing the foreskin several times each day is done when an infant has phimosis.

   D. Genetic counseling is not indicated. Ultrasound or transillumination is indicated for the diagnosis of a hydrocele.

   Ⓝ *NCLEX® Connection: Physiological Adaptation, Alterations in Body Systems*

2. A. **CORRECT:** A urethral opening on the dorsal surface of the penis is an expected finding of epispadias.

   B. An exposed bladder through the suprapubic area is an expected finding for bladder exstrophy.

   C. Ventral curvature of the penis is an expected finding of chordee.

   D. Foreskin of penis that does not retract is an expected finding of phimosis.

   Ⓝ *NCLEX® Connection: Physiological Adaptation, Basic Pathophysiology*

3. A. **CORRECT:** The nurse should prepare the newborn who has ambiguous genitalia for DNA analysis to confirm the newborn's sex.

   B. The nurse should avoid using sex-specific terminology until DNA analysis is complete.

   C. Immediate circumcision is not indicated. Newborns who have ambiguous genitalia might require reconstructive surgery. However, this might be delayed until the child is older.

   D. The nurse should promote bonding between the newborn and parents. Rooming-in is a method of promoting bonding.

   Ⓝ *NCLEX® Connection: Health Promotion and Maintenance, Aging Process*

4. A. Obstructive uropathy can occur in both males and females, but it is more common in males.

   B. **CORRECT:** The nurse should expect the infant who has obstructive uropathy to be at risk for urinary tract infections.

   C. The nurse should expect the infant who has obstructive uropathy to have concentrated urine.

   D. The nurse should expect the infant who has obstructive uropathy to have a prenatal history of oligohydramnios.

   Ⓝ *NCLEX® Connection: Health Promotion and Maintenance, Health Promotion/Disease Prevention*

PRACTICE Answer

Using the ATI Active Learning Template: Basic Concept

RELATED CONTENT

- Obstructive uropathy: Structural or functional obstruction in the urinary system.
- Chordee: Ventral curvature of the penis.
- Bladder exstrophy: Eversion of the posterior bladder through the anterior bladder wall and lower abdominal wall.
- Hypospadias: Urethral opening located just below the glans penis, behind the glans penis, or on the ventral surface of the penile shaft.
- Epispadias: Meatal opening located on the dorsal surface of the penis.

- Phimosis: Narrowing of the preputial opening of the foreskin.
- Cryptorchidism: One or both testes is undescended.
- Hydrocele: Fluid in the scrotum.
- Varicocele: Elongated, dilated, and tortuosity of the veins superior to the testicle.
- Testicular torsion: Testicle hangs free from the vascular structures.
- Ambiguous genitalia: Erroneous or abnormal sexual differentiation.

Ⓝ *NCLEX® Connection: Physiological Adaptation, Pathophysiology*

CHAPTER 25 *Renal Disorders*

This chapter includes acute glomerulonephritis, nephrotic syndrome, hemolytic uremic syndrome (HUS), acute kidney injury (AKI), and chronic kidney disease (CKD).

Acute glomerulonephritis

- Common features are oliguria, edema, hypertension, circulatory congestion, hematuria, and proteinuria.
- Acute poststreptococcal glomerulonephritis (APSGN) is an antibody-antigen disease that occurs as a result of certain strains of the group A beta-hemolytic streptococcal (GABHS) infection.

DATA COLLECTION

RISK FACTORS

- GABHS infection
- Sex: Most commonly seen in males.
- Age: Most common in children 5 to 8 years.

EXPECTED FINDINGS

Recent upper respiratory or streptococcal infection

PHYSICAL FINDINGS
- Cloudy, tea-colored urine
- Decreased urine output
- Irritability
- Pallor and ill appearance
- Lethargy
- Anorexia
- Vague reports of discomfort (headache, abdominal pain, dysuria)
- Periorbital edema
- Facial edema that is worse in the morning but then spreads to extremities and abdomen with progression of the day
- Mild to severe hypertension

LABORATORY/DIAGNOSTIC TESTS

Throat culture: To identify possible streptococcus infection (usually negative by the time of diagnosis)

Urinalysis: Proteinuria, smoky or tea-colored urine, hematuria, increased specific gravity

Kidney function: Elevated BUN and creatinine

Antistreptolysin O (ASO) titer: Positive indicator for the presence of streptococcal antibodies

Serum complement (C3): Decreased initially; increases as recovery takes place; returns to normal at 8 to 10 weeks after glomerulonephritis begins

Radiographs: Chest x-ray can indicate congestion of the pulmonary system, pleural effusion, and enlargement of the heart due to fluid retention.

PATIENT-CENTERED CARE

NURSING CARE

- Children who have blood pressure and urine output within the expected reference range can be managed at home.
- Monitor I&O.
- Monitor daily weights; weigh the child on the same scale with the same amount of clothing daily.
- Monitor vital signs.
- Monitor neurologic status and observe for behavior changes, especially in children who have edema, hypertension, and gross hematuria. Implement seizure precautions if indicated.
- Encourage adequate nutritional intake.
  - Possible restriction of sodium and fluid.
  - Restrict foods high in potassium during periods of oliguria.
  - Provide small, frequent meals of favorite foods due to a decrease in appetite.
  - Recommend the child for dietary consultation if indicated.
  - Avoid added salt and salty foods such as chips, which promote fluid retention.
- Manage fluid restrictions. Fluids can be restricted during periods of edema and hypertension.
- Monitor skin for breakdown. Qs
  - Encourage frequent turning and repositioning.
  - Keep skin dry.
  - Pad bony prominences, and use a specialty mattress.
  - Elevate edematous body parts.
- Evaluate tolerance for activity. Provide frequent rest periods.

- Provide for age-appropriate diversional activities.
- Cluster care to facilitate rest and tolerance of activity.
- Monitor and prevent infection.
  - Advise the child to turn, cough, and deep breathe to prevent pulmonary involvement.
  - Monitor vital signs, especially temperature, for changes secondary to infection.
  - Maintain good hand hygiene.
  - Administer antibiotic therapy (indicated for children who have evidence of persistent streptococcal infection).
- Provide emotional support.
- Reinforce teaching with the family about administration and adverse effects of diuretics and antihypertensive medications.
- Encourage follow-up care.

MEDICATIONS

Diuretics and antihypertensives

To remove accumulated fluid and manage hypertension

NURSING ACTIONS
- Monitor blood pressure.
- Monitor I&O.
- Monitor for electrolyte imbalances, such as hypokalemia.
- Observe for adverse effects of medications.

CLIENT EDUCATION
- Dizziness can occur with the use of antihypertensives.
- Take the medication as prescribed and notify the provider if adverse effects occur. Continue the medication unless instructed otherwise.

INTERPROFESSIONAL CARE

Assist in obtaining a dietary consult.

CLIENT EDUCATION

- Encourage the child to verbalize feelings related to body image.
- Follow appropriate dietary management.
- Maintain adequate rest.
- Monitor blood pressure and daily weight.
- Avoid contact with others who might be ill.

Nephrotic syndrome

- Alterations in the glomerular membrane allow proteins (especially albumin) to pass into the urine, resulting in decreased serum osmotic pressure.
- It can be primary, secondary, or congenital.

DATA COLLECTION

RISK FACTORS

Minimal change nephrotic syndrome (MCNS)
- Peak incidence is between 2 and 3 years of age.
- Cause is unknown, but it can have a multifactorial etiology (metabolic, biochemical, or physiochemical disturbance in the basement membrane of the glomeruli).

Secondary nephrotic syndrome: occurs after or is associated with glomerular damage due to a known cause

Congenital nephrotic syndrome: an inherited disorder

EXPECTED FINDINGS

PHYSICAL FINDINGS
- Weight gain over a period of days or weeks
- Facial and periorbital edema: decreased throughout the day
- Ascites
- Edema to lower extremities and genitalia
- Anorexia
- Diarrhea
- Irritability
- Lethargy
- Pallor
- Decreased frothy urine
- Blood pressure within expected reference range or slightly below

LABORATORY TESTS

Urinalysis/24-hr urine collection

- Proteinuria: protein greater than 2+ on dipstick
- Hyaline casts
- Few RBCs
- Oval fat bodies

Serum chemistry

Hypoalbuminemia: reduced serum protein and albumin

Hyperlipidemia: elevated serum lipid levels

Hemoconcentration: elevated Hgb, Hct, and platelets

Possible hyponatremia: reduced sodium level

Glomerular filtration rate: within or above the expected reference range

DIAGNOSTIC PROCEDURES

Kidney biopsy is indicated only if nephrotic syndrome is unresponsive to steroid therapy. Biopsy will show damage to the epithelial cells lining the basement membrane of the kidney.

PATIENT-CENTERED CARE

NURSING CARE

- Provide rest.
- Monitor I&O. Weigh diapers of infants and toddlers.
- Monitor urine for protein.
- Monitor vital signs.
- Monitor daily weights; weigh the child on the same scale with the same amount of clothing.
- Monitor edema and measure abdominal girth daily. Measure at the widest area, usually at or above the umbilicus. Check degree of pitting, color, and texture of skin.
- Monitor and prevent infection.
  - Assist the child to turn, cough, and deep breathe to prevent pulmonary involvement.
  - Monitor vital signs, especially temperature, for changes secondary to infection.
  - Maintain good hand hygiene.
  - Administer antibiotic therapy.
- Encourage nutritional intake within restriction guidelines. Salt can be restricted during the edematous phase.
- Cluster care to provide for rest periods.
- Inspect skin for breakdown areas.
  - Avoid use of urinary collection bags which can damage fragile skin.
  - Pad bony prominences, or use a specialty mattress to reduce breakdown of skin.
  - Encourage frequent turning and repositioning.
  - Keep the child's skin dry.
  - Elevate edematous body parts.
- Inform the family about administration and adverse effects of medication.
- Provide support to families and assist with referrals as needed. Relapses can cause physical, emotional, and financial stress for the child and family. Qᴛᴄ
- Encourage follow-up care.

MEDICATIONS

Corticosteroid: prednisone

NURSING ACTIONS

- Administer 60 mg/m²/day or 2 mg/kg/day for 4 to 6 weeks followed by 40 mg/m²/dose or 1.5 mg/kg/dose every other day for 2 to 5 months.
- Taper the dosage. Do not suddenly stop the medication. Qᴇʙᴘ
- Monitor for adverse effects (hirsutism, slowed linear growth, hypertension, GI bleeding, infection, hyperglycemia).
- Administer with meals.
- Educate the child and the family on the medication regime.

CLIENT EDUCATION

- Avoid large crowds (to decrease the risk of infection).
- Using corticosteroids can increase appetite, cause weight gain (especially in the face), and cause mood swings.
- Notify the provider of adverse effects.

Diuretic: furosemide

Eliminates excess fluid from the body

NURSING ACTIONS

- Encourage the child to eat foods that are high in potassium.
- Monitor serum electrolyte levels periodically.

Albumin

- Increases plasma volume and decreases edema
- Administered IV by an RN.

NURSING ACTIONS

- Monitor I&O.
- Monitor for anaphylaxis.

Cyclophosphamide

Form of immunosuppressant therapy for children who cannot tolerate prednisone or who have repeated relapses of MCNS.

INTERPROFESSIONAL CARE

Suggest a dietary consult.

CLIENT EDUCATION

- Encourage the child to verbalize feelings related to body image.
- Follow appropriate dietary management including restriction of sodium intake.
- Maintain adequate rest.
- Use strategies to decrease the risk of infection (good hand hygiene, up-to-date immunizations, avoidance of infected people).
- Monitor blood pressure, daily weight, and protein in urine. Notify the provider if manifestations worsen, which indicates relapse.

COMPLICATIONS

Circulation insufficiency

Thromboembolism

Sepsis/infection
- Steroid therapy increases the risk for infection.
- Keep the child away from potential infection sources. Qs
- Monitor for indications of infection.
- CLIENT EDUCATION
  - Complete the full dose of antibiotic.
  - Perform frequent hand hygiene.
  - Notify the provider of manifestations of infection.
  - Avoid potential infection sources including sick family members.

Hemolytic uremic syndrome

- HUS is an acute kidney disease characterized by AKI, hemolytic anemia, and thrombocytopenia.
- HUS is one of the main causes of acute kidney injury in early childhood.
- Breakdown of red blood cells clogs the kidneys.

DATA COLLECTION

RISK FACTORS

- Peak incidence is 6 months to 3 years.
- Toxins enter the bloodstream and destroy red blood cells.

Diarrhea-positive (D+) HUS: responsible for 90% of cases caused by ingestion of Shiga toxin producing *Escherichia coli*

Diarrhea-negative (D-) or atypical HUS: can be due to nonenteric infections, disturbances in the complement system, malignancies, or genetic disorders

EXPECTED FINDINGS

PHYSICAL FINDINGS
- Occurs after prodromal period of diarrhea and vomiting
- Occasionally occurs after varicella, measles, or a UTI
- Loss of appetite
- Irritability
- Lethargy
- Pallor
- Bruising, purpura, or rectal bleeding
- Anuria and hypertension in severe form
- Reduced or increased urinary output

LABORATORY TESTS

- CBC: decreased hemoglobin and hematocrit
- Elevated reticulocyte count
- Hematuria
- Proteinuria
- Elevated BUN and serum creatinine
- Fibrin split products in serum and urine (thrombocytopenia)

PATIENT-CENTERED CARE

NURSING CARE

SUPPORTIVE MEASURES
- Monitor I&O.
- Obtain daily weights.
- Assist with fluid replacement.
- Treat hypertension.
- Correct acidosis and electrolyte imbalances.
- Monitor for seizure activity and stupor.
- Provide seizure precautions.
- Monitor children receiving blood transfusions for severe anemia.
- Support the child and family regarding severity of the illness.
- **For child who has anuria for 24 hr, oliguria with uremia, or oliguria with hypertension and seizures** QEBP
  - Hemodialysis
  - Peritoneal dialysis
  - Continuous hemofiltration

NUTRITION
- Once vomiting and diarrhea resolves, enteral nutrition is initiated.
- Provide parenteral nutrition for children who have severe, persistent colitis and marked tissue catabolism

MEDICATIONS

- There is no evidence that heparin, corticosteroids, or fibrinolytic agents are beneficial.
- Plasma infusion is under study and can be useful.

INTERPROFESSIONAL CARE

Recommend a dietary consult.

CLIENT EDUCATION

- Avoid undercooked meat, especially ground beef. Internal temperature of meat should be at least 74° C (165° F).
- Avoid unpasteurized apple juice, unwashed raw vegetables, and alfalfa sprouts.
- Avoid public pools.
- Do not use antimotility medications for diarrhea.

Acute kidney injury

- AKI is the inability of the kidneys to excrete waste material, concentrate urine, and conserve electrolytes.
- The disorder affects most of the systems of the body.
- Causes are classified as prerenal, intrinsic renal, and postrenal. Prerenal are most common causes of AKI.

DATA COLLECTION

RISK FACTORS

Prerenal
- Dehydration secondary to diarrheal disease or persistent vomiting
- Shock, trauma, and burns

Intrinsic renal: Nephrotoxic substances

Postrenal: Obstructive uropathy

EXPECTED FINDINGS

PHYSICAL FINDINGS
- Oliguria: in reversible ARF, there is a period of severe low urinary output
- Abrupt diuresis: with return to normal urine volumes
- Edema
- Drowsiness
- Circulatory collapse
- Cardiac arrhythmia: from hyperkalemia
- Seizures: from hyponatremia or hypocalcemia
- Tachypnea: from metabolic acidosis
- CNS manifestations: from continued oliguria

LABORATORY/DIAGNOSTIC TESTS

- Hyperkalemia
- Hyponatremia
- Metabolic acidosis
- Hypocalcemia
- Anemia
- Azotemia
- Elevated plasma creatinine
- Elevated BUN
- ECG for cardiac arrhythmias

PATIENT-CENTERED CARE

NURSING CARE

- The child who has AKI is initially admitted to a pediatric intensive care unit. Prepare to assist with the care of the child following transfer to an acute care unit. Qrc
- Check and monitor kidney function.
- Treat underlying cause of AKI.
- Strictly monitor I&O. Client can have a urinary catheter.
- Monitor fluid and electrolyte balance.
- Limit fluid intake.
- Obtain daily weights.
- Monitor vital signs for hypertension.
- Limit activity.
- Observe for behavior changes or seizure activity.
- Implement seizure precautions if indicated.
- Monitor for infection.
- Keep family informed of child's progress.
- Encourage follow-up care.

MEDICATIONS

- Most medications used to provide initial treatment of AKI are administered IV by an RN.
  - **Mannitol and furosemide** to provoke a flow of urine in child who has oliguria and no lower tract obstruction.
  - **Calcium gluconate** to reduce serum potassium levels.
  - **Sodium bicarbonate** to reduce serum potassium levels.
  - **Glucose and insulin:** Insulin facilitates entry of glucose into cells and helps to reduce serum potassium levels.
  - **Antihypertensives** including labetalol and nitroprusside.
- Dialysis or continuous hemofiltration can be prescribed.
- Sodium polystyrene sulfonate 1 g/kg orally or rectally binds to potassium and excretes it from body.

NUTRITION

- Ingest concentrated foods without fluids.
- Maintain calories while minimizing tissue catabolism, metabolic acidosis, hyperkalemia, and uremia.
- Monitor for fluid overload in the child who is receiving parenteral nutrition.

INTERPROFESSIONAL CARE

Support the child and family.

CLIENT EDUCATION

- Maintain adequate rest.
- Follow therapeutic regimen.

Chronic kidney disease

- CKD begins when diseased kidneys can no longer maintain the normal chemical structure of body fluids under normal conditions.
- A variety of diseases and disorders can result in CKD.

DATA COLLECTION

RISK FACTORS

- Most common causes before 5 years of age are congenital kidney and urinary tract malformations and vesicoureteral reflux.
- Glomerular and hereditary kidney disease pare the main causes among the 5- to 15-year-old age group.

EXPECTED FINDINGS

PHYSICAL FINDINGS
- Loss of energy
- Increase fatigue on exertion
- Pallor
- Occasional elevated blood pressure
- Delayed growth
- Anorexia
- Nausea and vomiting
- Decrease interest in activities
- Decreased or increased urinary output and compensatory increase in fluid intake
- Anemia
- Headache
- Muscle cramps
- Nausea
- Weight loss
- Puffiness to face
- Malaise
- Bone or joint pain
- Itchy, bruised skin
- Amenorrhea in adolescents
- Circulatory overload manifested by hypertension, congestive heart failure, and pulmonary edema
- Confusion, dulling of sensorium, coma, tremors, muscle twitching, and seizures are findings of neurologic involvement.

LABORATORY/DIAGNOSTIC TESTS

Evaluate extent of kidney damage.
- Serum calcium
- CBC
- Serum creatinine

PATIENT-CENTERED CARE

NURSING CARE

- Provide rest.
- Monitor I&O.
- Monitor vital signs.
- Monitor daily weights.
- Manage hypertension.
- Monitor for infection.
- Monitor alertness and orientation.
- Maintain sodium restriction.
- Initiate fluid restriction if edema is present.
- Encourage reduction of dietary phosphorus.
- Keep family informed of child's progress.
- Encourage follow-up care.

MEDICATIONS

- Thiazides or furosemide for hypertension
- Beta blockers and vasodilators for severe hypertension
- Phosphorus binding agent
- Calcium
- Vitamin D: active form
- Water-soluble vitamins
- Sodium bicarbonate and potassium citrate to alleviate acidosis
- Folic acid and recombinant human erythropoietin for anemia
- Recombinant growth hormone for children who have growth retardation
- Antimicrobials for infection
- Antiepileptic for seizures
- Diphenhydramine for pruritus

NUTRITION

- Goal is to provide adequate calories and protein for growth. Qpcc
- Dietary phosphorus might need to be restricted.
- Potassium is restricted for oliguria or anuria.
- Ensure protein and milk intake is no greater than recommended daily allowance.
- Dietary sources of folic acid and iron.

INTERPROFESSIONAL CARE

- Obtain a dietary consult.
- Encourage dental care.

CLIENT EDUCATION

- Maintain adequate rest.
- Follow therapeutic regimen.

COMPLICATIONS

- Progressive deterioration
- End-stage kidney disease: irreversible
- Depression

Application Exercises

1. A nurse is collecting data from a child who has nephrotic syndrome. Which of the following findings should the nurse expect? (Select all that apply.)

   A. Dipstick protein of 1+

   B. Edema in the ankles

   C. Hyperlipidemia

   D. Weight loss

   E. Anorexia

2. A nurse is reviewing the laboratory and diagnostic test results of a 10-year-old child who has acute glomerulonephritis. Which of the following findings should the nurse expect?

   A. Decreased urine specific gravity

   B. Decreased serum creatinine

   C. Positive antistreptolysin O (ASO) titer

   D. Cardiac atrophy

3. A nurse is contributing to the plan of care for a toddler who has nephrotic syndrome. Which of the following interventions should the nurse recommend?

   A. Provide frequent play periods in the activity room.

   B. Place a urinary collection bag on the toddler.

   C. Measure abdominal girth daily.

   D. Keep lower extremities below the level of the heart.

4. A nurse is collecting data from a child who has chronic kidney disease. Which of the following findings should the nurse expect?

   A. Flushed face

   B. Hyperactivity

   C. Weight gain

   D. Delayed growth

5. A nurse is collecting data from a child who has poststreptococcal glomerulonephritis (APSGN). Which of the following manifestations should the nurse expect? (Select all that apply.)

   A. Frothy urine

   B. Periorbital edema

   C. Ill appearance

   D. Polyuria

   E. Hypertension

PRACTICE Active Learning Scenario

A nurse is reinforcing teaching with the parent of a child who has a new prescription for prednisone for nephrotic syndrome. Use the Active Learning Template: Medication to complete this item.

NURSING INTERVENTIONS: List three.

CLIENT EDUCATION: List four education points to reinforce.

Application Exercises Key

1. A. A client who has nephrotic syndrome is expected to have proteinuria of 2+ or greater.

   B. **CORRECT:** A client who has nephrotic syndrome is expected to have edema in the ankles.

   C. **CORRECT:** A client who has nephrotic syndrome is expected to have hyperlipidemia.

   D. A client who has nephrotic syndrome is expected to have weight gain.

   E. **CORRECT:** A client who has nephrotic syndrome is expected to have anorexia.

   Ⓝ *NCLEX® Connection: Physiological Adaptation, Basic Pathophysiology*

2. A. An increased urine specific gravity is an expected finding for a child who has acute glomerulonephritis.

   B. An increased serum creatinine level is an expected finding for a child who has acute glomerulonephritis.

   C. **CORRECT:** A positive ASO titer is an expected finding for a child who has acute glomerulonephritis. This finding is a positive indicator for the presence of streptococcal antibodies.

   D. An enlarged heart is an expected finding for a child who has acute glomerulonephritis.

   Ⓝ *NCLEX® Connection: Reduction of Risk Potential, Laboratory Values*

3. A. The nurse should promote rest and cluster care.

   B. The nurse should avoid the use of a urinary collection bag due to the risk of skin breakdown.

   C. **CORRECT:** The nurse should monitor the toddler's level of edema and measure abdominal girth daily.

   D. The nurse should elevate edematous areas, including the toddler's lower extremities, above the level of the heart.

   Ⓝ *NCLEX® Connection: Physiological Adaptation, Alterations in Body Systems*

4. A. The nurse should expect the child to exhibit pallor, not flushing.

   B. The nurse should expect the child to be fatigued, not hyperactive.

   C. The nurse should expect the child to have weight loss from anorexia, nausea, and vomiting.

   D. **CORRECT:** The nurse should expect the child to exhibit delayed growth.

   Ⓝ *NCLEX® Connection: Physiological Adaptation, Basic Pathophysiology*

5. A. A client who has APSGN is expected to have cloudy, tea-colored urine due to hematuria.

   B. **CORRECT:** A client who has APSGN is expected to have periorbital edema due to inadequate function of the kidneys resulting in fluid retention.

   C. **CORRECT:** A client who has APSGN is expected to have an ill appearance due to manifestations of inadequate functioning of the kidneys.

   D. A client who has APSGN is expected to have decreased urine output due to inadequate function of the kidneys.

   E. **CORRECT:** A client who has APSGN is expected to have hypertension due to inadequate function of the kidneys and edema.

   Ⓝ *NCLEX® Connection: Physiological Adaptation, Basic Pathophysiology*

PRACTICE Answer

Using the Active Learning Template: Medication

NURSING INTERVENTIONS

- Administer 60 mg/m²/day or 2 mg/kg/day for 4 to 6 weeks followed by 40 mg/m²/dose or 1.5 mg/kg/dose every other day for 2 to 5 months.
- Taper the dosage. Do not suddenly stop the medication. Monitor for adverse effects (hirsutism, slowed linear growth, hypertension, GI bleeding, infection, hyperglycemia).
- Administer with meals.

CLIENT EDUCATION

- Avoid large crowds to decrease the risk of infection.
- Using corticosteroids can increase appetite, cause weight gain (especially in the face), and cause mood swings.
- Follow the medication regimen.
- Notify the provider of adverse effects.

Ⓝ *NCLEX® Connection: Pharmacological and Parenteral Therapies, Medication Administration*

NCLEX® Connections

When reviewing the following chapters, keep in mind the relevant topics and tasks of the NCLEX outline, in particular:

Basic Care and Comfort

MOBILITY/IMMOBILITY: Provide care to an immobilized client (traction, bedridden).

Pharmacological Therapies

EXPECTED ACTIONS/OUTCOMES: Apply knowledge of pathophysiology when addressing client pharmacological agents.

Reduction of Risk Potential

POTENTIAL FOR COMPLICATIONS OF DIAGNOSTIC TESTS/TREATMENTS/PROCEDURES: Implement measures to prevent complication of client condition or procedure (circulatory complication, seizure, aspiration, potential neurological disorder).

POTENTIAL FOR COMPLICATIONS FROM SURGICAL PROCEDURES AND HEALTH ALTERATIONS: Provide care for the client before the surgical procedure and reinforce education.

THERAPEUTIC PROCEDURES: Assist with the performance of a diagnostic or invasive procedure.

Physiological Adaptation

ALTERATIONS IN BODY SYSTEMS: Reinforce education to the client regarding care and condition.

BASIC PATHOPHYSIOLOGY

Identify signs and symptoms related to an acute or chronic illness.

Consider general principles of client disease process when providing care (injury and repair, immunity, cellular structure).

Apply knowledge of pathophysiology to monitoring client for alterations in body systems.

UNIT 2 NURSING CARE OF CHILDREN WHO HAVE SYSTEM DISORDERS
SECTION: MUSCULOSKELETAL DISORDERS

CHAPTER 26 *Fractures*

A fracture occurs when the resistance between a bone and an applied stress yields to the stress, resulting in a disruption to the integrity of the bone. Bone healing and remodeling is faster in children than in adults due to a thicker periosteum and good blood supply.

Epiphyseal plate injuries can result in altered bone growth. Radiographic evidence of previous fractures in various stages of healing or in infants can be the result of physical abuse or osteogenesis imperfecta.

DATA COLLECTION

RISK FACTORS

- Obesity
- Poor nutrition
- Developmental characteristics, ordinary play activities, and recreation that place children at risk for injury (falls from climbing or running; trauma to bones from skateboarding, skiing, or playing soccer or basketball)

EXPECTED FINDINGS

PHYSICAL FINDINGS
- Pain
- Crepitus
- Deformity
- Edema
- Ecchymosis
- Warmth or redness
- Decreased use of affected area

COMMON TYPES OF FRACTURES IN CHILDREN (26.1)
- **Plastic deformation (bend):** The bone is bent no more than 45°.
- **Buckle (torus):** Compression of the bone resulting in a bulge or raised area at the fracture site.
- **Greenstick:** Incomplete fracture of the bone.
- **Transverse:** Break is straight across the bone. Q EBP
- **Oblique:** Break is diagonal across the bone.
- **Spiral:** Break spirals around the bone.
- **Physeal (growth plate):** Injury to the end of the long bone on the growth plate.

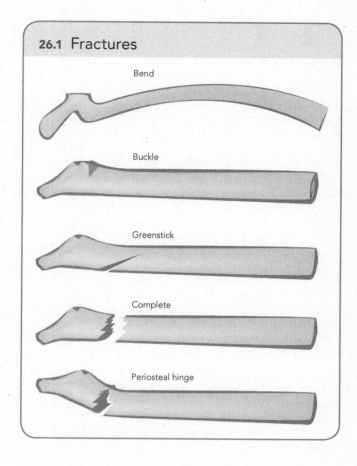

26.1 Fractures

Bend

Buckle

Greenstick

Complete

Periosteal hinge

- **Stress:** Small fractures/cracks in the bone due to repeated muscle contractions.
- **Complete:** Bone fragments are separated.
- **Incomplete:** Bone fragments are still attached.
- **Closed or simple:** The fracture occurs without a break in the skin.
- **Open or compound:** The fracture occurs with an open wound and bone protruding.
- **Complicated fracture:** The fracture results in injury to other organs and tissues.
- **Comminuted:** The fracture includes small fragments of bone that lie in surrounding tissue.

DIAGNOSTIC PROCEDURES

Radiograph

NURSING ACTIONS
- Instruct and assist the child to remain still during the procedure.
- Educate the child and parents about what to expect during the procedure.
- Provide emotional support.

PATIENT-CENTERED CARE

NURSING CARE

Provide emergency care at the time of injury.
- Maintain ABCs.
- Monitor vital signs, pain, and neurologic status.
- Determine the neurovascular status of the injured extremity.
- Position the child in a supine position for injuries to the distal arm, pelvis, and lower extremities.
- Position the child in a sitting position for injuries to the shoulder or upper arm.
- Remove jewelry or objects that can cause constriction on the affected extremity.
- Stabilize the injured area, avoiding unnecessary movement.
- If a pelvic fracture is suspected, monitor urine for blood and for development of hypovolemic shock
- Elevate the affected limb and apply ice packs (not to exceed 20 min).
- Administer analgesics.
- Keep the child warm.

GENERAL NURSING ACTIONS
- Assess pain frequently using an age-appropriate pain tool. Use appropriate pain management, both pharmacological and nonpharmacological.
- Monitor neurovascular status on a regular schedule. Report any change in status.
- Maintain proper alignment.
- Promote range of motion of fingers, toes, and unaffected extremities.
- Instruct the child and family regarding activity restrictions.

NEUROVASCULAR SYSTEM
- **Sensation:** Check for numbness or tingling sensation of the extremity. Loss of sensation can indicate nerve damage.
- **Skin temperature:** Monitor the temperature of the extremity. It should be warm, not cool, to touch.
- **Skin color:** Observe the color of the affected extremity. Compare the skin above and below the injury, and look for changes in pigmentation.
- **Capillary refill:** Press the nail beds of the affected extremity until blanching occurs, then release the nail. The nail bed should turn pink, indicating a return of blood flow, within 3 seconds.
- **Pulses:** Pulses should be palpable and strong. Pulses should also be equal to the pulses of the unaffected extremity.
- **Movement:** The child should be able to move the joints distal to the injury (fingers or toes).

MEDICATIONS

Analgesics

Administer analgesics for pain.

NURSING ACTIONS FOR OPIOID ANALGESIA: Monitor for respiratory depression and constipation.

CLIENT EDUCATION: Use techniques for adequate pain relief.

THERAPEUTIC PROCEDURES

Casting

TYPES OF CASTS: long-leg, short-leg, bilateral long-leg, long-arm, short-arm, shoulder spica, 1½ spica, full spica, and single spica
- Plaster of Paris casts are heavy, not water-resistant, and can take 10 to 72 hr to dry. Synthetic fiberglass casts are light, water-resistant, and dry quickly (5 to 20 min).
- Observe the skin integrity prior to casting. Cleanse and dry the skin. Pad bony prominences to prevent skin breakdown. The provider then applies the casting material.

NURSING ACTIONS
- Provide atraumatic care prior to cast application by showing the procedure on a doll or toy.
- Determine and monitor neurovascular status.
- Elevate the cast above the level of the heart during the first 24 to 48 hr to prevent swelling.
- Apply ice for the first 24 hr to decrease swelling.
- Turn and position the child every 2 hr so that dry air circulates around and under the cast for faster drying. This also will prevent pressure from changing the shape of the cast. Do not use heat lamps or warm hair dryers.
- Turn the child frequently while supporting all extremities and joints.
- Check for increased warmth or hot spots on the cast surface, which could indicate infection.
- Monitor for drainage on the cast. Outline any drainage on the outside of the cast with a marker (and note date and time) so it can be monitored for any additional drainage.
- Observe the general skin condition and the area around the cast edges.
- Provide routine skin care and thorough perineal care to maintain skin integrity.
- For plaster casts, use palms of hands to avoid denting when touching the cast, and expose the cast to air to promote drying.
- Use moleskin over any rough area of the cast that can rub against the child's skin.
- Cover areas of the cast with plastic to avoid soiling from urine or feces.
- Assist with proper crutch fitting, and reinforce proper use.
- Reinforce teaching with the child and parents about cast removal and cast cutter.

CLIENT EDUCATION
- Keep the affected extremity supported (with a sling) or elevated when sitting.
- When the cast is applied it will feel warm, but it will not burn the child.
- Report pain that is extremely severe or is not relieved 1 hr after the administration of pain medication.
- Perform neurovascular checks and know when to contact the provider.
- Use crutches for lower-extremity casts.
- Reinforce skin and perineal care with a spica cast.
- Do not place any foreign objects inside the cast to avoid trauma to the skin.
- Use proper restraints when transporting in any vehicle.
- Soak the extremity in warm water and then apply lotion following cast removal.

Traction care

Traction involves the use of a pulling force to reduce a fracture, maintain alignment, and provide muscle rest. The type of traction used depends on the fracture, age of the child, and associated injuries.

- **Skin traction** uses weights to apply a pulling force. Using tape and straps applied to the skin along with boots or cuffs, a rope connects the weights to the extremity (Buck, Russell, Bryant traction).
- **Skeletal traction** applies a continuous pulling force directly to the skeletal structure or specific bone **(26.2)**. When the fracture requires more pulling force than skin traction can withstand, the child will need skeletal traction. The provider inserts a pin or rod through or into the bone to connect the extremity to weights. The nurse should never remove the weights.
- **Halo traction (cervical traction)** uses a halo-type bar that encircles the head. The provider inserts screws into the child's outer skull. The bed or a vest worn by the child attaches to the halo and provides traction. **(26.3)**

NURSING ACTIONS

- Maintain body alignment.
- Provide pharmacological and nonpharmacological interventions for the management of pain and muscle spasms.
- Notify the provider if the child experiences severe pain from muscle spasms that is unrelieved with medications or repositioning.
- Monitor neurovascular status
- Routinely monitor skin integrity and document findings.
- Observe pin sites for pain, redness, swelling, drainage, or odor. Provide pin care per facility protocol.
- Monitor for changes in elimination, and promote usual patterns of elimination.
- Ensure that all the hardware is tight and that the bed is in the correct position.
- Ensure weights hang freely, the rope stays in the track, and the knots do not touch the pulley. Removing or adjusting weights requires a provider prescription and supervision.
- Consult with the provider for an overbed trapeze to assist the child to move in bed.
- Provide range of motion exercises and encourage activity of nonimmobilized extremities to maintain mobility and prevent contractures.
- Encourage deep breathing and use of incentive spirometry.
- Promote frequent position changing within restrictions of the traction.
- Remove sheets from the head of the bed to the foot of the bed, and remake the bed in the same manner.
- Review pin site care technique with the child and parents.
- Report any findings of compartment syndrome immediately.
- **For the client in a halo device**
  - Ensure that the wrench to release the rods is readily available in the event that CPR is necessary.
  - Move the child as a unit without applying pressure to the rods. This will prevent loosening of the pins and pain.
  - Inspect the pins regularly to ensure loosening does not occur.
  - Monitor integrity of the skin beneath the halo vest.

CLIENT EDUCATION

- Provide adequate hydration and nutrition while in traction.
- Use stool softeners.
- Report findings of infection to the provider.
- Do not use powder under the halo vest.

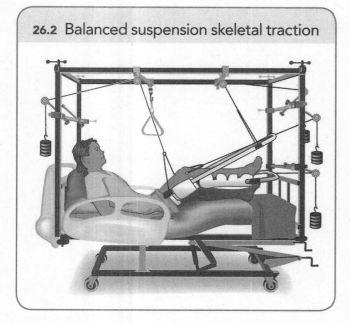

26.2 Balanced suspension skeletal traction

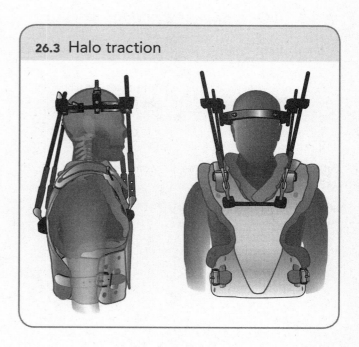

26.3 Halo traction

Surgical interventions

- Depending on the type of fracture, the child can require surgical intervention. The most common fractures requiring surgery include supracondylar fractures and fractures of the humerus and femur.
- Surgical reduction can be closed (no incision) or open (with incision), with or without pinning.

NURSING ACTIONS

- Monitor for findings of infection at the incision site.
- Encourage mobilization as soon as prescribed.
- Medicate for pain as needed.
- Provide crutch training for lower-extremity fractures.
- Instruct the child and parents about weight-bearing limitations to the affected extremity.
- Reinforce to the child and parents what to expect before and after the procedure, including NPO status.
- Review information about pain medication with the child and parents.

INTERPROFESSIONAL CARE

- Fracture care in children generally requires a consult with an orthopedic specialist.
- Notify social services in situations of suspected abuse.

CLIENT EDUCATION

CARE AFTER DISCHARGE

- Practice proper cast care, as well as pin care if indicated.
- Perform neurovascular checks and call or return to the provider if impairment occurs.
- Use antipruritic medications if prescribed.
- Maintain physical restrictions as prescribed.
- Use appropriate pain management strategies.
- Report increasing pain, redness, inflammation, and fever to the provider.
- Return to the provider for follow-up appointments as scheduled to prevent complications.

COMPLICATIONS

Compartment syndrome

- Compression of nerves, blood vessels, and muscle inside a confined place, resulting in neuromuscular ischemia; most commonly occurring in relation to tibial fractures or fractures involving the forearm.
- Untreated compartment syndrome can lead to deformity of the extremity, paralysis and infection.

Volkmann contracture: A permanent contracture of the forearm and hand

CAUSES: Tight dressing or cast, hemorrhage, burns, surgery, massive IV infiltration

FINDINGS (REMEMBER THE 5 P's) Qs

- **Pain** that is unrelieved with elevation or analgesics; increases with passive movement
- **Paresthesia** or numbness (early finding)
- **Pulselessness** distal to the fracture (late finding)
- **Paralysis** or an inability to move digits (nerve damage)
- **Pale**, cold skin and cyanosis to nail beds

NURSING ACTIONS

- Monitor the extremity every hour for the first 24 hr.
- The nurse should be able to place one finger in the space between the skin and the cast at all times.
- Notify the provider for suspected compartment syndrome.
- Place the affected extremity at heart level
- Loosen the dressing or assist with bivalving and opening the cast
- Prepare the child for fasciotomy.
- Complete dressing changes or maintain negative pressure wound therapy.

CLIENT EDUCATION: Report pain that is not relieved by analgesics, pain that continues to increase in intensity, numbness or tingling, or a change in color of the extremity.

Osteomyelitis

Infection within the bone secondary to a bacterial infection from an outside source, such as with an open fracture (endogenous) or from a bloodborne bacterial source (hematogenous)

MANIFESTATIONS

- Irritability
- Fever
- Tachycardia
- Edema
- Pain is constant but increases with movement
- Not wanting to use the affected extremity
- Site of infection tender, swollen, and warm to touch

NURSING ACTIONS

- Assist in diagnostic procedures, such as obtaining skin, blood, and bone cultures.
- Assist with joint or bone biopsy.
- Administer antibiotic therapy.
- Monitor hepatic, hematologic, and kidney function.
- Monitor for the development of superinfection (candidiasis, C. difficile infection).
- Immobilize and elevate the extremity.
- Administer pain medication.
- Consult with the parents and provider regarding home care needs. Qtc
- Talk with the child and parents about the length of treatment that can be needed and long-term antibiotic therapy.

CLIENT EDUCATION

- Monitor hearing due to ototoxicity of some antibiotics.
- Limit movement of the affected limb and avoid bearing any weight until cleared by the provider.
- Provide for diversional activities consistent with the child's level of development. Qpcc
- Maintain proper nutrition.

Application Exercises

1. A nurse is caring for a child who is in a plaster shoulder spica cast. Which of the following actions should the nurse take?

   A. Use a heat lamp to facilitate drying.

   B. Avoid turning the child until the cast is dry.

   C. Position the cast below heart level during while it dries.

   D. Apply moleskin to the edges of the cast.

2. A nurse is assisting with a group discussion about fractures. Which of the following information should the nurse include?

   A. "Children need a longer time to heal from a fracture than an adult."

   B. "Epiphyseal plate injuries can result in altered bone growth."

   C. "A greenstick fracture is a complete break in the bone."

   D. "Bones are unable to bend, so they break."

3. A nurse is caring for a child who sustained a fracture. Which of the following actions should the nurse take? (Select all that apply.)

   A. Place a heat pack on the site of injury.

   B. Elevate the affected limb.

   C. Check neurovascular status frequently.

   D. Encourage ROM of the affected limb.

   E. Stabilize the injury.

4. A nurse is caring for a child who has a fracture. Which of the following are manifestations of a fracture? (Select all that apply.)

   A. Crepitus

   B. Edema

   C. Pain

   D. Fever

   E. Ecchymosis

5. A nurse is caring for a child who is in skeletal traction. Which of the following actions should the nurse take? (Select all that apply.)

   A. Remove the weights to reposition the child.

   B. Check the child's position frequently.

   C. Observe pin sites every 4 hr.

   D. Ensure the weights are hanging freely.

   E. Ensure the rope's knot is in contact with the pulley.

PRACTICE Active Learning Scenario

A nurse is participating in an in-service about compartment syndrome with a group of nurses. What information should the nurse include? Use the ATI Active Learning Template: System Disorder to complete this item.

EXPECTED FINDINGS: List five.

NURSING CARE: List three nursing actions.

CLIENT EDUCATION: List one teaching point.

Application Exercises Key

1. A. The nurse can use a cool fan to facilitate drying of a plaster cast.

    B. The nurse should turn the child every 2 hr to expose all areas of the cast to air, which facilitates drying.

    C. The nurse should elevate a cast above heart level while it dries to prevent swelling of the extremity.

    D. **CORRECT:** The nurse should apply moleskin to the edges of the cast to prevent the cast from rubbing on the child's skin.

    (N) *NCLEX® Connection: Basic Care and Comfort, Mobility/Immobility*

2. A. Children heal from fractures quicker than adults due to a thicker periosteum and good blood supply.

    B. **CORRECT:** Detection and early treatment is crucial for an epiphyseal plate injury to prevent altered bone growth.

    C. A greenstick fracture is a partial break in the bone.

    D. Children's bones are soft and pliable, and can bend up to 45° before breaking.

    (N) *NCLEX® Connection: Physiological Adaptation, Basic Pathophysiology*

3. A. The nurse should place a cold pack on the site of injury to decrease swelling.

    B. **CORRECT:** Elevating the affected limb can decrease swelling at the injury site.

    C. **CORRECT:** Checking neurovascular status assists the nurse in determining if the affected limb has adequate blood supply.

    D. The nurse should encourage ROM of the nonaffected limb.

    E. **CORRECT:** Stabilizing the injury will prevent further injury and damage.

    (N) *NCLEX® Connection: Physiological Adaptation, Alterations in Body Systems*

4. A. **CORRECT:** A fracture can leave bone fragments that will exhibit a grating sound. Crepitus is a manifestation of a fracture.

    B. **CORRECT:** Swelling at the site occur related to the trauma. Edema is a manifestation of a fracture.

    C. **CORRECT:** A child who has a fracture will experience pain from the trauma.

    D. Fever following a fracture is unexpected, and can indicate infection, such as osteomyelitis.

    E. **CORRECT:** Bleeding under the skin can occur related to the trauma. Ecchymosis is a manifestation of a fracture.

    (N) *NCLEX® Connection: Physiological Adaptation, Basic Pathophysiology*

5. A. Only the provider should remove the weights, except in an emergency situation.

    B. **CORRECT:** The nurse should check the child's position frequently to ensure proper alignment is present. This avoids putting stress on the pinned areas and other areas of the body, which can worsen the child's pain.

    C. **CORRECT:** The nurse should observe the pin sites frequently to monitor for the development of infection or loosening of the pins. Follow facility protocol in providing pin site care.

    D. **CORRECT:** The nurse should ensure that the weights are hanging freely to allow for prescribed traction.

    E. The knot in the rope should not touch the pulley as this will alter the weight of the traction.

    (N) *NCLEX® Connection: Basic Care and Comfort, Mobility/Immobility*

PRACTICE Answer

Using the ATI Active Learning Template: System Disorder

EXPECTED FINDINGS
- Pain that is unrelieved with elevation or analgesics; increases with passive movement
- Paresthesia or numbness (early finding)
- Pulselessness distal to the fracture (late finding)
- Paralysis or an inability to move digits (nerve damage)
- Pale, cold skin and cyanosis to nail beds

NURSING CARE
- Monitor the extremity every hour for the first 24 hr.
- The nurse should be able to place one finger in the space between the skin and the cast at all times.
- Notify the provider of suspected compartment syndrome.
- Place the affected extremity at heart level.
- Loosen the dressing or open and bivalve the cast.
- Prepare the child for fasciotomy.
- Complete dressing changes or maintain negative pressure wound therapy.

CLIENT EDUCATION: Report pain that is not relieved by analgesics, pain that continues to increase in intensity, numbness, tingling, or a change in color of the extremity.

(N) *NCLEX® Connection: Reduction of Risk Potential, Potential for Complications from Surgical Procedures and Health Alterations*

UNIT 2   NURSING CARE OF CHILDREN WHO
HAVE SYSTEM DISORDERS
SECTION: MUSCULOSKELETAL DISORDERS

CHAPTER 27 # Musculoskeletal Congenital Disorders

Musculoskeletal congenital disorders can be identified at birth or might not be present until later in infancy, childhood, or adolescence. These disorders can involve a specific area of the body or affect the child's entire musculoskeletal system. Careful data collection and interprofessional collaboration assist in promoting the child's growth, development, and mobility.

Clubfoot

- A complex deformity of the ankle and foot (27.1)
- Can affect one or both feet, occur as an isolated defect, or in association with other disorders (cerebral palsy, spina bifida)
- Categorized as **positional** clubfoot (occurs from intrauterine crowding), **syndromic** (occurs in association with other syndromes), and **congenital** (idiopathic)

DATA COLLECTION

RISK FACTORS: presence of other syndromes, hereditary factors

EXPECTED FINDINGS
- Affected foot is smaller and shorter in length than the unaffected foot.
- Affected extremity can be shorter with less muscle mass than the unaffected extremity.
- Empty heel pad
- Transverse plantar crease

DIAGNOSTIC PROCEDURES: Prenatal ultrasound provides data for identification of the deformity.

PATIENT-CENTERED CARE

NURSING CARE

- Promote bonding. Encourage parents to hold and cuddle the child.
- Encourage parents to meet the developmental needs of the child.
- Perform neurovascular and skin integrity checks.

THERAPEUTIC PROCEDURES

Castings

- Series of castings starting shortly after birth and continuing until maximum correction is accomplished.
- Weekly manipulation of the foot to stretch the muscles with subsequent placement of a new cast. Q EBP
- Following serial casting, a percutaneous heel cord tenotomy is usually performed followed by a long leg cast for 3 weeks.
- A Denis Browne bar that connects specialized shoes can be applied to maintain the correction and prevent recurrence.
- Further surgical intervention is indicated if casting and heel cord tenotomy are unsuccessful.

NURSING CARE
- Check neurovascular status.
- Inspect skin.
- Perform cast care.
- Reinforce teaching about cast care including follow-up care for cast changes.

COMPLICATIONS

Growth and development delays

NURSING CARE
- Monitor growth and development.
- Recommend strategies to enhance normal growth and development.

Effects of casting

- Skin breakdown
- Neurovascular impairment

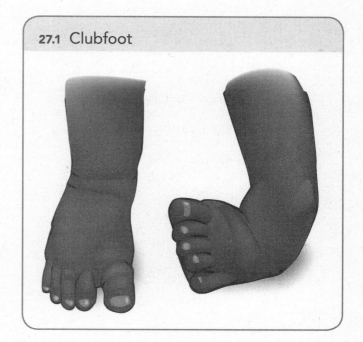

27.1 Clubfoot

Legg-Calve-Perthes disease

Aseptic necrosis of the femoral head can be unilateral or bilateral

DATA COLLECTION

RISK FACTORS

- Age: Affects children 2 to 12 years but more common between ages 4 to 8 years
- Sex: More common in males
- Trauma, inflammation to the femoral head

EXPECTED FINDINGS

- Intermittent painless limp, more noticeable with increased activity
- Hip stiffness
- Limited ROM
- Hip, thigh, knee pain
- Shortening of the affected leg
- Muscle wasting

DIAGNOSTIC PROCEDURES

- Radiograph of the hip and pelvis
- MRI

PATIENT-CENTERED CARE

NURSING CARE

- Treatment varies with the child's age and the appearance of the femoral head.
- Administer NSAIDs.
- Maintain rest and limited weight bearing. Advance to active motion as prescribed.
- Assist the child with physical therapy and ROM exercises.
- Provide care for abduction brace or casts.
- Maintain prescribed traction.
- Reinforce teaching about the limited weight bearing treatment prescribed.
- Offer developmentally appropriate strategies for learning and activities during the limited weight bearing periods. Qpcc

SURGICAL INTERVENTIONS

Osteotomy of the hip or femur

Developmental dysplasia of the hip (DDH)

A variety of disorders resulting in abnormal development of the hip structures that can affect infants or children
- **Acetabular dysplasia:** delay in acetabular development (acetabular roof is shallow and oblique)
- **Subluxation:** incomplete dislocation of the hip
- **Dislocation:** femoral head does not have contact with the acetabulum

DATA COLLECTION

RISK FACTORS

- Birth order (firstborn)
- Sex (female)
- Family history
- Breech intrauterine position
- Joint laxity
- Increased birth weight

EXPECTED FINDINGS

INFANT
- Asymmetry of gluteal and thigh folds
- Limited hip abduction
- Shortening of the femur
- Widened perineum
- Positive Ortolani test (hip is reduced by abduction)
- Positive Barlow test (hip is dislocated by adduction)

CHILD
- One leg shorter than the other
- Positive Trendelenburg sign (while bearing weight on the affected side, the pelvis tilts downward)
- Walking on toes on one foot
- Walks with a limp

DIAGNOSTIC PROCEDURES

Ultrasound: performed at 2 weeks of age to determine the cartilaginous head of the femur

X-ray: can diagnose DDH in infants older than 6 months of age

PATIENT-CENTERED CARE

NURSING CARE

- Treatment starts as soon as DDH is diagnosed and depends on the child's age and the extent of the dysplasia.
- Encourage parents to hold and cuddle the infant/child.
- Encourage parents to meet the developmental needs of the infant/child.

Newborn to 6 months

Pavlik harness
- Maintain harness placement for up to 12 weeks.
- Perform neurovascular and skin integrity checks.
- Removing the harness is dependent on the child's individual condition and needs.
- Show the family how to place the harness if removal is prescribed. Q̲s̲
- CLIENT EDUCATION
  - Do not adjust the straps.
  - Practice skin care (check skin, gently massage skin under straps, avoid lotions and powders, place diaper under the straps).

When adduction contracture is present

Bryant traction
- Skin traction
- Hips flexed at a 90° angle with the buttock raised off of the bed
- NURSING ACTIONS
  - Neurovascular checks
  - Maintain traction (ropes, boots, pulleys, and weights)
  - Ensure the child maintains alignment
  - Skin care

Hip spica cast
- Needs to be changed to accommodate growth
- NURSING ACTIONS
  - Check and maintain the hip spica cast.
  - Perform frequent neurovascular checks.
  - Perform range of motion with the unaffected extremities.
  - Perform frequent inspection of skin integrity, especially in the diaper area.
  - Check for pain control using an age-appropriate pain assessment tool. Intervene as indicated. Q̲ᴘᴄᴄ
  - Evaluate hydration status frequently.
  - Monitor elimination status daily.
  - Reinforce teaching regarding positioning, turning, neurovascular status, and care of the cast.

- CLIENT EDUCATION
  - Position casts on pillows. Q̲ᴇʙᴘ
  - Keep the casts elevated until dry.
  - Change position frequently to allow for drying.
  - Handle the casts with the palm of the hand until dry.
  - Note color and temperature of toes on casted extremity.
  - Give sponge baths to avoid wetting the cast.
  - Use a waterproof barrier around the genital opening of spica cast to prevent soiling with urine or feces.
  - Care after discharge includes using appropriate equipment (stroller, wagon, car seat) for maintaining mobility.

6 months to 2 years

Surgical closed reduction with placement of hip spica cast

NURSING ACTIONS
- Prepare family and child for surgery.
- Perform neurovascular checks.
- Manage postoperative pain.
- Provide skin care.
- Provide cast care.
- Reinforce teaching about spica cast and home care management.

Older children

- Surgical reduction with presurgical traction
- Femoral osteotomy, reconstruction, and tenotomy are often needed.

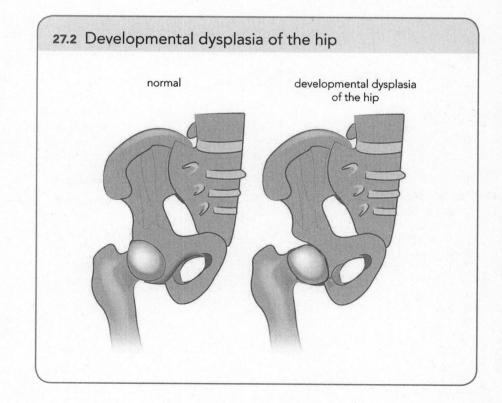

27.2 Developmental dysplasia of the hip

normal

developmental dysplasia of the hip

COMPLICATIONS

Postoperative complications: Atelectasis, ileus, infection

Effects of immobilization: Decreased muscle strength, bone demineralization, altered bowel motility

Effects of casting: Skin breakdown, neurovascular alterations

Infection
- Infection can be caused by bacteria such as *Staphylococcus aureus*.
- NURSING ACTIONS
  - Monitor vital signs. Observe changes in temperature that could be associated with complications of infection.
  - Keep the cast dry and intact.
  - Monitor for changes in neurovascular status (numbness; tingling; decreased mobility, sensation, or capillary refill).
  - Reposition the child frequently.
  - Maintain a high-fiber diet and promote adequate hydration.
  - Monitor bowel and bladder elimination. Report any changes, especially the decrease or absence of bowel sounds or distention.
  - Report any foul odor from cast or urine.
  - Observe changes in behavior, especially increasing irritability in infants.
  - Discuss possible complications of specific treatment or procedure with the child and family.
  - Advise the child and family about follow-up.
- CLIENT EDUCATION: Notify the provider with any concerns or indications of complications.

Osteogenesis imperfecta

An inherited condition that results in bone fractures and deformity along with restricted growth

DATA COLLECTION

RISK FACTORS

Parent who has osteogenesis imperfecta (OI)

EXPECTED FINDINGS

CLASSIC MANIFESTATIONS
- Multiple bone fractures
- Blue sclera
- Early hearing loss
- Small, discolored teeth

DIAGNOSTIC PROCEDURES

Bone biopsy

NURSING ACTIONS
- Prepare the child for the procedure.
- Assist with positioning the child.

PATIENT-CENTERED CARE

NURSING CARE

TREATMENT IS SUPPORTIVE.

MEDICATIONS

Pamidronate

Increase bone density

NURSING ACTIONS
- Administered IV by RN.
- Monitor for adverse effects (hypokalemia, hypomagnesemia, hypocalcemia, hypophosphatemia, thrombocytopenia, neutropenia, dysrhythmias, kidney failure, general malaise).
- Consult with physical therapy.
- Educate the parents on the child's limitations.
- Encourage support groups. Qᴛᴄ
- Assist child with meeting developmental milestones.

CLIENT EDUCATION
- Identify adverse effects and notify the provider.
- Practice low-impact exercises and safe handling to decrease the risk of fractures.
- Adhere to the medication regimen.
- Use braces and splints as prescribed.

SURGICAL INTERVENTIONS

- For severe cases
- Correct bone deformities, placement of rods.

COMPLICATIONS

Disuse osteoporosis
- Limit time in casts.
- Encourage activity.

Hearing loss

Permanent deformities

Scoliosis

- Scoliosis is a complex deformity of the spine that also affects the ribs.
- Characterized by a lateral curvature of the spine and spinal rotation that causes rib asymmetry.
- Idiopathic or structural scoliosis is the most common form of scoliosis and can be seen in isolation or associated with other conditions.

DATA COLLECTION

RISK FACTORS

- Genetic tendency
- Sex: more common in females
- Age: highest incidence from 8 to 15 years of age

EXPECTED FINDINGS

- Asymmetry in scapula, ribs, flanks, shoulders, and hips
- Improperly fitting clothing (one leg shorter than the other)

DIAGNOSTIC PROCEDURES

- Screen during preadolescence.
  - Observe the child, who should be wearing only underwear, from the back.
  - Have the child bend over at the waist with arms hanging down and observe for asymmetry of ribs and flank.
- An advance practice nurse or provider uses a scoliometer to measure truncal rotation. Radiography is used to determine the degree of curvature and skeletal maturity.

PATIENT-CENTERED CARE

NURSING CARE

Treatment depends on the degree, location, and type of curvature.

THERAPEUTIC PROCEDURES

Bracing: Customized braces slow the progression of the curve.

NURSING ACTIONS
- Assist with fitting the child with a brace.
- Inspect skin.
- Promote the child's positive self-image. Qpcc
- Reinforce teaching with the child on how to correctly apply the brace.

Surgical interventions

Spinal fusion with rod placement: Used for curvatures greater than 45°

PREOPERATIVE NURSING ACTIONS
- Inform and assist the adolescent to obtain autologous (self-donated) blood donations. Considerable blood loss is expected during spinal surgery.
- Obtain routine laboratory studies, including a type and cross match for blood.
- Reinforce with the adolescent and family about what can be expected during the postoperative period (monitoring equipment, NG tube, chest tubes, indwelling urinary catheters, patient-controlled analgesia [PCA] pumps).
- Discuss medical terms that are unfamiliar to the adolescent or family.

POSTOPERATIVE NURSING ACTIONS
- Perform standard postoperative care to prevent complications.
- Monitor pain using an age-appropriate pain assessment tool.
- Administer analgesia using a PCA pump. Adolescents often experience significant pain during the first few postoperative days.
- Perform frequent neurovascular checks.
- Use a log rolling technique when turning the adolescent to prevent damage to the spinal fusion.
- Inspect skin for pressure areas, especially if a brace has been prescribed. Qs
- Provide skin care by keeping skin clean and dry.
- Monitor surgical and drain sites for indications of infection. Provide wound care.
- Auscultate bowel sounds and monitor, observing for paralytic ileus.
- Monitor for decreases in Hgb and Hct. Observe for indications of bleeding.
- Encourage mobility as soon as tolerated. Ambulation is usually prescribed postoperative day 2 to 3.
- Monitor for infection.
- Perform range of motion exercises on unaffected extremities.
- Provide age-appropriate activities and opportunities to visit with friends and family during the hospital stay. Qpcc
- Emphasize the necessity of follow-up care.
- Reinforce the expected course of treatment and recovery.

CLIENT EDUCATION

PREOPERATIVE
- Use incentive spirometer, turning, coughing, and deep breathing to prevent complications.
- Use a PCA pump if age-appropriate.
- Log rolling will be used after surgery.
- Respiratory therapy techniques will be used postoperatively to reduce complications of anesthesia.

POSTOPERATIVE

- Practice physical therapy and proper positioning of the spine.
- Encourage independence following surgery for the adolescent who has a brace.
- Encourage the adolescent to contact friends when able.

CARE AFTER DISCHARGE: Arrange the environment to facilitate the adolescent's ability to be as independent as possible (keep favorite items within reach).

COMPLICATIONS

Breathing difficulties (with severe curvatures)

Spine or nerve damage

Lowered self-esteem: Assist the child with age-appropriate actions to promote positive self-esteem.

Infection following surgery

- Infection can be caused by bacteria, such as *Staphylococcus aureus*.
- NURSING ACTIONS
  - Monitor vital signs. Observe changes in temperature that could be associated with complications of infection.
  - Monitor for changes in neurovascular status (numbness; tingling; decreased mobility, sensation, or capillary refill).
  - Reposition the child frequently.
  - Maintain a high-fiber diet and promote adequate hydration.
  - Discuss possible complications of specific treatment or procedure with the child and family.
  - Educate the child and family about follow-up.
- CLIENT EDUCATION: Notify the provider with any concerns or indications of complications.

Application Exercises

1. A nurse is caring for a toddler who has dysplasia of the hip and a hip spica cast in place. The child's mother asks the nurse why a Pavlik harness is not being used. Which of the following responses should the nurse make?

   A. "The Pavlik harness is used for children with scoliosis, not hip dysplasia."

   B. "The Pavlik harness is used for school-age children."

   C. "The Pavlik harness cannot be used for your child because her condition is too severe."

   D. "The Pavlik harness is used for infants less than 6 months of age."

2. A nurse is reinforcing preoperative teaching with an adolescent client who is scheduled to receive spinal instrumentation for scoliosis. Which of the following information should the nurse include?

   A. "You will go home the same day of surgery."

   B. "You will have minimal pain after your surgery."

   C. "You will probably need to receive blood after surgery."

   D. "You will be assisted to walk 8 hours after surgery."

3. A nurse is caring for a child who is suspected of having Legg-Calve-Perthes disease. The nurse should prepare the child for which of the following diagnostic procedures?

   A. Bone biopsy

   B. Scoliometer measurement

   C. Ultrasound

   D. Radiographs

4. A nurse is collecting data from a child who has Legg-Calve-Perthes disease. Which of the following findings should the nurse expect? (Select all that apply.)

   A. Longer affected leg

   B. Hip stiffness

   C. Enlarged muscles in affected leg

   D. Limited range of motion

   E. Limp with walking

5. A nurse is collecting data from a preschool-age child for developmental dysplasia of the hip. Which of the following should the nurse include?

   A. Barlow test

   B. Check for Trendelenburg sign

   C. Manipulation of foot and ankle

   D. Ortolani test

PRACTICE Active Learning Scenario

A nurse is caring for a child in a hip spica cast. What should the nurse include in the care of this client? Use the ATI Active Learning Template: Therapeutic Procedure to complete this item.

NURSING INTERVENTIONS: List at least five actions the nurse should include in the child's care.

CLIENT EDUCATION: List at least six education points the nurse should include for the child and parents.

Application Exercises Key

1. A. The Pavlik harness is used for the treatment of dysplasia of the hip. However, another treatment is indicated for a toddler who has this disorder.

   B. The Pavlik harness is used for the treatment of dysplasia of the hip. However, another treatment is indicated for a toddler who has this disorder.

   C. The Pavlik harness is used for the treatment of dysplasia of the hip. However, another treatment is indicated for a toddler who has this disorder.

   D. **CORRECT:** The Pavlik harness is used for the treatment of an infant up to 6 months of age who has dysplasia of the hip. Surgical closed reduction with placement of a hip spica cast is the recommended treatment for a toddler who has this disorder.

   Ⓝ *NCLEX® Connection: Physiological Adaptation, Alterations in Body Systems*

2. A. Clients who have spinal instrumentation for scoliosis require acute postoperative care beyond the day of surgery.

   B. Clients who have spinal instrumentation for scoliosis experience significant pain that requires a PCA pump.

   C. **CORRECT:** Clients who have spinal instrumentation for scoliosis have a lengthy surgery with blood loss and often require postoperative blood transfusions.

   D. Clients who have spinal instrumentation for scoliosis are usually prescribed to ambulate postoperative day 2 or 3.

   Ⓝ *NCLEX® Connection: Reduction of Risk Potential, Potential for Complications from Surgical Procedures and Health Alterations*

3. A. A bone biopsy is used to diagnose cancer, infection, and other bone disorders. It does not diagnose Legg-Calve-Perthes.

   B. A scoliometer is used to measure truncal rotation for a child who is suspected of having scoliosis.

   C. An ultrasound is used to diagnose developmental dysplasia of the hip in infants less than 6 months of age.

   D. **CORRECT:** A child who has Legg-Calve-Perthes exhibits necrosis of the femoral head, which can be diagnosed by radiographs of the hip and pelvis.

   Ⓝ *NCLEX® Connection: Reduction of Risk Potential, Diagnostic Tests*

4. A. A child who has Legg-Calve-Perthes exhibits shortening of the affected leg.

   B. **CORRECT:** A child who has Legg-Calve-Perthes exhibits hip stiffness due to the necrosis of the femoral head.

   C. A child who has Legg-Calve-Perthes exhibits muscle wasting.

   D. **CORRECT:** A child who has Legg-Calve-Perthes exhibits limited range of motion due to the necrosis of the femoral head.

   E. **CORRECT:** A child who has Legg-Calve-Perthes exhibits an intermittent painless limp with walking due to the necrosis of the femoral head.

   Ⓝ *NCLEX® Connection: Physiological Adaptation, Basic Pathophysiology*

5. A. A provider or advanced practice nurse uses the Barlow test to assess developmental dysplasia of the hip for infants.

   B. **CORRECT:** A positive Trendelenburg sign is an indication of developmental dysplasia of the hip. The nurse should instruct the preschooler to bear weight on the affected leg while holding on to something for balance. The nurse observes from behind for abnormal downward tilting of the pelvis on the unaffected side.

   C. Manipulation of the foot and ankle checks for clubfoot.

   D. A provider or advanced practice nurse uses the Ortolani test assess developmental dysplasia of the hip for infants.

   Ⓝ *NCLEX® Connection: Health Promotion and Maintenance, Data Collection Techniques*

PRACTICE Answer

Using the ATI Active Learning Template: Therapeutic Procedure

NURSING INTERVENTIONS
- Check and maintain the hip spica cast.
- Perform frequent neurovascular checks.
- Perform range of motion with the unaffected extremities.
- Perform frequent inspection of skin integrity, especially in the diaper area.
- Check for pain control using an age-appropriate pain assessment tool. Intervene as indicated.
- Evaluate hydration status frequently.
- Monitor elimination status daily.
- Reinforce teaching regarding positioning, turning, neurovascular status, and care of the cast.

Ⓝ *NCLEX® Connection: Reduction of Risk Potential, Therapeutic Procedures*

CLIENT EDUCATION
- Position casts on pillows.
- Keep the casts elevated until dry.
- Encourage frequent position changes to allow for drying.
- Handle the casts with the palm of the hand until dry.
- Note color and temperature of toes on casted extremity.
- Give sponge baths to avoid wetting the cast.
- Use a waterproof barrier around the genital opening of spica cast to prevent soiling with urine or feces.
- Use appropriate equipment (stroller, wagon, car seat) for maintaining mobility after discharge.

CHAPTER 28 *Chronic Neuromusculoskeletal Disorders*

Chronic problems associated with mobility can reflect a problem with the musculoskeletal system or result from a disorder related to the neural pathway extending from the brain's cortex to the neuromuscular junction.

Cerebral palsy

- Cerebral palsy (CP) is a nonprogressive impairment of motor function, especially that of muscle control, coordination, and posture.
- CP can cause abnormal perception and sensation; visual, hearing, and speech impairments; seizures; and cognitive deficits.
- CP manifests differently in each child. Developmental outcomes vary and are dependent on the severity of the injury.

DATA COLLECTION

RISK FACTORS

The exact cause is not known. Prenatal, perinatal, and postnatal risk factors include the following.
- Existing brain anomalies, cerebral infections, head trauma (shaken baby syndrome), or anoxia to the brain
- Maternal chorioamnionitis
- Maternal infection
- Premature birth
- Multiple births
- Very low birth weights
- Inability of the placenta to provide the developing fetus with oxygen and nutrients
- Interruption of oxygen delivery to the fetus during birth

EXPECTED FINDINGS

Parents might describe concerns with development.

PHYSICAL FINDINGS
- Failure to meet developmental milestones
- Persistent primitive reflexes (Moro, tonic neck)
- Gagging or choking with feeding, poor suck reflex
- Tongue thrust
- Poor head control
- Rigid posture and extremities, abnormal posturing
- Asymmetric crawl
- Hyperreflexia
- Vision, speech, or hearing impairments
- Seizures
- Impaired social relationships

Spastic CP (pyramidal)
- Hypertonicity (muscle tightness or spasticity); increased deep tendon reflexes; clonus; and poor control of motion, balance, and posture
- Impairments of fine and gross motor skills
- Can present in all four extremities (tetraplegia); all extremities affected, lower more than upper (diplegia); three limbs (triplegia); one limb (monoplegia); or one side of the body (hemiplegia)
- Gait can appear crouched with a scissoring motion of the legs with feet plantar flexed.

Dyskinetic CP (nonspastic, extrapyramidal)
- **Athetoid:** Findings include involuntary jerking movements that appear slow, writhing, and wormlike. These movements involve the extremities, trunk, neck, face, and tongue.
- **Dystonic:** Slow, twisting movements affect the trunk or extremities with abnormal posturing from muscle contractions. Drooling and speech impairment related to involvement of the muscles of pharynx, larynx, and oral regions.

Ataxic CP (nonspastic, extrapyramidal)
- Evidence of wide-based gait and difficulty with coordination
- Poor ability to do repetitive movements
- Lack of coordination with purposeful movements (reaching for an object)

DIAGNOSTIC PROCEDURES

Complete check of the neurological system

Metabolic and genetic testing

Observation of general movements in children older than 2 years and younger than 5 years of age

MRI to evaluate structures or abnormal areas near bone
NURSING ACTIONS
- Assist the child to remain still during the procedure.
- Sedate the child.

PATIENT-CENTERED CARE

NURSING CARE

- Provide emotional support during diagnostic testing.
- Contribute to a plan of care that meets the child's individual needs.
- Monitor developmental milestones.
- Identify the need for hearing and speech evaluations.
- Promote independence with self-care activities as much as possible. Assist the child to maintain a positive self-image and a high level of self-esteem.
- Determine the extent of family coping and support.
- Identify the family's awareness of available resources.
- Collect data about the child's developmental level.
- Structure interventions and communications around the child's developmental level, rather than chronological age.
- Communicate with the child directly, but include parents as needed. Qpcc
- Help the child to use augmented communication, such as electronic devices for speech and other types of communication tools.
- Include the family in physical care during hospitalization.
  - Ask the family about routine care, and encourage them to provide it if appropriate.
  - Encourage the family to help verify the child's needs if communication is impaired.
- Maintain an open airway by elevating the head of the child's bed. (This is especially important if the child has increased oral secretions.) Qs
- Ensure suction equipment is available if required. Suction oral secretions as needed.
- Monitor for pain (especially with muscle spasms) using a developmentally appropriate pain tool.
- Administer medication for pain or spasms.
- Ensure adequate nutrition.
  - Check for aspiration in children who have severe disabilities.
  - Determine the child's ability to take oral nutrition.
  - Ascertain the correct positioning for feeding the child. Use head positioning and manual jaw control methods as needed.
  - Provide foods similar to those eaten at home when possible.
  - Administer supplements.
  - Administer feedings by gastric tube.
  - Maintain weight/height chart.
- Provide skin care.
  - Inspect skin under splints and braces.
  - Maintain skin integrity by turning the child to keep pressure off bony prominences.
  - Keep skin clean and dry.
- Provide rest periods as needed.
- Reinforce teaching about wound care.
- Reinforce teaching with the family and child about ankle-foot orthoses.
- Help the family identify resources needed (respite care).
- Suggest participation in a support group for CP.

MEDICATIONS

Baclofen

Used as a centrally acting skeletal muscle relaxant that decreases muscle spasm and severe spasticity

NURSING ACTIONS

- Administer orally. Baclofen can also be administered intrathecally via a specialized, surgically implanted pump by a qualified member of the health care team.
- Monitor effectiveness of the medication.
- Monitor for muscle weakness, increased fatigue, or less-common adverse effects (diaphoresis, constipation).
- Educate the family about expected responses of medications.
- Reinforce with the family the adverse effects of medications and when to call the provider.

Diazepam

Skeletal muscle relaxant used to decrease muscle spasms and severe spasticity

NURSING ACTIONS

- Use in older children and adolescents.
- Monitor for drowsiness and fatigue.
- Educate the family about expected responses to medications.
- Reinforce with the family the adverse effects of the medication and when to call the provider.

Botulinum toxin A

- Reduces spasticity in specific muscle groups
- Used primarily for children who have spasticity only in the lower extremities

NURSING ACTIONS: Monitor for temporary weakness.

CLIENT EDUCATION: Onset of the medication is 24 to 72 hr, with a peak of 2 weeks, lasting 3 to 6 months.

Antiepileptics

Control seizure activity

INTERPROFESSIONAL CARE

- Assist with the coordination of care with other professionals (speech, physical, and recreational therapists; education and medical specialists). Qtc
- Assist with referral for technical aids that can assist with coordination, speaking, mobility, and an increased level of independence. Some children benefit from the use of a voice-activated wheelchair.
- Surgical intervention is indicated for tendon release to correct contractures or other spastic deformities.

CLIENT EDUCATION

- Follow the therapeutic plan of care.
- Take rest periods as needed.
- Maintain changes made to feeding schedule and feeding techniques during hospitalization.
- Adhere to the medication regimen.
- Engage in regular dental care.
- Provide developmental stimulation.
- Perform self-urinary catheterization if needed.
- Use pulmonary hygiene techniques.
- Work with the interprofessional team.

COMPLICATIONS

Aspiration

NURSING ACTIONS
- Keep the child's head elevated.
- Keep suction available if copious oral secretions are present or the child has difficulty with swallowing foods or fluids. Qs

CLIENT EDUCATION
- Use feeding techniques to decrease the risk of aspiration.
- Take CPR classes.

Potential for injury

NURSING ACTIONS
- Raise the child's bed rails to prevent falls from the bed.
- Pad side rails and wheelchair arms to prevent injury from seizure activity.
- Secure the child in mobility devices, such as wheelchairs.
- Encourage the child to receive adequate rest to prevent injury at times of fatigue.
- Encourage the use of helmets, seat belts, and other safety equipment.
- Reinforce safety precautions with the child and family.

Spina bifida

Spinal bifida is failure of the osseous spine to close. Neural tube defects (NTDs) are present at birth and affect the CNS and osseous spine.

Spina bifida occulta mostly affects the lumbosacral area and is not visible.

Spina bifida cystica: Protrusion of the sac is visible
- **Meningocele:** The sac contains spinal fluid and meninges.
- **Myelomeningocele:** The sac contains spinal fluid, meninges, and nerves.

DATA COLLECTION

RISK FACTORS

- Medications/substances taken during pregnancy
- Maternal malnutrition
- Insufficient folic acid intake during pregnancy
- Exposure to radiation or chemicals during pregnancy

EXPECTED FINDINGS

- Presence of risk factors in prenatal history
- Family history of neural tube defects

PHYSICAL FINDINGS
- Protruding sac midline of the osseous spine (cystica)
- Dimpling in the lumbosacral area (occulta)
- Port wine angioma (occulta)
- Dark hair tufts (occulta)
- Subcutaneous lipoma (occulta)

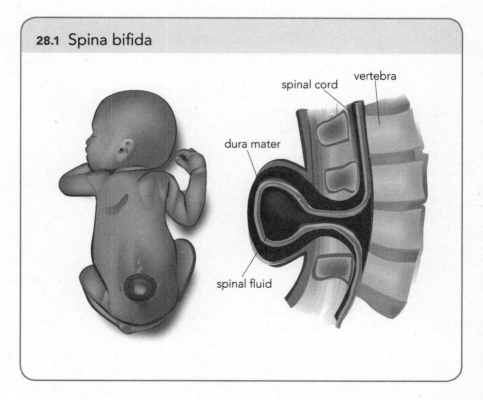

28.1 Spina bifida

vertebra

spinal cord

dura mater

spinal fluid

LABORATORY TESTS

MATERNAL BLOOD TESTS: Serum alpha-fetoprotein between 16 and 18 weeks of gestation indicate possible NTD.

INFANT BLOOD TESTS: Blood cultures determine causative pathogen if appropriate.

DIAGNOSTIC PROCEDURES

PRENATAL
- **Ultrasound** can show visual defect.
- **Amniocentesis** following elevated alpha-fetoprotein levels detects anencephaly or myelomeningocele.

POSTNATAL: MRI, ultrasonography, and CT to evaluate spinal cord and brain

PATIENT-CENTERED CARE

NURSING CARE

- Promote infant-parent attachment.
- Inspect the sac.
- Perform routine data collection of the newborn.
- Check the level of neurologic involvement.
- Obtain accurate output measurements.
- Measure head circumference and inspect fontanels.

INTERPROFESSIONAL CARE

Neurosurgery, neurology, urology, orthopedics, pediatrics, physical therapy, occupational therapy, and social services

THERAPEUTIC PROCEDURES

Closure of a myelomeningocele sac is done as soon as possible to prevent complications of injury and infection.

PREOPERATIVE NURSING ACTIONS
- Prepare the family for surgery (within 24 to 72 hr after birth).
- Protect the sac from injury.
- Place infant in a warmer, without clothing.
- Apply a sterile, moist, nonadhering dressing with 0.9% sodium chloride on the sac, changing it every 2 hr. Q𝐄𝐁𝐏
- Inspect the sac closely for leaks, irritation, abrasions and localized indications of infection.
- Monitor for systemic indications of infection (fever, irritability, lethargy).
- Place infant in the prone position with hips flexed and legs abducted.
- Assist with administration of IV antibiotic.
- Avoid rectal temperatures.
- Avoid cuddling or putting pressure on the sac.

POSTOPERATIVE NURSING ACTIONS
- Monitor vital signs.
- Monitor I&O.
- Monitor for indications of infection.
- Assist in providing pain management.
- Assist with incision care.

- Observe for CSF leakage.
- Maintain prone position until other positions are prescribed.
- Resume oral feedings.
- Reinforce teaching on postoperative care at home.
- Depending on disability, reinforce ROM techniques.
- Address body image concerns.
- Offer support to the family.
- Assist the family with obtaining medical equipment/services needed at home.

ONGOING NURSING CARE
- Measure head circumference.
- Inspect skin integrity.
- Check for allergies, such as latex allergy.
- Monitor cognitive development.
- Monitor bladder and bowel functioning.
- Monitor motor development.
- Monitor for infections.

CLIENT EDUCATION

- Assist the child with range of motion (ROM) exercises.
- Assist the child with independence throughout the lifespan.

COMPLICATIONS

Skin ulceration

Caused by prolonged pressure in one area

NURSING ACTIONS
- Monitor skin for breakdown.
- Reposition frequently to prevent pressure on bony prominences.
- Monitor skin under splints and braces.

CLIENT EDUCATION: Monitor skin integrity.

Latex allergy

The child is at an increased risk for a latex allergy. Allergy responses range from urticaria to wheezing, which can progress to anaphylaxis. A latex allergy is linked to allergies to some foods (bananas, avocados, kiwi, chestnuts).

NURSING ACTIONS
- Assist with testing for allergy.
- Reduce exposure.
- Provide the family with a list of household items that can contain latex (water toys, pacifiers, plastic storage bags).
- Educate the family about how to identify indications of allergic reaction and report them to the provider.
- Reinforce instruction about the use of epinephrine. Q𝐬

CLIENT EDUCATION: Avoid exposing the child to latex.

Increased intracranial pressure

Caused by shunt malfunction or hydrocephalus.

MANIFESTATIONS
- INFANTS: high-pitched cry, lethargy, vomiting, bulging fontanels, widening cranial suture lines, increased head circumference
- CHILDREN: headache, lethargy, nausea, vomiting, double vision, decreased school performance of learned tasks, decreased level of consciousness, seizures

NURSING ACTIONS
- Assist with preparation for surgery for shunt or shunt revision.
- Use gentle movements when performing ROM exercises.
- Minimize environmental stressors (noise, frequent visitors).
- Monitor and manage pain.
- Inform the child and parents about manifestations of shunt malfunction and hydrocephalus and when to notify the provider.

Bladder issues

The child is at an increased risk for bladder dysfunction (either spasms or flaccidity).

NURSING ACTIONS
- Monitor for indications of bladder dysfunction or infection.
- Monitor for blood in the urine.
- Assist with preparation of the family and child for surgery if needed.
- Reinforce teaching with the child and family about care of stoma (vesicostomy).

Orthopedic issues

Corrections of associated potential problems, such as clubfoot, scoliosis, and other malformations of the feet and legs

NURSING ACTIONS
- Monitor for indications of infection.
- Administer pain medications.
- Assist with preparation of the family and child for surgery.
- Provide cast care.
- Monitor for neurosensory deficits.
- Reinforce teaching with the family about indications of infection.
- Reinforce teaching with the family about cast and splint care.

Juvenile idiopathic arthritis

Juvenile idiopathic arthritis (JIA) is a chronic autoimmune inflammatory disease affecting joints and other tissues.
- The chronic inflammation of the synovium of the joints leads to wearing down and damage to the articular cartilage.
- JIA is rarely life-threatening. It can subside over time, but it can result in residual joint deformities and altered joint function.
- There are multiple classifications of JIA with or without a rheumatoid factor.

DATA COLLECTION

RISK FACTORS

- Immunogenic susceptibility
- Environmental triggers

EXPECTED FINDINGS

PHYSICAL FINDINGS
- Joint swelling, stiffness, redness, and warmth that tend to be worse in the morning or after inactivity
- Mobility limitations
- Fever
- Rash
- Limp in the morning
- Delayed growth

LABORATORY TESTS

- Elevated C-reactive protein can be present.
- Erythrocyte sedimentation rate (ESR) can be elevated.
- CBC with differential can show elevated WBCs, especially during exacerbations.
- Antinuclear antibodies (ANA) indicate an increased risk for uveitis.
- Rheumatoid factor is rarely detected in children.

DIAGNOSTIC PROCEDURES

- Radiographic studies can be used for baseline comparison. X-rays can demonstrate increased synovial fluid in the joint, which causes soft tissue swelling or widening of the joint. Later findings can include narrowed joint spaces.
- Slit lamp eye examination is used to diagnosis uveitis.

PATIENT-CENTERED CARE

NURSING CARE

- Care is primarily in an outpatient setting.
- Assist the child with an exercise program.
- Reinforce teaching about relaxation techniques and nonpharmacological pain management.
- Evaluate pain and response to analgesics.
- Encourage a support group.
- Encourage the child to participate in a physical therapy program to increase mobility and prevent deformities.
- Encourage activity as tolerated.
- Encourage full ROM exercises.
- Apply heat or warm moist packs to the affected joints prior to exercise.
- Encourage warm baths.
- Identify alternate ways to meet developmental needs, especially during periods of exacerbation.
- Encourage self-care by allowing adequate time for completion. Qpcc
- Encourage a well-balanced diet with adequate fluid intake.
- Encourage participation in school and contact with peers.
- Collaborate with the school nurse and teachers to arrange for care during the school day (medication administration, in-school physical therapy, extra sets of books, split days).
- Inform the family that exacerbation worsens with illnesses.
- Advise the family about routine follow-up with providers and regular eye exams.

MEDICATIONS

Nonsteroidal anti-inflammatory drugs (NSAIDs)

Ibuprofen, naproxen, diclofenac, indomethacin, and tolmetin control pain and inflammation.

CLIENT EDUCATION
- Take NSAIDs as prescribed.
- NSAIDs should be taken with food to minimize gastric irritation.
- Report changes in stool, GI discomfort, or increase in bruising immediately.

Methotrexate

A cytotoxic disease-modifying antirheumatic drug (DMARD) that slows joint degeneration and progression of rheumatoid arthritis when NSAIDs do not work alone

NURSING ACTIONS: Monitor liver function tests and CBC regularly.

CLIENT EDUCATION
- Avoid alcohol.
- Use effective birth control to avoid birth defects while taking this medication.
- Immune suppression is a possible adverse effect.

Corticosteroids

Prednisone provides relief of inflammation and pain. It is reserved for life-threatening complications, severe arthritis, pericarditis, and uveitis.

NURSING ACTIONS
- Administer as eye solution or PO. Assist with IV administration.
- An injection by the provider into the intra-articular space can provide effective pain relief.
- Administer at the lowest effective dose for short-term therapy and then discontinue by tapering the dose.

CLIENT EDUCATION
- Weight gain, especially in the face, is a common adverse effect.
- Monitor height and weight.
- An alteration in growth is a possible long-term complication.
- Avoid exposure to potentially infectious agents.
- Practice healthy eating habits.

Etanercept

Etanercept is a tumor necrosis factor alpha-receptor blocker, a DMARD that is used when methotrexate is not effective for immunosuppressive action.

NURSING ACTIONS
- Administer a tuberculin skin test prior to starting etanercept and yearly while the client takes the medication. Qs
- Administer etanercept once or twice each week by subcutaneous injection.

CLIENT EDUCATION
- There is a potential for allergic reactions.
- Avoid exposure to infectious agents.

INTERPROFESSIONAL CARE

Physical therapist, occupational therapist, ophthalmologist, dentist, dietitian, social worker, school nurse

COMPLICATIONS

Joint deformity and functional disability

NURSING ACTIONS
- Reinforce the individualized therapeutic plan of care.
- Advocate for the child when treatments are not producing expected results.

CLIENT EDUCATION
- Adhere to the treatment regimen.
- Engage in self-care and active participation in an exercise program.

Muscular dystrophy

Muscular dystrophy (MD) is a group of inherited disorders with progressive degeneration of symmetric skeletal muscle groups causing progressive muscle weakness and wasting.

Onset of disease, pace of progression, and muscle group affected depend on the type of MD.

- **Duchenne (pseudohypertrophic) muscular dystrophy** (DMD) is the most common form of MD. Inherited as an X-linked recessive trait, DMD has an onset between 3 and 5 years of age. Progressive disease with life expectancy with current technology for DMD reaches into early adulthood.
- **Facioscapulohumeral muscular dystrophy** is an autosomal dominant inherited disorder with the age of onset occurring during early adolescence. Progression is slow with normal life span.
- **Limb-girdle muscular dystrophy** is an autosomal dominant and recessive, heterogeneous disorder. It appears later in childhood with a slow progression.

DATA COLLECTION

RISK FACTORS

Family history

EXPECTED FINDINGS

PHYSICAL FINDINGS

- Fatigue
- Muscle weakness beginning in the lower extremities
- Unsteady gait, with a waddle
- Lordosis
- Delayed motor skill development
- Frequent falling
- "Walks" hands up legs to push torso to an upright position when rising to a standing position (Gowers' sign)
- Difficulty getting out of bed or climbing stairs
- Learning difficulties
- Mild cognitive delays that do not worsen with disease progression
- Progressive difficulty walking with possible loss of ability to walk often occurs by age 12 years (DMD)
- Progressive muscle atrophy
- Respiratory and cardiac difficulties as the disease progresses

LABORATORY TESTS

- Serum polymerase chain reaction to detect the dystrophin gene mutation
- Elevated serum creatine kinase (can be elevated prior to manifestations)

DIAGNOSTIC PROCEDURES

- Muscle biopsy
- Electromyography

PATIENT-CENTERED CARE

NURSING CARE

- Encourage and provide for genetic counseling.
- Check and monitor the following.
  - Ability to perform ADLs
  - Respiratory function (depth, rhythm, rate of respirations) during sleep and daytime hours
  - Cardiac function
  - Child's and parents' understanding of long-term effects
  - Child's and parents' coping and support systems
- Maintain optimal physical function for as long possible.
  - Encourage the child to be independent for as long as possible and to perform ADLs.
  - Perform ROM exercises and provide appropriate physical activity (stretching exercises, strength and muscle training, breathing exercises). Q̲EBP
  - Maintain proper body alignment and encourage the child to reposition frequently to avoid skin breakdown.
  - Assist with orthoses and braces.
- Maintain respiratory functioning.
  - Encourage the use of incentive spirometry.
  - Position the child to enhance expansion of lungs.
  - Reinforce teaching on how to use a mechanical cough device.
  - Provide oxygen.
  - Provide noninvasive ventilation.
- Encourage adequate fluid intake.
- Monitor and encourage adequate nutritional intake.
- Encourage routine physical exams and immunizations.
- Facilitate discussion of end-of-life decisions.

MEDICATIONS

Corticosteroids

Prednisone increases muscle strength

NURSING ACTIONS
- Monitor for infection.
- Monitor for adverse effects.
- Inform the family about adverse effects and when to notify the provider.

CLIENT EDUCATION
- Avoid potentially infectious agents.
- Practice healthy eating habits.

INTERPROFESSIONAL CARE

Neurologist; genetic counselor; physical, occupational, and respiratory therapists; dietitian; social worker; nurse; school teacher
- Encourage parents to consider assistance with care as disease progresses (respite, long-term, palliative, and home health care).
- Assist with a referral for the child and parents to support groups for MD. Qᴛᴄ

THERAPEUTIC PROCEDURES

Surgery can be indicated for release or repair of contractures or for insertion of a gastrostomy tube or tracheostomy.

COMPLICATIONS

Respiratory compromise

Progressive weakening of respiratory muscles decrease the child's ability to maintain adequate respirations.

NURSING ACTIONS
- Help the child turn hourly or more frequently.
- Have the child use deep breathing and coughing.
- Suction as needed. Qₛ
- Administer oxygen.
- Assist with intermittent positive pressure ventilation and mechanically-assisted cough devices.
- Administer antibiotics.
- Promote discussion of mechanical ventilation options with the child and parents.

Application Exercises

1. A nurse is caring for a child who has cerebral palsy. Which of the following medications should the nurse expect to administer to treat painful muscle spasms? (Select all that apply.)

   A. Baclofen

   B. Diazepam

   C. Indomethacin

   D. Methotrexate

   E. Prednisone

2. A nurse is contributing to a plan of care for a toddler who has cerebral palsy. Which of the following actions should the nurse recommend?

   A. Structure interventions according to chronological age.

   B. Identify the need for an evaluation of hearing ability.

   C. Monitor pain level routinely using a numeric rating scale.

   D. Provide total care for daily hygiene activities.

3. A nurse is caring for a school-age child who has juvenile idiopathic arthritis. Which of the following home care actions should the nurse recommend? (Select all that apply.)

   A. Provide extra time for completion of ADLs.

   B. Use cold compresses for joint pain.

   C. Take ibuprofen on an empty stomach.

   D. Consider home schooling

   E. Perform range of motion exercises.

4. A nurse is collecting data from a child who has muscular dystrophy (MD). Which of the following findings should the nurse expect? (Select all that apply.)

   A. Purposeless, involuntary, abnormal movements

   B. Spinal defect and saclike protrusion

   C. Muscular weakness in lower extremities

   D. Unsteady, waddling gait

   E. Kyphosis of the back

5. A nurse is caring for an infant who has a myelomeningocele and is scheduled for surgical repair. Which of the following actions should the nurse take?

   A. Encourage the parents to cuddle the infant.

   B. Check the infant's temperature rectally.

   C. Place the infant in a supine position.

   D. Apply a sterile, moist dressing on the sac.

PRACTICE Active Learning Scenario

A nurse is caring for a child who has a new prescription for baclofen. Use the ATI Active Learning Template: Medication to complete this item.

THERAPEUTIC USES

MEDICATION ADMINISTRATION

COMPLICATIONS: List adverse effects.

CLIENT EDUCATION: Include two education points.

Application Exercises Key

1. A. **CORRECT:** Baclofen is a centrally acting skeletal muscle relaxant that decreases muscle spasm and severe spasticity.

   B. **CORRECT:** Diazepam is a skeletal muscle relaxant that decreases muscle spasms and severe spasticity.

   C. Indomethacin is a non-steroidal anti-inflammatory (NSAID) medication used to decrease pain and inflammation in children who have juvenile idiopathic arthritis (JIA).

   D. Methotrexate is a cytotoxic disease-modifying antirheumatic drug that slows joint degeneration and progression of rheumatoid arthritis. It is used for children who have juvenile idiopathic arthritis (JIA).

   E. Prednisone is a corticosteroid that increases muscle strength for children who have muscular dystrophy. It also decreases inflammation in children who have JIA.

   Ⓝ *NCLEX® Connection: Pharmacological Therapies, Expected Actions/Outcomes*

2. A. The nurse should structure interventions according to the toddler's developmental level, rather than chronological age.

   B. **CORRECT:** The toddler who has CP has an increased risk for hearing impairment. The nurse should identify the toddler's need for a hearing evaluation.

   C. The nurse should routinely monitor the toddler's pain level using a developmentally appropriate pain tool, such as a FACES pain rating scale. The numeric rating scale is appropriate for children as young as 5 years of age who have a concept of numbers.

   D. Though a preschooler requires assistance and supervision with hygiene activities, the nurse should promote as much independence as possible.

   Ⓝ *NCLEX® Connection: Reduction of Risk Potential, Potential for Alterations in Body Systems*

3. A. **CORRECT:** Providing extra time for the completion of ADLs promotes independence in the child and provides a means to maintain mobility.

   B. Using a warm compress or moist pack can provide comfort and relieve stiffness.

   C. Ibuprofen should be taken with food to prevent GI distress.

   D. The child should be encouraged to attend school and have contact with peers to meet developmental needs.

   E. **CORRECT:** Range of motion exercises will assist in maintaining function of the joints.

   Ⓝ *NCLEX® Connection: Physiological Adaptation, Alterations in Body Systems*

4. A. A child who has cerebral palsy exhibits purposeless, involuntary, abnormal movements.

   B. An infant who has the spinal defect myelomeningocele will exhibit a saclike protrusion.

   C. **CORRECT:** A child who has MD will exhibit muscular weakness in the lower extremities as one of the first manifestations.

   D. **CORRECT:** A child who has MD will exhibit an unsteady, waddling gait due to the progressive muscle weakness.

   E. A child who has MD is expected to have lordosis of the back.

   Ⓝ *NCLEX® Connection: Physiological Adaptation, Basic Pathophysiology*

5. A. Cuddling the infant could cause pressure on the sac, which could cause rupture.

   B. Rectal temperatures could cause irritation or rectal prolapse.

   C. Placing the infant in supine position could cause pressure on the sac, which could cause rupture.

   D. **CORRECT:** The nurse should apply a sterile, moist, nonadhering dressing on the sac to keep it moist until surgery.

   Ⓝ *NCLEX® Connection: Physiological Adaptation, Alterations in Body Systems*

PRACTICE Answer

Using the ATI Active Learning Template: Medication

THERAPEUTIC USES: Used as a centrally acting skeletal muscle relaxant that decreases muscle spasm and severe spasticity. Indicated for the treatment of cerebral palsy.

NURSING ADMINISTRATION
- Administer orally. It can also be administered intrathecally via a specialized, surgically implanted pump by a qualified member of the health care team.
- Monitor effectiveness of the medication.

COMPLICATIONS
- Muscle weakness
- Increased fatigue
- Less common adverse effects (diaphoresis, constipation)

CLIENT EDUCATION
- Expected responses of medications
- Adverse effects of medications and when to call the provider

Ⓝ *NCLEX® Connection: Pharmacological and Parenteral Therapies, Medication Administration*

NCLEX® Connections

When reviewing the following chapters, keep in mind the relevant topics and tasks of the NCLEX outline, in particular:

Pharmacological Therapies

MEDICATION ADMINISTRATION: Administer medication by ear, eye, nose, inhalation, rectum, vagina, or skin route.

Reduction of Risk Potential

LABORATORY VALUES: Monitor diagnostic or laboratory test results.

Physiological Adaptation

ALTERATIONS IN BODY SYSTEMS
Identify signs and symptoms of an infection (temperature changes, swelling, redness, mental confusion, foul smelling urine).

Provide care to the correct client alteration in body system.

Reinforce education to the client regarding care and condition.

BASIC PATHOPHYSIOLOGY
Identify signs and symptoms related to an acute or chronic illness.

Consider general principles of client disease process when providing care (injury and repair, immunity, cellular structure).

Apply knowledge of pathophysiology to monitoring the client for alterations in body systems.

FLUID AND ELECTROLYTE IMBALANCES: Provide interventions to restore the client's fluid and/or electrolyte balance.

CHAPTER 29 *Skin Infections
and Infestations*

Skin infections are bacterial, viral, or fungal. Flies, mosquitoes, chiggers, bees, fire ants, mites, ticks, spiders, and scorpions are the frequent cause of arthropod bites and stings. Skin infestations include scabies and lice.

Skin infections

Bacterial infections include impetigo contagiosa, pyoderma, folliculitis, furuncle, carbuncle, cellulitis, and staphylococcal scalded skin syndrome.

Viral infections include verruca, verruca plantaris, herpes simplex virus, varicella zoster virus, and molluscum contagiosum.

Fungal infections include tinea capitis, tinea corporis, tinea cruris, tinea pedis, and candidiasis.

DATA COLLECTION

RISK FACTORS

BACTERIAL
- Contact with infected person
- Congenital or acquired immunodeficiency disorders
- Immunosuppression
- Generalized malignancy

VIRAL: Contact with infected person

FUNGAL
- Contact with infected person
- Geographic area

EXPECTED FINDINGS

History of causative agent/exposure
BACTERIAL (29.1)
VIRAL (29.2)
FUNGAL (29.3)

LABORATORY TESTS

Cultures (bacterial, viral, fungal)

PATIENT-CENTERED CARE

NURSING CARE

- Observe the general condition of the affected area.
- Check for evidence of associated infection.
- Assist in preventing the child from scratching or touching the affected areas.
- Reinforce the importance of proper hand hygiene
BACTERIAL (29.1)
VIRAL (29.2)
FUNGAL (29.3)

CLIENT EDUCATION

Avoid the spread of infections.
- Use effective hand hygiene.
- Avoid sharing clothing, hats, combs, brushes, or towels.
- Keep the child from touching the affected area by using distraction.
- Do not squeeze vesicles.
- Apply topical medications as prescribed.
- Administer oral medications as prescribed.

Arthropod bites and stings

Scorpions, black widow, and brown recluse spiders inject venom that requires immediate attention.

DATA COLLECTION

RISK FACTORS

Geographic area

EXPECTED FINDINGS

History of causative agent/exposure **(29.4)**

PATIENT-CENTERED CARE

NURSING CARE (29.4)

CLIENT EDUCATION

- Prevent secondary infections.
- Children at risk for or who have a history of severe reactions should wear a medical alert bracelet. **Qs**
- Inspect skin after possible exposure.
- Prevent bites.
  ○ Avoid areas of tall grass.
  ○ Use insect repellent.
  ○ Avoid contact with insects.
  ○ Avoid wood piles.
  ○ Inspect and treat pets, carpets, and furniture.
  ○ Avoid flowery prints and bright clothing.
  ○ Avoid perfumes and colognes.

29.1 Bacterial skin infections

	CAUSATIVE ORGANISM	MANIFESTATIONS	MANAGEMENT
Impetigo contagiosa	Staphylococcus	Reddish macule becomes vesicular Erupts easily and becomes purulent and oozes then forms dry crusts Spreads peripherally and by direct contact Pruritus common	Topical bactericidal or triple antibiotic ointment Oral or parenteral antibiotics for severe cases Wash crusts with soap and water.
Pyoderma	Staphylococcus Streptococcus	Deeper infection into the dermis Possible systemic effects (fever, lymphangitis)	Cleanse with soap and water. Bathe using antibacterial soap. Launder washcloths and towels separately to prevent bacterial spread. Apply mupirocin to lesions. Systemic antibiotics.
Folliculitis (pimple)	*Staphylococcus aureus* Methicillin-resistant *Staphylococcus aureus* (MRSA)	Infection of a hair follicle	Apply warm moist compresses. Clean skin often. Topical antibiotic medications Systemic antibiotics for severe cases
Furuncle (boil)	*Staphylococcus aureus* MRSA	Larger swollen, red lesion of a single hair follicle	Incision, draining, and irrigation of severe lesions
Carbuncle (multiple boils)	*Staphylococcus aureus* MRSA	More extensive swollen, red lesions involving multiple hair follicles Systemic effects: malaise	For MRSA infections, soak in diluted bleach solution. Mupirocin to nares twice daily
Cellulitis	Streptococcus Staphylococcus *Haemophilus influenzae*	Firm, swollen, red area of the skin and subcutaneous tissue Skin warm to the touch Possible systemic effects (fever, malaise)	Oral or parenteral antibiotics Rest and immobilize affected area. Warm soaks as needed Acute care for systemic manifestations
Staphylococcal scalded skin syndrome (Ritter disease)	*Staphylococcus aureus*	Rough-textured skin with macular erythema Epidermis becomes wrinkled within 2 days with large bullae appearing then separates leaving a raw, red, glistening, scaled appearance to skin	Systemic antibiotics Burow's solution or saline for gentle cleansing Compresses of 0.25% silver nitrate

29.2 Viral skin infections

	CAUSATIVE ORGANISM	MANIFESTATIONS	MANAGEMENT
Verruca (warts)	Human papillomavirus	Elevated, rough, flesh colored firm papules Can occur anywhere on the skin Can be single or in groups	Individualized destructive therapy (surgical removal, electrocautery, cryotherapy, laser)
Verruca plantaris (plantar warts)	Human papillomavirus	Flat warts on the plantar surface of the feet, which are painful when walking Possibly surrounded by hyperkeratosis	Caustic solution applied to wart Wear insoles with holes to decrease pressure for 2 to 3 days Soak affected area for 20 min Repeat treatment until wart falls off
Cold sore (fever blister)	Herpes simplex virus type 1	Near a mucocutaneous area (lips, nose, buttocks, genitalia). Group of painful vesicles that itch and burn surrounded by erythematous base	Apply Burow's solution during weeping stage Soft and acid-free foods Oral antiviral (acyclovir) to reduce duration Oral antiviral (valacyclovir) for genital herpes
Genital herpes	Herpes simplex virus type 2	After drying, form a crusty area followed by exfoliation Healing occurs in 8 to 10 days Possible lymphadenopathy	
Herpes zoster (shingles)	Varicella zoster virus	Neurologic pain, hyperesthesias, or itching. Vesicular lesions along the lumbar and thoracic spine with deep nagging pain. Same virus as chicken pox	Use oral or topical analgesics Apply moist compresses Oral antiviral (acyclovir)
Molloscum contagiosum	*Poxvirus*	Flesh-colored papules on stalks (extremities, face, trunk)	Resolves spontaneously in 18 months Complicated cases: remove pox chemically or with curettage, cryotherapy, or electrodessication.

29.3 Fungal skin infections

	CAUSATIVE ORGANISM	MANIFESTATIONS	MANAGEMENT
Tinea capitis (ringworm of the scalp)	*Trichophyton tonsurans* *Microsporum audouinii* *Microsporum canis*	Scaly, circumscribed lesion with alopecia on the scalp Pruritus	Use of selenium sulfide shampoos Oral griseofulvin Complicated cases: oral ketoconazole Treat infected pets (especially cats).
Tinea corporis (ringworm of the body)	*Trichophyton rubrum* *Trichophyton mentagrophytes* *Microsporum canis*	Round erythematous scaling epidermal patch Spreads peripherally and clears centrally	Oral griseofulvin Topical antifungal (tolnaftate, clotrimazole)
Tinea cruris (jock itch)	*Epidermophyton floccosum* *Trichophyton rubrum* *Trichophyton mentagrophytes*	Medial and proximal aspect of the thigh and crural folds May include the scrotum Pruritus Round erythematous scaling patch	Apply wet compresses or take sitz bath Wear light-colored socks, well-ventilated shoes (tinea pedis) Treat infected pets (tinea corporis)
Tinea pedis (athlete's foot)	*Trichophyton rubrum* *Trichophyton interdigitale* *Epidermophyton floccosum*	Between toes or on the plantar surface of the feet. Maceration and fissuring lesions between the toes and patches with tiny vesicles on the plantar surface of the foot	
Candidiasis (moniliasis)	*Candida albicans*	Found in moist areas of the skin surface White exudate, peeling inflamed areas that bleed easily Pruritus	Topical antifungal ointment (miconazole, nystatin)

Skin infestations

Scabies mite (*Sarcoptes scabiei*) spreads by direct contact with an infected person. The mite burrows into the skin and lays eggs.

Pediculosis capitis (head lice), *Pediculus humanus capitis*, spreads by direct contact with an infected person, bedding, and objects (hair brush, clothing). The life span of the adult louse is 1 month, and they can live up to 48 hr without a human host. The female lays eggs at night, close to the skin surface and at the junction of the hair shaft. The nits hatch in 7 to 10 days.

DATA COLLECTION

RISK FACTORS

SCABIES: long-term care facilities, nursing facilities, day care settings

HEAD LICE: day care; schools; overcrowded conditions; sharing combs, brushes, or hats

EXPECTED FINDINGS

Itching (29.5)

DIAGNOSTIC TESTS

SCABIES: examination under a microscope or skin biopsy

PATIENT-CENTERED CARE

NURSING CARE (29.5)

- Check for infestation.
  - SCABIES: Pencil-like marks on skin
  - HEAD LICE: Adult lice are hard to see: small, grayish-tan, and no wings. Nits look like dandruff on the hair shaft and are firmly attached.
- Inspect for a secondary skin infection.
- Instruct the child and parents about medications. Qᴾᶜᶜ

CLIENT EDUCATION

- Avoid home remedies, as they can worsen infection.
- Practice correct laundering of potentially infected clothing and bedding.
- Contain unwashable items in a tightly sealed bag for 14 days.
- Boil combs, brushes, and hair accessories for 10 min, or soak in lice-killing products for 1 hr.
- Do not share personal items.

COMPLICATIONS

Secondary infections

Examples include staphylococcus, streptococcus, and *Haemophilus influenzae*.

NURSING ACTIONS

- Ensure the family understands the prescribed plan of care to prevent secondary infections.
- Monitor for secondary infections.
- Administer medications as prescribed for secondary infection.
- Review manifestations of secondary infections.

29.4 Arthropod bites and stings

	MANIFESTATIONS	MANAGEMENT
Mosquitoes, fleas, flies	Variable, from no reaction to hypersensitivity reaction Papular urticaria Firm papules	Use antipruritic agent. Administer oral and topical antihistamines. Take baths.
Bees, wasps, hornets, fire ants, yellow jackets	Local reaction: small red itchy wheal that is warm to the touch Systemic reaction (mild to severe): generalized edema, pain, nausea and vomiting, confusion, respiratory problems, and shock	Remove the stinger. Cleanse with soap and water. Apply cool compresses. Apply home products (baking soda, lemon juice). Administer topical and oral antihistamines. Epinephrine and corticosteroids for severe cases.
Chiggers	Bites on warm parts of the body Variable, from no reaction to hypersensitivity reaction Papular urticaria Firm erythematous papules	Systemic steroids for severe cases
Ticks	Attaches to the skin with head embedded Firm, discrete, pruritic nodule at site Possible urticaria or persistent localized edema	Remove by pulling straight up with steady, even pressure with tweezers to remove the tick. Remove any remaining parts using a sterile needle. Cleanse site with soap and disinfectant.
	LYME DISEASE: tick infected with *Borrelia burgdorferi* Can appear in any of these stages: **Stage 1: 3 to 30 days following bite** • Erythema migrans at site • Chills, fever, itching, headache, fainting, stiff neck, muscle weakness; bull's eye rash at the site of the bite **Stage 2: occurs 3 to 10 weeks following bite** • Systemic involvement begins (neurologic, cardiac and musculoskeletal) • Paralysis or weakness in the face, muscle pain, swelling in large joints (knees), fever, fatigue, splenomegaly **Stage 3: 2 to 12 months following bite** • Systemic involvement is advanced (musculoskeletal pain that includes the muscles, tendons, bursae and synovia); possible arthritis, deafness, cardiac complications and encephalopathy. • Abnormal muscle movement and weakness, numbness and tingling, speech problems	Observe clients bitten by a tick for 30 days Antibiotic (single dose) for clients who meet criteria Antibiotic (2- to 3-week course) for clients who have confirmed disease Doxycycline for children older than 8 years and amoxicillin or cefuroxime for children under 8 years. Cefuroxime for children who have an allergy to penicillin
Brown recluse spiders	Mild sting leads to transient erythema and blister Pain 2 to 8 hr following bite Star-shaped purple area in 3 to 4 days Necrotic ulceration in 7 to 14 days Systemic: elevated temperature, nausea, vomiting, malaise, joint pain	Cool compresses Antibiotic, corticosteroids Analgesic for pain Possible skin graft
Black widow spiders	Mild sting leads to swollen, painful, and erythematous site Dizziness, weakness, and abdominal pain Possible delirium, paralysis, seizures, and death	Cleanse bite with antiseptic. Apply cool compresses. Administer antivenin. Administer muscle relaxant.
Scorpions	Intense pain Erythema, burning, numbness Restlessness and vomiting Ascending paralysis: seizures, weakness, increase in pulse, thirst, salivation, dysuria, pulmonary edema leading to coma and death Death for children less than age 4 in the first 24 hr	Position site in dependent position. Keep child calm. Administer antivenin. Analgesic for pain. Admit to intensive care unit for close monitoring.

29.5 Skin infestations

	MANIFESTATIONS	MANAGEMENT
Scabies mite: Sarcoptes scabiei	Intense itching especially at night Rash, especially between fingers Thin, pencil-like marks on the skin **INFANTS** • Widespread on the body • Pimples on the trunk • Blisters on the palms of the hands and soles of the feet **YOUNG CHILDREN:** Most common on head, neck, shoulders, palms, and soles **OLDER CHILDREN:** Most common on hands, wrists, genitals, and abdomen	Apply a scabicide such as 5% permethrin cream over the entire body to remain on the skin for 8 to 14 hr; repeat in 1 to 2 weeks. Treat entire family and persons that have been in contact with infected person during and 60 days after infection. Wash underwear, towels, clothing, and sleepwear in hot water. Vacuum carpets and furniture. Apply calamine lotion or cool compresses until itching subsides following treatment. Difficult cases: May use oral ivermectin.
Pediculosis capitis (head lice): Pediculus humanus capitis	Intense itching Small, red bumps on the scalp Nits (white specks) on the hair shaft	1% permethrin shampoo Spinosad 0.9% topical suspension Remove nits with a nit comb, repeat in 7 days after shampoo treatment Wash clothing and bedding in hot water with detergent Difficult cases: use malathion 0.5%

Application Exercises

1. A nurse is collecting data from an infant who has scabies. Which of the following findings should the nurse expect? (Select all that apply.)

   A. Nits on the hair shaft

   B. Pencil-like marks on hands

   C. Blisters on soles of the feet

   D. Small, red bumps on the scalp

   E. Pimples on the trunk

2. A nurse is reviewing insect bite prevention with a group of parents. Which of the following information should the nurse include? (Select all that apply.)

   A. Wear perfumes when outside.

   B. Avoid areas of tall grass.

   C. Wear bright-colored clothing.

   D. Wear insect repellent.

   E. Check pets frequently.

3. A nurse is reinforcing teaching with a parent of a child who has pediculosis capitis. Which of the following instructions should the nurse include?

   A. Apply mayonnaise to the affected area at night.

   B. Treat all pets.

   C. Use an over-the-counter medication containing 1% permethrin.

   D. Discard the child's stuffed animals.

4. A nurse is caring for a child who has cellulitis on the hand. Which of the following actions should the nurse take?

   A. Administer oral antibiotics.

   B. Cleanse area using Burow's solution.

   C. Prepare for cryotherapy.

   D. Apply a topical antifungal medication.

5. A nurse is contributing to the plan of care for a child who has tinea capitis. Which of the following actions should the nurse recommend? (Select all that apply.)

   A. Treat infected pets.

   B. Use selenium sulfide shampoo.

   C. Cleanse area with silver nitrate.

   D. Administer antiviral medication.

   E. Use moist, warm compresses.

Application Exercises Key

1. A. Nits on the hair shaft are a manifestation of pediculosis capitis.

    B. **CORRECT:** Pencil-like marks on hands are a manifestation of scabies.

    C. **CORRECT:** Blisters on the soles of the feet are a manifestation of scabies.

    D. Small, red bumps on the scalp are a manifestation of pediculosis capitis.

    E. **CORRECT:** Pimples on the trunk are a manifestation of scabies.

    Ⓝ *NCLEX® Connection: Physiological Adaptation, Basic Pathophysiology*

2. A. Perfumes can attract insects.

    B. **CORRECT:** Insects live in tall grasses.

    C. Bright-colored clothing attracts insects.

    D. **CORRECT:** The parents should apply insect repellent to prevent insect bites.

    E. **CORRECT:** The parents should inspect pets for insects to prevent exposing family members.

    Ⓝ *NCLEX® Connection: Health Promotion and Maintenance, Health Promotion/Disease Prevention*

3. A. Home remedies such as mayonnaise increase the risk of infection; the parent should avoid their use.

    B. Pediculosis capitis involves person-to-person transmission; pets are not hosts.

    C. **CORRECT:** The parent should treat pediculosis capitis with 1% permethrin, which can be purchased over the counter.

    D. The parent should place the stuffed animals in a sealed bag for 14 days to kill the lice.

    Ⓝ *NCLEX® Connection: Physiological Adaptation, Alterations in Body Systems*

4. A. **CORRECT:** Oral antibiotics are a component of treating cellulitis.

    B. Cleansing with Burow's solution is part of treatment for staphylococcal scalded skin syndrome or herpes simplex virus.

    C. Cryotherapy is a therapy for human papillomavirus.

    D. Topical antifungal medications are part of the treatment of candidiasis or tinea corporis.

    Ⓝ *NCLEX® Connection: Physiological Adaptation, Alterations in Body Systems*

5. A. **CORRECT:** Pets, especially cats, can transmit tinea capitis to persons. The client should treat infected pets.

    B. **CORRECT:** Selenium sulfide shampoo is indicated for children who have tinea capitis.

    C. Silver nitrate compresses are indicated for the treatment of staphylococcal scalded skin syndrome.

    D. Tinea capitis is a fungal infection. The client requires an antifungal medication.

    E. Warm compresses are indicated for the treatment of bacterial skin infections.

    Ⓝ *NCLEX® Connection: Physiological Adaptation, Alterations in Body Systems*

A nurse is reinforcing teaching with a group of parents about preventing skin infections. What instructions should the nurse include? Use the ATI Active Learning Template: System Disorder to complete this item.

CLIENT EDUCATION: Describe five education points that the nurse should reinforce.

Using the ATI Active Learning Template: System Disorder

CLIENT EDUCATION
- Use effective hand hygiene.
- Avoid sharing clothing, hats, combs, brushes, and towels.
- Keep the child from touching the affected area by using distraction.
- Do not squeeze vesicles.
- Apply topical medications as prescribed.
- Administer oral medications as prescribed.

Ⓝ *NCLEX® Connection: Health Promotion and Maintenance, Health Promotion/Disease Prevention*

UNIT 2 NURSING CARE OF CHILDREN WHO
HAVE SYSTEM DISORDERS
SECTION: INTEGUMENTARY DISORDERS

CHAPTER 30 *Dermatitis and Acne*

Common skin conditions of the pediatric population include contact dermatitis, atopic dermatitis, and acne.

Contact dermatitis

Contact dermatitis is an inflammatory reaction of the skin. It is caused when the skin comes into contact with chemicals or other irritants (feces, urine, soaps, poison ivy, animals, metals, dyes, medications).

Diaper dermatitis can be caused by urine, feces, detergents, soaps, or chemicals that come in contact with the genital area. It can also be a result of *Candida albicans*.

Seborrheic dermatitis (cradle cap, blepharitis, otitis externa) has an unknown etiology but is most common during infancy and puberty.

DATA COLLECTION

RISK FACTORS

- Use of cloth or disposable diapers that are not superabsorbent.
- Exposure to an irritant

EXPECTED FINDINGS

Pruritus

PHYSICAL FINDINGS
Depends on the cause of the irritant and the client
- **Contact dermatitis**
  ○ Red bumps that can form moist, weeping blisters
  ○ Skin warm and tender to the touch
  ○ Presence of oozing, drainage, or crusts
  ○ Skin becomes scaly, raw, or thickened
- **Seborrheic dermatitis**
  ○ Thick lesions
  ○ Yellowish, scaly, oily patches
  ○ Mildly pruritic
- **Diaper dermatitis**
  ○ Bright red rash that extends gradually
  ○ Fiery red and scaly areas on the scrotum and penis
  ○ Red or scaly areas on the labia
  ○ Pimples, blisters, ulcers, large bumps, or pustules
  ○ Smaller red patches that blend together

PATIENT-CENTERED CARE

NURSING CARE

Diaper dermatitis
- Promptly remove the soiled diaper.
- Clean the perineal area with a nonirritating cleanser.
- Expose the affected area to air.
- Use superabsorbent disposable diapers to reduce skin exposure.
- Apply a skin barrier (zinc oxide, petrolatum ointment). Do not wash it off with each diaper change. Q℮ʙᴾ

Contact dermatitis: Remove irritant, and limit further exposure.

Poisonous plant exposure
- Cleanse exposed area as soon as possible with cold running water, then shower with soap and water.
- Wash clothes and shoes in hot water with detergent.
- Apply calamine lotion, Burow's solution compresses, or natural colloidal oatmeal baths.
- Use topical corticosteroid gel.
- Administer oral corticosteroids for severe reactions or for irritation on the face, neck, or genitalia.

Seborrheic dermatitis
- Treat by gently scrubbing the scalp to remove scales and crusted areas. Petrolatum, vegetable oil, or mineral oil can be helpful.
- Use a fine-tooth comb to remove the loosened crusts from the hair.
- Shampoo daily with antiseborrheic shampoo.

MEDICATIONS

Antihistamines

Hydroxyzine or diphenhydramine
Administer in cases of allergic/medication reactions.

NURSING ACTIONS: Instruct the family on the importance of the medication and administering on schedule.

CLIENT EDUCATION: Some antihistamines have a sedating effect. Monitor the child and provide for safety during use. Qs

Antibiotics

Used to treat secondary infections.

CLIENT EDUCATION: Continue the medication until the course of treatment is complete.

Antifungal ointments

Clotrimazole
Used to treat *Candida albicans*.

NURSING ACTIONS: Review the importance of the medication and administering schedule with the family.

CLIENT EDUCATION

- Change diapers frequently.
- Avoid bubble baths and harsh soaps.
- Encourage children to wear long sleeves and pants when there is risk of possible exposure to irritants.
- Remove an offending agent as soon as exposure takes place.
- Practice proper hand hygiene.
- Avoid use of wipes containing alcohol or detergents. Cleanse the diaper area with a soft cloth and warm water, cold cream, or other nonsoap cleanser.
- Do not use talcum powder.

COMPLICATIONS

Bacterial infections

Caused by breaks in the skin from scratching.

NURSING ACTIONS
- Monitor the area for indications of infection.
- Cleanse the area with mild soap and water.
- Administer antipruritics and antibiotics.

CLIENT EDUCATION
- Avoid offending agents.
- Keep fingernails trimmed short.

Atopic dermatitis

- Atopic dermatitis (AD) is a type of eczema that is characterized by pruritus and associated with a history of allergies that are of an inherited tendency (atopy). (Eczema describes a category of integumentary disorders, not a specific disorder with a determined etiology.)
- Classifications of atopic dermatitis are based on the child's age, how the lesions are distributed, and the appearance of the lesions.
- AD cannot be cured but can be well controlled.

DATA COLLECTION

RISK FACTORS

- Allergic condition and family history of atopy
- Previous skin disorder and exacerbation of present skin disorder
- Exposure to irritating or causative agents

EXPECTED FINDINGS

- Recent exposure to any irritant (medication, food, soap, animals)
- Intense pruritus

PHYSICAL FINDINGS
- Unaffected skin that can appear dry and rough
- Hypopigmentation of skin in small, diffuse areas
- Pallor surrounding the nose, mouth, and ears.
- Bluish discoloration underneath the eyes
- Numerous infections of the nails
- Lymphadenopathy, especially around affected areas
- Indications of a wound infection (swelling, purulent drainage, pain, increased temperature, redness extending beyond the wound margin)

Infants

Onset at 2 to 6 months of age with spontaneous remission by 3 years of age

DISTRIBUTION: Generalized distribution of lesions on cheeks, scalp, trunk, hands and feet, as well as extensor surfaces of extremities

LESIONS
- Symmetrical
- Erythema
- Vesicles, papules
- Weeping, oozing, crusting, scaling

Children

- Onset at 2 to 3 years of age with 90% of children having manifestations by 5 years of age
- Can follow infantile eczema

DISTRIBUTION: Lesions in the flexural areas (antecubital and popliteal fossae, neck), wrists, ankles, and feet with symmetric involvement

LESIONS
- Clusters
- Erythematous or flesh-colored papules
- Dry
- Hyperpigmented
- Lichenification
- Keratosis pilaris

Adolescents

Onset at age 12 and can continue into adulthood

DISTRIBUTION: Similar distribution to children

LESIONS
- Same as for children (clusters; erythematous or flesh-colored papules; dry; hyperpigmented; lichenification; keratosis pilaris)
- Dry, thick
- Confluent papules

PATIENT-CENTERED CARE

NURSING CARE

- Keep skin hydrated with tepid baths (with or without mild soap or emulsifying oil), then apply an emollient within 3 min of bathing. Two or three baths may be given daily with one prior to bedtime. Q EBP
- Dress the child in cotton clothing. Avoid wool and synthetic fabrics.
- Avoid excessive heat and perspiration, which increases itching.
- Avoid irritants (bubble baths, soaps, perfumes, fabric softeners).
- Provide support to the child and family.
- Wash skin folds and genital area frequently with water.
- Assist in identifying and minimizing exposure to the causative agent.

MEDICATIONS

Antihistamines

Hydroxyzine or diphenhydramine
CLIENT EDUCATION
- Some antihistamines have a sedating effect. Monitor the child during use.
- Ensure safety of the child when using sedating antihistamines. Qs

Loratadine or fexofenadine
- Oral antihistamine for antipruritic effect
- Less likely to cause sedation.
- CLIENT EDUCATION: Use during the daytime.

Antibiotics

Antibiotics are used to treat secondary infections.

Topical corticosteroids

Topical corticosteroids may be used intermittently to reduce or control flare-ups. They can be low-, moderate-, or high-potency and are prescribed based on the degree of skin involvement (extremity vs. eyelids), age of the child, and consequences from adverse effects.

Topical immunomodulators (nonsteroidal)

Tacrolimus or pimecrolimus to decrease inflammation during flare-ups

NURSING ACTIONS
- Use for children older than 2 years of age.
- Use at the start of an exacerbation of AD when skin turns red and starts to itch.

CLIENT EDUCATION
- Monitor for indications of infection.
- Change diapers when wet or soiled.
- Keep nails short and trimmed.
- Place gloves or cotton socks over hands for sleeping.
- Dress young children in soft, cotton, one-piece, long-sleeve, long-pant outfits.

- Remove items that can promote itching (woolen blankets, scratchy fabrics). Use cotton items whenever possible.
- Use mild detergents to wash clothing and linens. The wash cycle can be repeated without soap.
- Avoid latex products, tobacco smoke, furry pets, dust, and molds.
- Encourage tepid baths without the use of soap. Avoid oils and powders.
- Follow specific directions regarding topical medications, soaks, and baths. Emphasize the importance of understanding the sequence of treatments to maximize the benefit of therapy and prevent complications.
- Avoid overheating the bedroom during winter months.
- Use a room humidifier.
- Maintain treatment to prevent flare-up.
- Follow up with the provider as directed.
- Participate in support groups.

COMPLICATIONS

Infection

Caused by breaks in the skin from scratching

NURSING ACTIONS
- Keep nails trimmed.
- Administer antipruritics.
- Monitor the area for indications of infection.
- Cleanse the area with mild soap and water.

CLIENT EDUCATION: Avoid offending agents. Q PCC

Acne

- Acne is the most common skin condition during adolescence.
- Acne is self-limiting and not life-threatening. However, it poses a threat to self-image for adolescents.
- Acne involves the pilosebaceous follicles (hair follicle and sebaceous gland complex) of the face, neck, chest, and upper back.
- *Propionibacterium acnes* is the bacteria associated with inflammation in acne.

DATA COLLECTION

RISK FACTORS

- Acne has a genetic link.
- Acne affects both males and females.
- Hormonal fluctuations can result in acne flares in females.
- Cosmetic products containing ingredients such as petrolatum and lanolin can increase acne outbreaks.
- Adolescents working at fast-food restaurants can have an increased incidence of acne due to exposure to cooking grease.
- There is a possible dietary link with acne and high-glycemic-index foods and dairy products.

EXPECTED FINDINGS

Report of exacerbations and remissions

PHYSICAL FINDINGS

- Lesions (comedones) are either open (blackheads) or closed (whiteheads). Both are most often found on the face, neck, back, and chest.
- *P. acnes* can lead to inflammation manifesting as papules, pustules, nodules, or cysts.

PATIENT-CENTERED CARE

NURSING CARE

- Discuss the process of acne with the adolescent and family.
- Discuss the importance of adherence with the plan of care.
- Provide written instructions to accompany verbal instructions.
- Instruct the adolescent to gently wash the face and other affected areas, avoiding scrubbing and abrasive cleaners.
- Inform the adolescent and family about medications, especially adverse effects.
- Determine if the adolescent female is sexually active prior to beginning treatment with isotretinoin (pregnancy category X). **Qs**
- Monitor for indications of depression or suicidal ideation in adolescents who are taking isotretinoin.
- Provide support and encouragement to the adolescent and family.
- Encourage family support of the adolescent to assist in coping with body-image changes. **Qpcc**

MEDICATIONS

Tretinoin

Decreases keratin formation and clogging of the ducts

CLIENT EDUCATION

- Tretinoin can irritate the skin. Wait 20 to 30 min after washing the face before application in order to decrease skin irritation.
- Use a pea-size amount of medication and apply at night.
- Avoid sun exposure.
- Use sunscreen (SPF 15 or greater) daily to avoid sunburn.

Benzoyl peroxide

Antibacterial agent
- Inhibits growth of *P. acnes*
- Can bleach bed linens, towels, and clothing, but not skin

Topical and oral antibacterial agents

Inhibits growth of *P. acnes*

CLIENT EDUCATION

- Various topical antibacterial agents are available (clindamycin, azelaic acid, dapsone). Monitor for allergic reactions.
- Every-other-day application decreases adverse effects (drying of the skin, burning sensations, erythema).
- Oral antibacterial medications (tetracycline, doxycycline, erythromycin, minocycline) are indicated for severe acne that is unresponsive to topical agents.
- Avoid sun exposure due to photosensitivity.
- Use sunscreen with an SPF of 15 or greater when exposure to sun is unavoidable.

Isotretinoin

Affects factors involved in the development of acne
- Only prescribed by dermatologists for severe acne that is unresponsive to other therapies
- Isotretinoin is teratogenic. It is contraindicated in clients of childbearing age who are not taking oral contraceptives. If sexually active, the client must agree to use two forms of effective contraception for 1 month before and during treatment, and at least 1 month following treatment.

NURSING ACTIONS: Monitor for behavioral changes.

CLIENT EDUCATION: Adverse effects include dry skin and mucous membranes, dry eyes, decreased night vision, headaches, photosensitivity, elevated cholesterol and triglycerides, depression, suicidal ideation, and violent behaviors.

Oral contraceptive pills

- Decreases endogenous androgen production and bioavailability, resulting in decreased acne development
- Indicated only for adolescent females.

CLIENT EDUCATION

- Therapeutic effects can take 4 to 6 months to achieve.
- Therapy is combined with a topical acne treatment.
- There is a risk for phlebitis and embolism.

CLIENT EDUCATION

- Adherence to the therapeutic plan is essential to preventing acne flares.
- Eat a balanced, healthy diet.
- Get adequate sleep, rest, and daily exercise.
- Wash the affected area gently with a mild cleanser once or twice daily. Do not pick or squeeze comedones.
- Shampoo frequently.
- Wear protective clothing and sunscreen when outside.
- Avoid the use of tanning beds.
- If taking isotretinoin, follow up and monitor cholesterol and triglycerides.
- Use effective contraception while taking isotretinoin.

COMPLICATIONS

Infection and cellulitis

Caused by lesions of dermatitis and acne or breaks in the skin from scratching

NURSING ACTIONS
- Monitor the area for indications of infection.
- Cleanse the area with mild soap and water.
- Check the skin for redness, swelling, and pain, which can indicate cellulitis.
- Monitor for fever.
- Observe the face, back, and chest for scarring.

CLIENT EDUCATION Qpcc
- Notify the provider if indications of cellulitis occur.
- Loss of skin tissue due to acne formation causes scarring.
- Avoid vigorous scrubbing of the skin.
- Avoid squeezing or picking at acne.
- Possible treatments for scarring include chemical peels and laser therapy.

PRACTICE Active Learning Scenario

A nurse is reinforcing teaching with a parent of a child who has eczema. What information should the nurse include? Use the ATI Active Learning Template: System Disorder to complete this item.

ALTERATION IN HEALTH (DIAGNOSIS)

CLIENT EDUCATION: Include at least five education points.

Application Exercises

1. A nurse is reinforcing teaching with the parent of an infant who has seborrheic dermatitis of the scalp. Which of the following instructions should the nurse include?

   A. "You can use petrolatum to help soften and remove patches from your infant's scalp."

   B. "When patches are present, you should keep your infant away from others."

   C. "You should avoid washing your infant's hair while patches are present on the scalp."

   D. "When patches are present, it indicates that your infant has a systemic infection."

2. A nurse is caring for a child who has contact dermatitis due to poison ivy. Which of the following actions should the nurse take? (Select all that apply.)

   A. Remove the clothing over the rash.

   B. Initiate contact isolation precautions while the rash is present.

   C. Expose the rash to a heat lamp for 15 min.

   D. Cleanse the affected skin with hydrogen peroxide solution.

   E. Apply calamine lotion to the skin.

3. A nurse is caring for an adolescent who has acne and a prescription for isotretinoin from the dermatologist. Which of the following laboratory findings should the nurse plan to monitor?

   A. Cholesterol and triglycerides

   B. BUN and creatinine

   C. Serum potassium

   D. Serum sodium

4. A nurse is reviewing the plan of care for an infant who has diaper dermatitis. Which of the following actions should the nurse expect to include? (Select all that apply.)

   A. Apply talcum powder with every diaper change.

   B. Allow the buttocks to air-dry.

   C. Use mild soap baby wipes to cleanse the area.

   D. Use cloth diapers until the rash is gone.

   E. Apply zinc oxide ointment to the affected area.

5. A nurse is collecting data from an infant who has eczema. Which of the following findings should the nurse expect? (Select all that apply.)

   A. Generalized distribution of lesions

   B. Papules

   C. Ecchymosis in flexural areas

   D. Crusting lesions

   E. Keratosis pilaris

Application Exercises Key

1. A. **CORRECT:** The nurse should recommend that the parent use petrolatum, vegetable oil, or mineral oil to help soften and remove scales and crusted areas.

    B. Seborrheic dermatitis is not contagious, so it is not necessary to keep the infant away from others.

    C. Washing the infant's hair daily with an antiseborrheic shampoo can help remove scales and crusted areas and can help prevent recurrence.

    D. The cause of seborrheic dermatitis is unknown and is not associated with a systemic infection.

    Ⓝ NCLEX® Connection: Physiological Adaptation, Alterations in Body Systems

2. A. **CORRECT:** Removing the irritant from the skin will decrease the child's exposure. The nurse should remove the clothing over the affected area.

    B. Poison ivy is not spread by contact with the rash. Once the plant oils are removed, it cannot be transmitted to others.

    C. The nurse should avoid using a heat lamp, which can cause skin burns.

    D. The nurse should cleanse the affected area with cold running water, followed by soap and water as soon as possible following exposure.

    E. **CORRECT:** The nurse should apply calamine lotion to assist in relieving discomfort.

    Ⓝ NCLEX® Connection: Physiological Adaptation, Alterations in Body Systems

3. A. **CORRECT:** Adverse effects of isotretinoin include elevated cholesterol and triglycerides. The nurse should plan to monitor these laboratory values during treatment.

    B. Medications such as cephalosporins and furosemide can alter serum BUN and creatinine levels. However, they do not need to be monitored in clients taking isotretinoin.

    C. Medications such as diuretics and corticosteroids can alter serum potassium levels. However, they do not need to be monitored in clients taking isotretinoin.

    D. Medications such as IV fluids and corticosteroids can alter the serum sodium level. However, they do not need to be monitored in clients taking isotretinoin.

    Ⓝ NCLEX® Connection: Pharmacological Therapies, Adverse Effects/ Contraindications/Side Effects/Interactions

4. A. Talcum powder can cake and cause inhalation injury.

    B. **CORRECT:** Allowing the buttocks to air-dry facilitates thorough drying of the skin.

    C. Commercial baby wipes often contain chemicals, such as alcohol and soap, that can irritate the skin. The nurse should cleanse the diaper area with a soft cloth and warm water, cold cream or other nonsoap cleanser.

    D. Disposable superabsorbent diapers should be used for infants who have diaper dermatitis to assist in keeping the skin dry.

    E. **CORRECT:** Zinc oxide ointment protects the skin from moisture and irritation.

    Ⓝ NCLEX® Connection: Basic Care and Comfort, Elimination

5. A. **CORRECT:** Generalized distribution of lesions is an expected finding in infants who have eczema.

    B. **CORRECT:** Papules are an expected finding in infants who have eczema.

    C. Lesions, rather than ecchymosis, in the flexural areas are an expected finding in children 2 years of age and older.

    D. **CORRECT:** Crusting lesions are an expected finding in infants who have eczema.

    E. Keratosis pilaris is an expected finding in children 2 years of age and older.

    Ⓝ NCLEX® Connection: Physiological Adaptation, Basic Pathophysiology

PRACTICE Answer

Using ATI Active Learning Template: System Disorder

ALTERATION IN HEALTH (DIAGNOSIS): Eczema describes a category of integumentary disorders, not a specific disorder with a determined etiology. They are characterized by pruritus and associated with a history of allergies that are of an inherited tendency (atopy).

CLIENT EDUCATION
- Monitor for indications of infection
- Change diapers when wet or soiled.
- Keep nails short and trimmed.
- Place gloves or cotton socks over hands for sleeping.
- Dress young children in soft, cotton, one-piece, long-sleeve, long-pant outfits.
- Remove items that can promote itching (woolen blankets, scratchy fabrics). Use cotton items whenever possible.

- Use mild detergent to wash clothing and linens, or wash clothes a second time without soap.
- Avoid latex products, tobacco smoke, furry pets, dust, and mold.
- Encourage tepid baths without the use of soap. Avoid oils and powders.
- Follow specific directions regarding topical medications, soaks, and baths.

- Emphasize the importance of understanding the sequence of treatments to maximize the benefit of therapy and prevent complications.
- Avoid overheating the bedroom during winter months. Use a room humidifier.
- Maintain treatment to prevent flare-ups.
- Follow up with the provider as directed.
- Participate in support groups.

Ⓝ NCLEX® Connection: Physiological Adaptation, Illness Management

UNIT 2   NURSING CARE OF CHILDREN WHO
HAVE SYSTEM DISORDERS
SECTION: INTEGUMENTARY DISORDERS

CHAPTER 31   *Burns*

Thermal, chemical, electrical, and radioactive agents can cause burns, which result in cellular destruction of the skin layers and underlying tissue. The type and severity of the burn affect the treatment plan.

Thermal burns occur when there is exposure to flames, hot surfaces, hot liquids, or cold (frostbite). Chemical burns occur when there is exposure to a caustic agent (acid, alkali, organic compound). Cleaning agents used in the home and industrial setting cause chemical burns.

Electrical burns occur when an electrical current passes through the body. This type of burn can result in severe damage, including loss of organ function, tissue destruction with the subsequent need for amputation of a limb, and cardiac and respiratory arrest.

HEALTH PROMOTION AND DISEASE PREVENTION

- Provide adequate supervision.
- Establish a safe play area.
- Keep hot liquids, electrical cords, and chemicals out of reach.

DATA COLLECTION

RISK FACTORS

- Maltreatment, neglect, or lack of supervision
- Developmental growth of the child

EXPECTED FINDINGS

SUBJECTIVE DATA
- Type of burning agent (dry heat, moist heat, chemical, electrical, ionizing radiation, cold temperatures)
- Duration of contact
- Area of the body in which the burn occurred

PHYSICAL FINDINGS (31.1)

31.1 Stages of burns

FIRST-DEGREE	SECOND-DEGREE		THIRD-DEGREE	FOURTH-DEGREE
Superficial	**Superficial partial-thickness**	**Deep partial-thickness**	**Full-thickness**	**Deep full-thickness**
Damage to epidermis	Damage to the entire epidermis. Dermal elements are intact	Damage to the entire epidermis and some parts of the dermis. Sweat glands and hair follicles remain intact	Damage to the entire epidermis and dermis and possible damage to the subcutaneous tissue. Nerve endings, hair follicles, and sweat glands are destroyed	Damage to all layers of the skin that extends to muscle, fascia, and bones
APPEARANCE	**APPEARANCE**	**APPEARANCE**	**APPEARANCE**	**APPEARANCE**
Pink to red in color with no blisters. Blanches with pressure	Painful, moist, red in color with blisters, mild to moderate edema, and no eschar. Blanches with pressure	Mottled, red to white in color, with blisters and moderate edema. Blanches with pressure	Red to tan, black, brown, or waxy white in color. Dry, leathery appearance. No blanching	Color variable. Dull and dry. Charring. Possible visible ligaments, bone or tendons
SENSATION/HEALING	**SENSATION/HEALING**	**SENSATION/HEALING**	**SENSATION/HEALING**	**SENSATION/HEALING**
Painful. Heals within 3 to 7 days. No scarring	Painful. Heals in less than 21 days. Variable amounts of scarring. Sensitive to temperature changes, exposure to air, and light touch	Painful. Sensitive to temperature changes and light touch. Healing time can extend beyond 21 days. Scarring is likely	As burn heals, painful sensations return and severity of pain increases. Heals within weeks to months. Scarring is present. Grafting is required	No pain is present. Heals within weeks to months. Scarring is present. Grafting is required. Amputation possible

EXTENT OF INJURY

Total body surface area (TBSA)

- Age-related charts determine the extent of injury to body surface, which is expressed in percentages.
- Infants' skin is thin, so injury is likely to be deeper.
- A smaller TBSA places the child at risk for an increased severity of burns

Classification

The provider assesses and classifies wounds as minor, moderate, or major. The severity of the injury depends on the child's age, causative agent, body area (face, torso, extremities) and TBSA involved, and the extent and depth of the burn.

Minor: treated in outpatient setting

Moderate: treated in a hospital with expertise in burn care

Major: requires medical services of a burn center

LABORATORY TESTS

MAJOR BURNS: CBC, serum electrolytes, BUN, ABGs, random glucose levels, liver enzymes, urinalysis

PATIENT-CENTERED CARE

NURSING CARE

Minor burns

- Stop the burning process.
  - Place the child in a horizontal position and roll him in a blanket to extinguish the fire.
  - Run cool water over the area to stop the burning process.
  - Remove clothing or jewelry that can conduct heat.
  - Apply compresses soaked with tepid water over the injury. Do not use ice.
  - Flush chemical burns with large amounts of water.
- Cover the burn with a clean cloth to prevent contamination.
- Cleanse with mild soap and tepid water. (Avoid excess friction.)
- Removing blisters is controversial.

- Use antimicrobial ointment.
- Apply dressing and change as prescribed (often daily or twice daily).
  - Nonadherent: fine-mesh gauze
  - Hydrocolloid: occlusive dressing
- Keep the child warm.
- If necessary, child is seen in a health care facility for medical care.
- Provide mild analgesia.
- Check immunization status, and determine the need for immunization. Administer tetanus vaccine if it has been more than 5 years since last immunization.

CLIENT EDUCATION
- Avoid using greasy lotions or butter on burns.
- Monitor for indications of infection.

Moderate burns

- Avoid rupturing blistered areas due to risk for infection.
- Apply topical antibiotic and cover with a bulky dressing to prevent further damage to the burned area.
- Assist with scheduling a return visit to the provider within 24 hr to check for adequate pain control and indications of infection.

Major burns

- Maintain airway and ventilation.
- Provide humidified 100% supplemental oxygen.
- Monitor vital signs.
- Maintain cardiac output.
- Assist with initiation of IV access with large-bore catheter. Multiple access points might be necessary.
- Fluid replacement is important during the first 24 hr.
- Be prepared to monitor the child if blood products are prescribed.
- Monitor for manifestations of septic shock, and notify the provider of findings.
  - Alterations in sensorium (confusion)
  - Prolonged capillary refill time
  - Spiking fever
  - Mottled or cool extremities
  - Decreased bowel sounds
  - Tachycardia
  - Tachypnea
  - Decreased urine output

31.2 Severity grading system

Adopted by the American Burn Association

	MINOR	MODERATE	MAJOR
Partial-thickness burns	Less than 10% of TBSA	10% to 20% of TBSA	Greater than 20% of TBSA
Full-thickness burns	Usually outpatient Can require 1- to 2-day admission	Admission to hospital, preferably one with expertise in burn care	Admission to a burn center

- Manage pain.
  - Establish ongoing monitoring of pain and effectiveness of pain management.
  - Avoid IM or subcutaneous injections.
  - Expect IV opioid analgesics (morphine sulfate, midazolam, fentanyl) to be prescribed. Monitor for respiratory depression. Qs
  - Collaborate with the RN for administration of IV pain medications prior to dressing changes or procedures.
  - Use nonpharmacologic methods for pain control (guided imagery, music therapy, therapeutic touch) to enhance the effects of analgesics and promote improved pain management.
- Prevent infection.
  - Follow standard precautions when performing wound care.
  - Change dressings.
  - Restrict plants and flowers due to the risk of contact with pseudomonas.
  - Change position frequently to prevent contractures and prolonged pressure.
  - Limit visitors.
  - Use reverse isolation.
  - Monitor for manifestations of infection, and report to the charge nurse and provider.
  - Use client-designated equipment (blood pressure cuffs, thermometers).
  - Administer tetanus toxoid.
  - Administer antibiotics.
- Provide nutritional support.
  - Increase caloric intake to meet increased metabolic demands and prevent hypoglycemia.
  - Increase protein intake to prevent tissue breakdown and promote healing.
  - Provide enteral therapy if necessary due to decreased gastrointestinal motility and increased caloric needs. Total parenteral nutrition can be indicated.
  - Administer vitamins A and C to facilitate cell growth, and zinc for wound healing.
- Restore mobility.
  - Maintain correct body alignment, splint extremities, and facilitate position changes to prevent contractures.
  - Maintain active and passive range of motion.
  - Assist with ambulation as soon as the child is stable.
  - Apply pressure dressings to prevent contractures and scarring.
  - Closely monitor areas at high risk for pressure sores (heels, sacrum, back of head).
- Provide psychological support.
  - Provide developmentally appropriate support for the child.
  - Assist with coping.
  - Use a family-centered approach.
  - Recommend and assist with referrals as needed.

MEDICATIONS

Topical antibiotics

Silver sulfadiazine, mafenide
- Use with partial- and full-thickness wounds.
- Apply to cleansed, debrided area.
- Wear sterile gloves for application.

Bacitracin: Use for prevention of secondary infection.

Morphine sulfate

Analgesia administered by the RN via continuous IV infusion with boluses prior to procedures

NURSING ACTIONS
- Monitor for respiratory depression.
- Monitor pain relief.
- Educate the child and family on the safety precautions needed with opioid administration.

Midazolam, fentanyl , propofol , and nitrous oxide

Sedation and analgesia administered IV by the RN, advanced practice nurse, or provider just prior to the start of a procedure

NURSING ACTIONS
- Monitor the need for sedation prior to a procedure.
- Monitor pain relief.
- Monitor for adverse effects
- Educate the child and family about safety precautions needed with administration.

THERAPEUTIC PROCEDURES

Wound care

NURSING ACTIONS
- Premedicate prior to wound care.
  - Administer analgesics.
  - Administer hydroxyzine or diphenhydramine for pruritus.
- Remove previous dressings.
- Check for odors, drainage, and discharge.
- Cleanse the wound.
- Assist with debridement.
  - Provide hydrotherapy (place child or affected extremity in a warm tub of water or use warm running water, as if to shower) to cleanse the wound. Use once or twice a day. Use mild soap or detergent to gently wash burns, and then rinse with tepid water.
  - Encourage active range of motion during hydrotherapy.
  - Monitor for cold stress and hypothermia.

Skin coverings

Biologic skin coverings can be used to promote healing of large burns. Requires repeated surgical application.
- **Allograft (homograft):** Skin from human cadavers that is used for partial- and full-thickness burn wounds
- **Xenograft:** Obtained from animals, such as pigs, for partial-thickness burn wounds
- **Synthetic skin coverings:** Used for partial-thickness burn wounds
- **Artificial skin:** A biologic product that allows the dermis to regenerate; used for partial- and full-thickness burns (healing is faster)

Permanent skin coverings can be the treatment of choice for burns covering large areas of the body.
- **Autograft:** Client's skin
- **Sheet graft:** Sheet of skin used to cover the wound
- **Mesh graft:** Sheet of skin placed in a mesher so skin graft has small slits in it; allows graft to cover larger areas of burn wound
- **Cultured epithelium:** Epithelial cells cultured for use when grafting sites are limited

NURSING ACTIONS
- Maintain immobilization of the graft site.
- Elevate the extremity.
- Provide wound care to the donor site.
- Administer analgesics. Collaborate with the RN for IV administration.
- Monitor for infection before and after skin coverings or grafts are applied.
  - Discoloration of unburned skin surrounding burn wound
  - Green color to subcutaneous fat
  - Degeneration of granulation tissue
  - Development of subeschar hemorrhage
  - Hyperventilation indicating systemic involvement of infection
  - Unstable body temperature

CLIENT EDUCATION
- Keep the extremity elevated.
- Report evidence of infection.

INTERPROFESSIONAL CARE

Recommend and assist with referral to services (nutrition; child life; social support; respiratory, occupational, or physical therapy; individual and family counseling) as needed.

CLIENT EDUCATION Qᴛᴄ

- Continue to perform range-of-motion exercises and work with a physical therapist to prevent contractures.
- Monitor the wound for infection and perform wound care.
- Use age-appropriate safety measures for the home. Qs
  - Cover electrical outlets.
  - Supervise children when in the bath.
  - Keep irons out of reach of children.
  - Teach the dangers of playing with matches.
- Avoid sun exposure between 1000 and 1500, wear protective clothing, and apply sunscreen to prevent sunburn.

CARE AFTER DISCHARGE
- Assist with a referral for home health services.
- Assist with a referral to occupational therapy for evaluation of the home environment and assistance to relearn how to perform ADLs.
- Assist with a referral to social services for community support services.

COMPLICATIONS

Inhalation injury

Direct thermal injury
- Occurs with burns to the face and lips. Damage occurs to the tracheobronchial tree after inhalation of heated gases and toxic chemicals produced during combustion.
- Can be delayed 24 to 48 hr.
- Findings include wheezing, increased secretions, hoarseness, wet rales in the lungs, singed nasal hairs, laryngeal edema, and carbonaceous secretions.

Carbon monoxide injury
- Occurs when inhalation takes place in an enclosed area.
- Findings include mucosal erythema and edema followed by sloughing of the mucosa.

NURSING ACTIONS: Maintain airway and ventilation, and provide 100% oxygen.

Shock/systemic sepsis

NURSING ACTIONS
- Assist with the administration of IV fluids.
- Monitor I&O.
- Monitor laboratory findings, noting indications of anemia and infection.
- Monitor vital signs.
- Check sensorium.
- Check capillary refill in extremities.

Pulmonary problems

Edema, bacterial pneumonia, aspiration, embolus, pulmonary insufficiency

NURSING ACTIONS
- Maintain airway via intubation, sometimes tracheostomy.
- Administer oxygen.

Wound infections

NURSING ACTIONS
- Check for discoloration, edema, odor, and drainage.
- Check for fluctuations in temperature and heart rate.
- Obtain a wound culture.
- Administer antibiotics.
- Monitor laboratory findings, noting indications of anemia and infection.
- Maintain surgical aseptic technique with dressing changes.

Application Exercises

1. A nurse is caring for a school-age child who has a minor burn. Which of the following actions should the nurse take?
   - A. Keep the wound open to air.
   - B. Apply cool, wet compresses to the affected area.
   - C. Clean the affected area using a soft-bristle brush.
   - D. Apply lotion twice a day to the affected area.

2. A nurse is assisting with data collection from a preschooler who has major burns and suspected septic shock. Which of the following findings should the nurse expect? (Select all that apply.)
   - A. Increased body temperature
   - B. Altered sensorium
   - C. Decreased capillary refill
   - D. Decreased urine output
   - E. Increased bowel sounds

3. A nurse is assisting with the care of an adolescent who has a major burn and is experiencing severe pain. Which of the following prescriptions should the nurse expect for management of the adolescent's pain?
   - A. Morphine sulfate IV via continuous infusion
   - B. Meperidine IM as needed
   - C. Acetaminophen PO every 4 hr
   - D. Hydrocodone PO every 6 hr

4. A nurse is contributing to the plan of care for an adolescent who has a major burn. Which of the following interventions should the nurse recommend? (Select all that apply.)
   - A. Advise visitors to bring cut flowers instead of live plants.
   - B. Implement reverse isolation precautions.
   - C. Administer tetanus toxoid vaccine if more than 5 years since last immunization.
   - D. Encourage visits from the adolescent's peers.
   - E. Use client-designated equipment.

5. A nurse is assisting with the care of a school-age child who has a major burn. Which of the following actions should the nurse take?
   - A. Maintain immobilization of the affected area.
   - B. Position the child supine without pillows.
   - C. Initiate a high-protein, high-calorie diet.
   - D. Limit the child's intake of zinc.

PRACTICE Active Learning Scenario

A nurse is reinforcing teaching with a newly licensed nurse about manifestations of burns. Use the ATI Active Learning Template: Basic Concept to complete this item.

UNDERLYING PRINCIPLES: List the depth, appearance, sensation, and healing of partial-thickness, deep partial-thickness and full-thickness burns.

Application Exercises Key

1. A. The nurse should cover the burn wound to prevent contamination.

   B. **CORRECT:** The nurse should apply cool, wet compresses to stop the burning process.

   C. The nurse should use gentle cleansing with tepid water and a mild soap and avoid the use of friction.

   D. The nurse should avoid the use of lotions to burned areas.

   Ⓝ *NCLEX® Connection: Physiological Adaptation, Alterations in Body Systems*

2. A. **CORRECT:** Increased body temperature is a manifestation of septic shock.

   B. **CORRECT:** Altered sensorium is a manifestation of septic shock.

   C. Prolonged capillary refill time is a manifestation of septic shock.

   D. **CORRECT:** Decreased urine output is a manifestation of septic shock.

   E. Decreased bowel sounds are a manifestation of septic shock.

   Ⓝ *NCLEX® Connection: Physiological Adaptation, Basic Pathophysiology*

3. A. **CORRECT:** Opioids administered IV via continuous infusion are recommended for adolescents who have major burns. The nurse should collaborate with the RN for administration of the prescribed pain medication.

   B. IM medications are contraindicated for adolescents who have major burns.

   C. Mild analgesics, such as acetaminophen, are recommended for adolescents who have minor burns.

   D. IV opioid medications are recommended for adolescents who have major burns.

   Ⓝ *NCLEX® Connection: Pharmacological Therapies, Pharmacological Pain Management*

4. A. The nurse should recommend restriction of both plants and flowers to reduce the adolescent's risk of contact with pseudomonas.

   B. **CORRECT:** The nurse should recommend implementation of reverse isolation precautions to reduce the adolescent's risk of infection.

   C. **CORRECT:** The nurse should recommend administration of the tetanus toxoid vaccine to reduce the risk of infection if it has been more than 5 years since the adolescent last received the immunization.

   D. The nurse should recommend limiting visitors to reduce the adolescent's risk of infection.

   E. **CORRECT:** The nurse should recommend using client-designated equipment, such as a blood pressure cuff and thermometer, to reduce the adolescent's risk of infection.

   Ⓝ *NCLEX® Connection: Reduction of Risk Potential, Potential for Alterations in Body Systems*

5. A. The nurse should use active and passive range of motion on the child's affected area to prevent contractures.

   B. The nurse should facilitate position changes and prevent pressure to areas at risk for pressure sores.

   C. **CORRECT:** The nurse should initiate a high-protein, high-calorie diet to meet the child's increased metabolic demands and promote healing.

   D. The nurse should promote the child's intake of vitamins A and C to facilitate cell growth, and zinc to promote wound healing.

   Ⓝ *NCLEX® Connection: Physiological Adaptation, Alterations in Body Systems*

PRACTICE Answer

Using the ATI Active Learning Template: Basic Concept

UNDERLYING PRINCIPLES

Superficial	Superficial partial-thickness	Deep partial-thickness	Full-thickness	Deep full-thickness
• Damage to the epidermis • Pink to red in color with no blisters • Blanches with pressure • Painful • Heals within 3 to 7 days with no scarring	• Damage to the entire epidermis with intact dermal elements • Moist • Red in color with blisters • Blanches with pressure • Mild to moderate edema • No eschar • Painful • Sensitive to temperature changes and light touch • Heals in less than 21 days with variable scarring	• Damage to the entire epidermis and some parts of the dermis • Sweat glands and hair follicles remain intact • Mottled • Red to white in color with blisters • Blanches with pressure • Moderate edema • Painful • Sensitive to temperature changes and light touch • Healing can go beyond 21 days with scarring	• Damage to the entire epidermis and dermis with possible damage to the subcutaneous tissue • Nerve endings, hair follicles, and sweat glands are destroyed • Red to tan, black, brown, or waxy white in color • Dry, leathery appearance • No blanching • As burn heals, painful sensations return and severity of pain increases • Heals within weeks to months • Scarring is present • Grafting is required	• Damage to all layers of the skin that extends to the muscle, tendons, and bones • Color variable, dull, and dry with charring • Possible visible ligaments, bone, or tendons • No pain is present • Heals within weeks to months • Scarring is present and grafting is required • Amputation possible

Ⓝ *NCLEX® Connection: Physiological Adaptation, Pathophysiology*

NCLEX® Connections

When reviewing the following chapters, keep in mind the relevant topics and tasks of the NCLEX outline, in particular:

Pharmacological Therapies

DOSAGE CALCULATIONS: Use clinical decision making when calculating doses.

EXPECTED ACTIONS/OUTCOMES: Apply knowledge of pathophysiology when addressing pharmacological agents.

MEDICATION ADMINISTRATION: Reinforce client teaching on client self-administration of medications.

Reduction of Risk Potential

DIAGNOSTIC TESTS: Perform diagnostic testing (blood glucose, oxygen saturation, testing for occult blood).

THERAPEUTIC PROCEDURES: Assist with the performance of a diagnostic or invasive procedure.

Physiological Adaptation

ALTERATIONS IN BODY SYSTEMS
Identify and/or intervene to control signs of hypoglycemia or hyperglycemia.

Reinforce education to client regarding care and condition.

BASIC PATHOPHYSIOLOGY
Identify signs and symptoms related to an acute or chronic illness.

Apply knowledge of pathophysiology to monitoring client for alterations in body systems.

CHAPTER 32   Diabetes Mellitus

Diabetes mellitus is characterized by a partial or complete metabolic deficiency of insulin. Type 1 is characterized by destruction of pancreatic beta cells. Type 2 arises when the body fails to use insulin properly combined with insulin insufficiency.

Diabetes mellitus is a contributing factor for the development of cardiovascular disease, hypertension, renal failure, blindness, and stroke as individuals age.

DATA COLLECTION

RISK FACTORS

- Genetics can predispose a person to type 1 and type 2 diabetes mellitus.
- Toxins and viruses can predispose an individual to diabetes by destroying the beta cells, leading to type 1 diabetes mellitus.
- Obesity, physical inactivity, triglycerides greater than 250 mg/dL, and hypertension can lead to insulin resistance and type 2 diabetes mellitus.

EXPECTED FINDINGS

BLOOD GLUCOSE ALTERATIONS
- **Hypoglycemia:** blood glucose less than 60 mg/dL
  - Hunger, lightheadedness, and shakiness
  - Headache
  - Anxiety and irritability
  - Pale, cool skin
  - Diaphoresis
  - Irritability
  - Normal or shallow respirations
  - Tachycardia and palpitations
  - Strange or unusual feelings
  - Decreasing level of consciousness
  - Difficulty in thinking and inability to concentrate
  - Change in emotional behavior
  - Slurred speech
  - Headache and blurred vision
  - Seizures leading to coma

- **Hyperglycemia:** blood glucose usually greater than 250 mg/dL
  - Thirst
  - Polyuria (early), oliguria (late)
  - Nausea, vomiting, abdominal pain
  - Skin that is warm, dry, and flushed with poor turgor
  - Dry mucous membranes
  - Confusion
  - Weakness
  - Lethargy
  - Weak pulse
  - Diminished reflexes
  - Rapid, deep respirations with acetone/fruity odor due to ketones (Kussmaul respirations)

LABORATORY TESTS

DIAGNOSTIC CRITERIA FOR DIABETES
- 8-hr fasting blood glucose level of 126 mg/dL or greater
- Random blood glucose of 200 mg/dL or greater with classic signs of diabetes
- Oral glucose tolerance test of 200 mg/dL or greater in the 2-hr sample

Fasting blood glucose

CLIENT EDUCATION: Fast (no food or drink other than water) for 8 hr prior to the blood draw. Postpone antidiabetic medications until after the level is drawn.

Oral glucose tolerance test

A fasting blood glucose level is drawn at the start of the test. The client is instructed to consume a specified amount of glucose. Blood glucose levels are drawn every 30 min for 2 hr. The child must be monitored for hypoglycemia throughout the procedure.

CLIENT EDUCATION: Consume a balanced diet for the 3 days prior to the test. Fast for 8 hr prior to the test.

Glycosylated hemoglobin (HbA1c)

The expected reference range is 4% to 6%, but an acceptable target for children who have diabetes can be 6.5% to 8%.

DIAGNOSTIC PROCEDURES

Self-monitored blood glucose (SMBG) Qᴘᴄᴄ

- Blood glucose monitoring is essential to management of diabetes. Measurements should be checked at a minimum before meals and at bedtime.
- Ensure that the child follows the proper procedure for blood sample collection and use of a glucose meter.

CLIENT EDUCATION
- Check the accuracy of the strips with the control solution provided.
- Keep a record of the SMBG that includes time, date, serum glucose level, insulin dose, food intake, and other events that can alter glucose metabolism (activity level, illness).

PATIENT-CENTERED CARE

NURSING CARE Q_{Tc}

- Monitor the following.
  - Vital signs
  - Blood glucose levels and factors affecting levels (other medications, diet, activity)
  - I&O and weight
  - Skin integrity and healing status of any wounds, paying close attention to the feet and folds of the skin
  - Sensory alterations (tingling, numbness)
  - Visual alterations
  - Presence of recurrent infections
  - Dietary practices
  - Exercise patterns
  - The child's proficiency at SMBG
  - The child's proficiency at self-administering medication
- Follow facility policy for nail care. Some protocols allow for trimming toenails straight across with clippers and filing edges with a nail file. If clippers or scissors are contraindicated, the child should file nails straight across.
- Discuss personal hygiene.
- Caution the child against wearing sandals, walking barefoot, or wearing shoes without socks.
- Instruct the child to cleanse cuts with warm water and mild soap, gently dry, and apply a dry dressing. Instruct the child and parents to monitor healing and seek intervention promptly.
- Tell the child the importance of having medical identification.
- Examine the child's eyes yearly.
- Emphasize the importance of regular dental and health care visits.
- Provide nutritional guidelines.
  - Read labels for nutritional value.
  - Meal planning is based on growth and development requirements.
  - Plan meals to achieve accurate timing of food intake, activity, onset, and peak of insulin. Calories and food composition should be similar each day.
  - Eat at regular intervals and do not skip meals.
  - Count grams of carbohydrates consumed.
  - Recognize that 15 g of carbohydrates are equal to 1 carbohydrate exchange.
  - Avoid high-fat and high-carbohydrate food items.
  - Use artificial sweeteners in moderation.
- Discuss techniques for SMBG (obtaining blood samples; recording and responding to results; correctly handling supplies and equipment).
- Assist with an exercise plan.
  - Children active with team sports require a snack 30 min prior to activity.
  - Prolonged activities require food intake every 45 to 60 min.
  - Adjustment in diet and insulin can be required with changes in activities.

- Discuss child illness management guidelines.
  - Monitor blood glucose and urinary ketone levels every 3 hr.
  - Continue to take insulin or oral antidiabetic agents. However, dosages can differ.
  - Encourage sugar-free, noncaffeinated liquids to prevent dehydration.
  - Meet carbohydrate needs by eating soft foods if possible. If not, consume liquids equal to the usual carbohydrate content.
  - Rest.
  - Call the provider for the following.
    - Blood glucose greater than 240 mg/dL
    - Positive ketones in the urine
    - Disorientation or confusion occurs
    - Rapid breathing is experienced
    - Vomiting occurs more than once
    - Liquids cannot be tolerated
- Discuss manifestations of hypoglycemia (shakiness, diaphoresis, anxiety, nervousness, chills, headache, confusion, difficulty focusing, hunger, dizziness, pallor, palpations).
  - Check blood glucose levels.
  - Follow guidelines outlined by the provider or diabetes educator. Q_s
    - Treat with 10 to 15 g simple carbohydrate (1 tbsp sugar). Examples are 4 oz orange juice, 8 oz milk, 3 to 4 glucose tablets, or 4 oz regular soft drink.
    - For mild reactions, use milk or fruit juice.
    - Monitor blood glucose frequently.
    - Follow with complex carbohydrates.
    - If the child is unconscious or unable to swallow, administer glucagon SC or IM and notify the provider. Administer simple carbohydrate as soon as tolerated. Watch for vomiting, and take precautions against aspiration.
- Discuss manifestations of hyperglycemia (lethargy, confusion, thirst, nausea, vomiting, abdominal pain, manifestations of dehydration, rapid respirations, fruity breath).
  - Encourage oral fluid intake.
  - Administer insulin.
  - Test urine for ketones, and report if present.
  - Consult the provider if manifestations persist or progress.

MEDICATIONS

- Insulin is used to manage type 1 diabetes.
- The rate of onset, peak, and duration of action varies for each type of insulin. (32.1)

Insulin pumps
- Regular insulin
- Delivers a programmed amount of insulin on a consistent basis
- Boluses can be administered before meals.

Insulin injections
- Self-administered injections two or more times per day.
- Mixing insulin (usually rapid- and intermediate-acting)

32.1 Rate of onset, peak, and duration of action by insulin type

	TYPE	ONSET	PEAK	DURATION
Rapid-acting	Insulin lispro	15 to 30 min	30 min to 2.5 hr	3 to 6.5 hr
Short-acting	Regular insulin	30 min	20 min to 7 hr	4 to 12 hr
Intermediate-acting	NPH insulin	1 to 2 hr	6 to 14 hr	18 to 24 hr
Long-acting	Insulin glargine	3 to 4 hr	None	24 hr

NURSING ACTIONS

- Do not mix insulin glargine with other insulin due to incompatibility.
- Provide information regarding self-administration of insulin.
- Observe the child and parent drawing up and administering the insulin injection, and offer additional instruction as indicated.
- Observe the child and parent using the insulin pump and offer additional instruction as indicated.

CLIENT EDUCATION

- Rotate injection sites (to prevent lipohypertrophy) within one anatomic site four or five injections before switching to another anatomic site (to prevent day-to-day changes in absorption rates).
- Inject at a 90° angle. Use pinch technique if skin is thin. Aspiration for blood is not necessary.
- When mixing a rapid- or short-acting insulin with a longer-acting insulin, draw up the shorter-acting insulin into the syringe first. (This reduces the risk of introducing the longer-acting insulin into the vial of the shorter-acting insulin.)

INTERPROFESSIONAL CARE Q℠

- Refer the child and family to a diabetes nurse educator for comprehensive education in diabetes management.
- Referrals often include a pediatric endocrinologist, nutritionist, and exercise physiologist.
- School teachers, school nurses, guidance counselors, and coaches should also be involved.

COMPLICATIONS

Diabetic ketoacidosis (DKA)

- DKA is an acute, life-threatening condition characterized by hyperglycemia (glucose greater than 330 mg/dL), ketonemia, glycosuria, ketonuria, and acidosis (pH 7.30 and bicarbonate 15 mmol/L), resulting in the breakdown of body fat for energy and an accumulation of ketones in the blood, urine, and lungs. The onset is rapid, and the mortality rate is high.
- Causes of DKA include insufficient insulin, acute stress, and poor management of acute illness.

NURSING ACTIONS

- Admit the client to an intensive care unit.
- Place the client on a cardiac monitor.
- Obtain venous access for administration of fluids, electrolytes, and insulin.
- Collect subjective and objective data for DKA.
  - Ketone levels in the blood and urine
  - Blood glucose levels
  - Labs: electrolytes, BUN, ABG, CBC
  - Fruity scent to the breath
  - Mental confusion
  - Dyspnea
  - Nausea and vomiting
  - Dehydration
  - Weight loss
  - Electrolyte imbalances
  - Untreated: Coma, which can progress to death
- Provide rapid isotonic fluid (0.9% sodium chloride) replacement to maintain perfusion to vital organs. Large quantities are often required to replace losses. Monitor for fluid volume excess and cerebral edema.
- When serum glucose levels approach 250 mg/dL, glucose is added to IV fluids to maintain 120 to 240 mg/dL blood glucose levels. Regular insulin is infused continuously through an IV by trained personnel.
- Monitor glucose levels hourly, or more frequently if required.
- Monitor serum potassium levels. Potassium levels are initially elevated. With insulin therapy, potassium shifts into cells and the child needs to be monitored for hypokalemia. Provide potassium replacement therapy in all replacement IV fluids as indicated by lab values. Make sure urinary output is adequate before administering potassium.
- Sodium bicarbonate is administered by slow IV infusion for severe acidosis (pH less than 7.0) by trained personnel. Monitor potassium levels because a correction of acidosis that occurs too quickly can lead to hypokalemia. Monitor closely for changes in level of consciousness
- Administer oxygen to clients who are cyanotic and whose arterial oxygen level is less than 80%.
- Reinforce instructions to manage diabetes. Q℘c

Long-term complications

- Kidney disease
- Eye disease
- Neurologic complications

Application Exercises

1. A nurse is reviewing sick-day management with a parent of a child who has type 1 diabetes mellitus. Which of the following instructions should the nurse include in the teaching? (Select all that apply.)

    A. Monitor blood glucose levels every 3 hr.

    B. Discontinue taking insulin until feeling better.

    C. Drink 8 oz of fruit juice every hour.

    D. Test urine for ketones.

    E. Call the provider if blood glucose is greater than 240 mg/dL.

2. A nurse is reinforcing teaching about self-care with a child who has type 1 diabetes mellitus. The nurse should identify which of the following statements by the child indicates understanding?

    A. "I should skip breakfast when I am not hungry."

    B. "I should increase my insulin with exercise."

    C. "I should drink a glass of milk when I am feeling irritable."

    D. "I should draw up the NPH insulin into the syringe before the regular insulin."

3. A nurse is caring for a child who has type 1 diabetes mellitus. The nurse should identify which of the following findings are manifestations of diabetic ketoacidosis? (Select all that apply.)

    A. Blood glucose 58 mg/dL

    B. Weight gain

    C. Dehydration

    D. Mental confusion

    E. Fruity breath

4. A nurse is reinforcing teaching with a school-age child who has diabetes mellitus about insulin administration. Which of the following instructions should the nurse include?

    A. "You should inject the needle at a 30-degree angle."

    B. "You should combine glargine and regular insulin in the same syringe."

    C. "You should aspirate for blood before injecting the insulin."

    D. "You should give four or five injections in one area before switching sites."

5. A nurse is reinforcing teaching with an adolescent who has diabetes mellitus about manifestations of hypoglycemia. Which of the following findings should the nurse include? (Select all that apply.)

    A. Increased urination

    B. Hunger

    C. Manifestations of dehydration

    D. Irritability

    E. Sweating and pallor

    F. Kussmaul respirations

PRACTICE Active Learning Scenario

A nurse is caring for child who has type 1 diabetes mellitus. What nursing interventions should the nurse include? Use the ATI Active Learning Template: System Disorder to complete this item.

ALTERATION IN HEALTH (DIAGNOSIS)

MEDICATIONS: List the types of insulin used for children who have type 1 diabetes mellitus.

NURSING CARE: Describe eight interventions.

CLIENT EDUCATION: Describe three client outcomes.

Application Exercises Key

1. A. **CORRECT:** A client who is experiencing illness can have waning blood glucose levels. Frequent monitoring of blood glucose levels is done to identify hyperglycemic or hypoglycemic episodes.

    B. A client who is experiencing illness should continue taking insulin during to prevent hyperglycemic episodes.

    C. A client who is experiencing illness should drink fluids without sugars.

    D. **CORRECT:** A client who is experiencing illness should test urine for ketones to assist in early detection of ketoacidosis.

    E. **CORRECT:** A client who is experiencing illness should notify the provider of blood glucose levels greater than 240 mg/dL to obtain further instructions in caring for hyperglycemia.

    Ⓝ *NCLEX® Connection: Physiological Adaptation, Alterations in Body Systems*

2. A. A client who has diabetes should eat three meals per day with snacks and avoid skipping meals to prevent hypoglycemic episodes.

    B. The insulin requirements of a client who has type 1 diabetes decrease with exercise. Increasing the amount of insulin with exercise could precipitate a hypoglycemic episode.

    C. **CORRECT:** An early manifestation of hypoglycemia is irritability. Drinking a glass of milk, which is approximately 15 g of carbohydrates, indicates understanding of the teaching.

    D. Regular insulin should be drawn up into the syringe prior to drawing up NPH to avoid altering the regular insulin.

    Ⓝ *NCLEX® Connection: Physiological Adaptation, Alterations in Body Systems*

3. A. Diabetic ketoacidosis is classified as a blood glucose level greater than 300 mg/dL.

    B. Clients who have diabetic ketoacidosis display weight loss.

    C. **CORRECT:** Clients who have diabetic ketoacidosis experience osmotic diuresis because of the electrolyte shift.

    D. **CORRECT:** Clients who have diabetic ketoacidosis experience mental confusion because of the electrolyte shift.

    E. **CORRECT:** Clients who have diabetic ketoacidosis experience fruity breath because of the body's attempt to eliminate ketones.

    Ⓝ *NCLEX® Connection:*
    Physiological Adaptation, Medical Emergencies

4. A. The client should inject the needle at a 90° angle.

    B. The client should not mix glargine with any other medication due to incompatibility.

    C. It is not necessary to aspirate for blood prior to administering insulin.

    D. **CORRECT:** The client should administer four or five injections about 2.5 cm (1 in) apart before switching to another site.

    Ⓝ *NCLEX® Connection:*
    Pharmacological Therapies, Medication Administration

5. A. An increase in urination is a manifestation of hyperglycemia.

    B. **CORRECT:** Hunger is a manifestation of hypoglycemia because of the increased adrenergic nervous system activity.

    C. Dehydration is a manifestation of hyperglycemia.

    D. **CORRECT:** Irritability is a manifestation of hypoglycemia because of the depleted glucose in the CNS.

    E. **CORRECT:** Sweating and pallor are manifestations of hypoglycemia because of the increased adrenergic nervous system activity.

    F. Kussmaul respirations are a manifestation of hyperglycemia.

    Ⓝ *NCLEX® Connection:*
    Physiological Adaptation, Alterations in Body Systems

PRACTICE Answer

Using the ATI Active Learning Template: System Disorder

ALTERATION IN HEALTH (DIAGNOSIS):
Diabetes mellitus is characterized by a partial or complete metabolic deficiency of insulin.

MEDICATIONS
- Insulin lispro: Rapid-acting
- Regular insulin: Short-acting
- NPH insulin: Intermediate-acting
- Insulin glargine: Long-acting

NURSING CARE
- Monitor manifestations of hyperglycemia and hypoglycemia.
- Provide nail care.
- Discuss wound care.
- Provide nutritional guidelines.
- Encourage yearly eye exams.
- Encourage dental and medical follow-up.
- Discuss self-monitoring of blood glucose.
- Discuss guidelines to follow when sick.
- Discuss hypoglycemia and hyperglycemia.
- Reinforce teaching about medications.

CLIENT EDUCATION
- The child will have blood glucose levels within an acceptable range.
- The child will maintain a glycosylated hemoglobin of 8% or less.
- The child and family will be able to self-administer insulin.
- The child and family will be able to monitor for complications and intervene as necessary.
- The child and family will maintain adequate dietary intake to support growth and development.

Ⓝ *NCLEX® Connection: Physiological Adaptation, Alterations in Body Systems*

UNIT 2 NURSING CARE OF CHILDREN WHO HAVE SYSTEM DISORDERS
SECTION: ENDOCRINE DISORDERS

CHAPTER 33 *Growth Hormone Deficiency*

Human growth hormone (GH), somatotropin, is a naturally occurring substance secreted by the pituitary gland. GH is important for normal growth, development, and cellular metabolism. A deficiency in GH prevents somatic growth throughout the body.

Other hormones that work with GH to control metabolic processes include adrenocorticotropic hormone (ACTH), thyroid-stimulating hormone (TSH), and the gonadotropins (follicle-stimulating hormone and luteinizing hormone).

Hypopituitarism is the diminished or deficient secretion of pituitary hormones (primarily GH). Consequences of the condition depend on the degree of the deficiency.

DATA COLLECTION

RISK FACTORS

- Structural factors (tumors, trauma, structural defects, surgery)
- Heredity disorders
- Other pituitary hormone deficiencies (deficiencies of TSH or ACTH)
- GH deficiencies are usually idiopathic.

EXPECTED FINDINGS

PHYSICAL FINDINGS
- Short stature but proportional height and weight
- Delayed epiphyseal closure
- Increased insulin sensitivity
- Delayed dentition
- Underdeveloped jaw
- Delayed sexual development

LABORATORY TESTS

Plasma insulin–like growth factor–1 (IGF–1) and IGF binding protein–3 (IGFBP–3) levels

Further evaluation is indicated if the values are one standard deviation below the mean for age.

NURSING ACTIONS
- Collect the indicated amount of blood for the test.
- Explain the laboratory procedure to the family and child.

CLIENT EDUCATION: Fast the night before the test. Qpcc

DIAGNOSTIC PROCEDURES

GH stimulation

GH stimulation testing is generally done for children who have short stature and low levels of IGF–1 and IGFBP–3.

NURSING ACTIONS
- Assist with insertion of peripheral IV. Used for administration of medication and for obtaining blood samples throughout the test.
- Draw baseline blood samples for glucose, cortisol, and GH.
- Assist with the administration of medication that triggers the release of GH (arginine or GH-releasing hormone).
- Assist with administration of insulin. The intended hypoglycemic response stimulates secretion of GH.
- Obtain blood sample every 30 min for 3 hr following medication administration
- Check blood glucose levels every 15 to 30 min.
- Give ice chips during the procedures.
- Observe for manifestations of hypoglycemia (somnolence, diaphoresis, postural hypotension, nervousness).

CLIENT EDUCATION: NPO after midnight on the morning of the test.

Radiologic assessments

- The provider evaluates skeletal maturity by comparing epiphyseal centers on an x-ray to published age-appropriate standards.
- The provider performs a general skeletal survey on children younger than 3 years of age, or surveys the hands and wrists in older children. This provides information about growth as well as epiphyseal function.

NURSING ACTIONS: Assist in positioning the child.

Computed tomographic scanning, magnetic resonance imaging, and skull x-rays

Used to identify tumors or other structural defects

NURSING ACTIONS
- Monitor the child and assist with positioning during the procedure.
- Provide emotional support. Qpcc

Evaluation of the growth curve

NURSING ACTIONS
- Measure and plot height and weight.
- Check height velocity (height over time.)
- Determine height-to-weight relationship.
- Project target height in context of genetic potential.

PATIENT-CENTERED CARE

NURSING CARE

- Measure and mark the child's height and weight on a growth chart as part of every visit to the provider.
  - The height of a child is more affected than weight. Bone age usually matches height age.
  - Measure children who are younger than 3 years of age at least every 6 months, and children older than 3 years of age every year.
- Check and monitor effectiveness of GH replacement. GH is supplied by recombinant DNA technology.
- Administer other hormone replacements as indicated (thyroid hormone).
- Provide support to the child and family regarding psychosocial concerns (altered body image, depression). Reassure the child and family that there are no cognitive delays or deficits. Qpcc
- Stress the importance of maintaining realistic expectations based on the child's age and abilities.
- Instruct the child and parents how to administer medication by subcutaneous injection for home use.

MEDICATIONS

Somatropin

Used as a human growth hormone that is a replacement for deficiency in growth hormones

NURSING ACTIONS
- Administer the medication via subcutaneous injections.
- Use cautiously in children who are receiving insulin.

INTERPROFESSIONAL CARE

- Consult with an endocrinologist.
- Psychological counseling can be indicated to help the child and family cope during this period of time.

CLIENT EDUCATION

- There should not be any significant adverse effects when GH replacement therapy is used in prescribed doses for GH deficiency.
- GH assists with muscle growth and helps improve self-esteem.
- GH should be administered 6 to 7 days a week.
- Comply with prescribed schedule of injections.
- GH usually is continued until bone maturation takes place. Radiologic evidence of epiphyseal closure is a criterion for ending therapy. This can be 16 years of age or older for males and 14 years of age or older for females. Qebp
- Seek evaluation during early adulthood. Children who have GH deficiency in childhood should be evaluated in early adulthood to determine the need for continued replacement therapy.

COMPLICATIONS

GH deficiency without hormone replacement can result in disruption of vertical growth, delayed epiphyseal closure, retarded bone age, delayed sexual development, and premature aging later in life.

Application Exercises

1. A nurse is caring for a child who has short stature. The nurse should expect which of the following diagnostic tests to be completed to confirm growth hormone (GH) deficiency? (Select all that apply.)

   A. CT scan of the head

   B. Bone age scan

   C. GH stimulation test

   D. Serum IGF-1

   E. DNA testing

2. A nurse is reinforcing teaching with a parent of a child who has a growth hormone deficiency. The nurse should identify which of the following as complications of untreated growth hormone deficiency? (Select all that apply.)

   A. Delayed sexual development

   B. Premature aging

   C. Advanced bone age

   D. Short stature

   E. Premature epiphyseal closure

3. A parent of a school-age child who has GH deficiency asks the nurse how long the child will need to take injections for growth delay. Which of the following responses should the nurse make?

   A. "Injections are usually continued until age 10 for girls and age 12 for boys."

   B. "Injections continue until your child reaches the fifth percentile on the growth chart."

   C. "Injections should be continued until there is evidence of epiphyseal closure."

   D. "Injections will need to be continued throughout your child's entire life."

4. A nurse is collecting data from a child who has short stature. The nurse should identify which of the following findings as an indication of growth hormone deficiency?

   A. Decreased height that is proportionally equal to weight.

   B. Increased height that is proportionally greater than weight.

   C. Increased weight that is proportionally greater than height.

   D. Decreased weight that is proportionally less than height.

PRACTICE Active Learning Scenario

A nurse is assisting with the plan of care for a child who is to undergo a growth hormone (GH) stimulation test. What interventions should the nurse include? Use the ATI Active Learning Template: Diagnostic Procedure to complete this item.

NURSING INTERVENTIONS: Include one preprocedure nursing action and three intraprocedure actions.

Application Exercises Key

1. A. **CORRECT:** A CT scan of the head is conducted to determine whether there is a structural component to the short stature.

   B. **CORRECT:** A bone age scan is conducted to determine the development of the bones.

   C. **CORRECT:** A GH stimulation test is conducted to confirm diagnosis of GH deficiency.

   D. **CORRECT:** A serum IGF-1 is obtained as a preliminary test to determine GH deficiency.

   E. DNA testing is not a diagnostic test to determine GH deficiency.

   Ⓝ *NCLEX® Connection: Reduction of Risk Potential, Diagnostic Tests*

2. A. **CORRECT:** Complications of untreated growth hormone deficiency include delayed sexual development.

   B. **CORRECT:** Complications of untreated growth hormone deficiency include premature aging.

   C. Complications of untreated growth hormone deficiency include retarded bone age.

   D. **CORRECT:** Complications of untreated growth hormone deficiency include short stature.

   E. Complications of untreated growth hormone deficiency include delayed epiphyseal closure.

   Ⓝ *NCLEX® Connection: Physiological Adaptation, Basic Pathophysiology*

3. A. Injections are continued until there is evidence of epiphyseal closure; age is variable among clients.

   B. Injections are continued until there is evidence of epiphyseal closure; growth is variable among clients.

   C. **CORRECT:** Injections are continued until there is evidence of epiphyseal closure on radiographic tests.

   D. Injections are continued until there is evidence of epiphyseal closure; age is variable among clients.

   Ⓝ *NCLEX® Connection: Pharmacological Therapies, Expected Actions/Outcomes*

4. A. **CORRECT:** Children who have growth hormone deficiency present with short stature with proportional height and weight.

   B. Children who have growth hormone deficiency present with short stature with proportional height and weight.

   C. Children who have growth hormone deficiency present with short stature with proportional height and weight.

   D. Children who have growth hormone deficiency present with short stature with proportional height and weight.

   Ⓝ *NCLEX® Connection: Physiological Adaptation, Basic Pathophysiology*

PRACTICE Answer

Using the ATI Active Learning Template: Diagnostic Procedure

NURSING INTERVENTIONS

Preprocedure
- Ensure the child is NPO after midnight on the morning of the test.
- Assist with the insertion of a peripheral IV site.

Intraprocedure
- Draw baseline blood samples for glucose, cortisol, and GH.
- Assist with the administration of medication that triggers the release of GH (arginine or GH-releasing hormone).
- Assist with the administration of insulin to produce a hypoglycemic response.
- Obtain blood sample every 30 min for 3 hr following medication administration.
- Check blood glucose levels every 15 to 30 minutes.
- Provide ice chips during the procedures.
- Observe for manifestations of hypoglycemia (somnolence, diaphoresis, postural hypotension, nervousness).

Ⓝ *NCLEX® Connection: Reduction of Risk Potential, Diagnostic Tests*

NCLEX® Connections

When reviewing the following chapters, keep in mind the relevant topics and tasks of the NCLEX outline, in particular:

Safety and Infection Control

STANDARD PRECAUTIONS/TRANSMISSION-BASED PRECAUTIONS/SURGICAL ASEPSIS
Identify communicable diseases and modes of transmission (airborne, droplet, contact).

Identify the client's knowledge of infection control procedures.

Identify the need for and implement appropriate isolation techniques.

Health Promotion and Maintenance

HEALTH PROMOTION/DISEASE PREVENTION
Identify clients in need of immunizations (required and voluntary).

Identify precautions and contraindications to immunizations.

HIGH RISK BEHAVIORS: Reinforce client teaching related to client high risk behavior (unprotected sexual relations, needle sharing).

Pharmacological Therapies

MEDICATION ADMINISTRATION: Administer a subcutaneous, intradermal, or intramuscular medication.

Reduction of Risk Potential

THERAPEUTIC PROCEDURES: Reinforce client teaching on treatments and procedures.

Physiological Adaptation

ALTERATIONS IN BODY SYSTEMS: Reinforce education to client regarding care and condition.

BASIC PATHOPHYSIOLOGY

Identify signs and symptoms related to an acute or chronic illness.

Consider general principles of client disease process when providing care (injury and repair, immunity, cellular structure).

Apply knowledge of pathophysiology to monitoring client for alterations in body systems.

UNIT 2 NURSING CARE OF CHILDREN WHO
HAVE SYSTEM DISORDERS
SECTION: IMMUNE AND INFECTIOUS DISORDERS

CHAPTER 34 *Immunizations*

Administration of a vaccine stimulates the immune system to produce antibodies against a specific disease. Vaccines have the same antigen as the disease, but it is either killed or weakened and therefore not strong enough to cause the disease. Antibodies disappear after they destroy the infection/antigen, but memory cells are formed to protect from future exposures to that same infection. This is called immunity.

The Advisory Committee on Immunization Practices makes recommendations and creates guidelines regarding immunizations. Children who are born preterm should receive the dose of each vaccine according to the immunization schedule. Recommendations for immunizations change periodically. Check the CDC website (www.cdc.gov) for the most up-to-date recommendations.

CHILDHOOD IMMUNIZATIONS

For children who have missed scheduled immunizations, use the "catch-up" schedule located on the CDC website. (34.1)

PURPOSE

- Decrease or eliminate certain infectious diseases in society.
- Prevent infectious diseases and their complications.

COMPLICATIONS, CONTRAINDICATIONS, AND PRECAUTIONS

- A severe allergic reaction, such as anaphylaxis, can occur in response to any vaccine and is a contraindication for receiving further doses of that vaccine or other vaccines containing that substance. QEBP
- The common cold and other minor illnesses are not contraindications to immunizations.
- Severe febrile illness is a contraindication to all immunizations.
- Do not administer live virus vaccines (varicella, MMR) to a child who is severely immunocompromised.
- Precautions to immunizations require providers to analyze data and weigh the risks that come with immunizing or not immunizing. (34.2)

34.1 Childhood immunizations

MINIMUM AGE	NUMBER OF DOSES	SCHEDULE	CONSIDERATIONS
Hepatitis B (HepB)			
Birth	Three	Birth 1 to 2 months 6 to 18 months	Minimum of 4 weeks between doses one and two. Minimum of 8 weeks between doses two and three. Final dose no earlier than 24 weeks of age and at least 16 weeks after first dose. Should be withheld for infants born prematurely and weighing less than 2,000 g if the mother is negative for hepatitis B.
Rotavirus (RV)			
6 weeks	Two (RV1) or Three (RV5)	2 and 4 months (Rotarix [RV1]) or 2, 4, and 6 months (RotaTeq [RV5])	Maximum age for the first dose is 14 weeks, 6 days. Maximum age for the last dose is 8 months, 0 days. Series should not be initiated for children 15 weeks, 0 days or older.
Diphtheria, tetanus, and acellular pertussis (DTaP)			
6 weeks	Five	2 months 4 months 6 months 15 to 18 months 4 to 6 years	Minimum of 6 months between doses three and four. Dose four can be given as early as 12 months of age. Dose five is not needed if dose four was given at 4 years of age or older.

MINIMUM AGE	NUMBER OF DOSES	SCHEDULE	CONSIDERATIONS
Tetanus, diphtheria, and acellular pertussis (Tdap); tetanus and diphtheria (Td)			
10 years	One (Tdap) Every 10 years (Td)	11 to 12 years then Booster every 10 years (Td)	Administer one dose to adolescents who are pregnant (with each pregnancy) regardless of timing of previous Td or Tdap vaccine (27 to 36 weeks of gestation). Booster with Td every 10 years after administration of Tdap. Administer Tdap or Td according to recommendations for wounds other than clean, minor if 5 years, or longer since previous dose of tetanus toxoid.
Haemophilus influenzae type b (Hib)			
6 weeks (all except Hiberix) 12 months (Hiberix)	Four (ActHIB, MenHibrix, or Pentacel) or Three (PedvaxHib or COMVAX)	2 months 4 months 6 months (only if four-dose series) 12 to 15 months (booster dose with any Hib-containing vaccine)	Administer Hiberix as a booster dose at 12 months to 4 years of age only if a prior dose of Hib was received. Only 1 dose is recommended for children who are 15 months of age or older, and not immunized.
Pneumococcal conjugate (PCV13)			
6 weeks	Four	2 months 4 months 6 months 12 to 15 months	Administer a one-time dose of PCV13 to children who are 14 to 59 months of age and received age-appropriate dosing with PCV7. Follow current recommendations for dual vaccination series with PCV13 and PPSV23 for children who have high-risk conditions.
Inactivated poliovirus (IPV)			
6 weeks	Four	2 months 4 months 6 to 18 months 4 to 6 years	Final dose should be administered on or after the age of 4 years and at least 6 months from the previous dose.
Inactivated influenza vaccine (IIV)			
6 months	Yearly	Yearly	Administer starting with availability, usually in early fall. Administration recommendations can change yearly because the vaccine is created with different influenza strains each year.
Measles, mumps, rubella (MMR)			
12 months	Two	12 to 15 months 4 to 6 years	Administer one dose to infants age 6 to 11 months if traveling internationally. However, a two-dose series is still recommended starting at 12 to 15 months. Dose two of the series can be given prior to the age of 4 years if it has been at least 4 weeks since the first dose.
Varicella (VAR)			
12 months	Two	12 to 15 months 4 to 6 years	Dose two of the series can be given prior to the age of 4 years if it has been at least 3 months since the first dose.
Hepatitis A (HepA)			
12 months	Two	12 to 23 months 6 to 18 months after first dose	Administer the final dose 6 to 18 months after the first. Two-dose series is recommended for anyone over the age of 2 years who needs immunity to hepatitis A virus.
Meningococcal conjugate (MenACWY)			
2 months (MenACWY-CRM) 9 months (MenACWY-D)	One	11 to 12 years 16 years (booster)	Follow recommendations for earlier administration to children who have high-risk conditions or who travel to areas with hyperendemic or epidemic rates of meningococcal disease.
Human papillomavirus (HPV)			
9 years	Three	11 to 12 years 1 to 2 months after first dose 24 weeks after first dose	HPV2, HPV4, and HPV9 are approved for females. HPV4 and HPV9 are approved for males.

NURSING ADMINISTRATION

- Obtain informed consent from the child's parent or legal guardian prior to administration.
- Provide vaccine information sheets (VIS), and review the content with parents and older children. Include the publication date of each VIS given in documentation.
- Give IM immunizations in the vastus lateralis or ventrogluteal muscle in infants and young children, and into the deltoid muscle for older children and adolescents.
- Give subcutaneous injections in the outer aspect of the upper arm or anterolateral thigh.
- Use strategies to provide atraumatic care.
  - Allow the parent to remain with the child during immunization.
  - Use an appropriately sized needle for the route, site, age, and amount of medication. Adequate needle length reduces the incidence of swelling and tenderness at the injection site. Qpcc
    - Provide distraction.
    - Apply a topical anesthetic prior to injection.
    - Encourage breastfeeding during immunization or give infants a concentrated oral sucrose solution 2 min prior to, during, and 3 min after immunization administration
- Monitor the child for adverse effects following administration according to facility policy and Advisory Committee on Immunization Practices recommendations. Have emergency medications and equipment on standby in case the child experiences an allergic response, such as anaphylaxis (rare).
- Encourage caregivers to use comforting measures.
  - During the procedure: cuddling, pacifiers
  - After the procedure: cool compresses to injection site, gentle movement of involved extremity
- Provide praise afterward.
- Apply a colorful bandage, if appropriate.
- Document the administration of the vaccine.
  - Date, route, and site of immunization
  - Type, manufacturer, lot number, and expiration date of the vaccine
  - Evidence of informed consent from the parent or legal guardian
  - Name, address, and title of administering nurse
- Encourage parents to maintain up-to-date immunizations for the child.
- Instruct parents to avoid administering aspirin to the child to treat fever or local reaction following administration of a live virus vaccine due to the risk of Reye syndrome.
- Instruct the parents and child to observe for complications and notify the provider if adverse effects occur.
- Report any adverse reactions to the Vaccine Adverse Event Reporting System.

NURSING EVALUATION OF MEDICATION EFFECTIVENESS

Depending on therapeutic intent, effectiveness can be evidenced by the following.
- Improvement of local reaction to immunization with absence of pain, fever, and swelling at the site of injection
- Development of immunity

34.2 Immunization considerations

ADVERSE EFFECTS	CONTRAINDICATIONS	PRECAUTIONS
DTaP		
Mild • Redness, swelling, and tenderness at the injection site • Low fever • Behavioral changes (drowsiness, irritability, anorexia) Moderate • Inconsolable crying for 3 hr or more • Fever 40.6° C (105° F) or higher • Seizures (with or without fever) • Shock-like state Severe: Acute encephalopathy (rare)	Encephalopathy within 7 days following prior doses of the vaccine	Guillain-Barré syndrome within 6 weeks of prior dose of tetanus toxoid Progressive neurologic disorders; uncontrolled seizures Fever 40.6° C (105° F) or higher within 48 hr of prior dose Shock-like state within 48 hr of prior dose Seizures within 3 days of prior dose Inconsolable crying for 3 hr or more within 48 hr of prior dose
Hib		
Redness, swelling, warmth, and tenderness at the injection site Fever greater than 37.8° C (101° F), vomiting, diarrhea, and crying	Age younger than 6 weeks	

ADVERSE EFFECTS	CONTRAINDICATIONS	PRECAUTIONS
RV		
Irritability Mild, temporary diarrhea or vomiting Intussusception	History of intussusception Severe combined immunodeficiency (SCID), which is a rare disorder that is inherited	Chronic gastrointestinal disease Spina bifida Bladder exstrophy Immunocompromised (other than SCID)
IPV		
Tenderness at the injection site	Anaphylactic reaction to neomycin, streptomycin or polymyxin B,	Pregnancy
MMR		
Mild: Local reactions (rash; fever; swollen glands in cheeks and/or neck) Moderate • Joint pain and stiffness lasting for days to weeks • Febrile seizure • Low platelet count Severe • Transient thrombocytopenia • Deafness • Long-term seizures • Brain damage	Pregnancy	History of thrombocytopenia or thrombocytopenic purpura Anaphylactic reaction to eggs, gelatin, or neomycin Transfusion with blood product containing antibodies within the prior 11 months Simultaneous tuberculin skin testing
VAR		
Mild • Tenderness and swelling at injection site • Fever • Rash (mild) possible for up to 1 month after vaccination Moderate: Seizures Severe • Pneumonia • Low blood count (extremely rare) • Severe brain reactions (extremely rare)	Pregnancy Anaphylactic reaction to gelatin or neomycin	Transfusion with blood product containing antibodies within the prior 11 months Treatment with antiviral medication within 24 hr prior to immunization (avoid taking antivirals for 14 days following immunization) Treatment with corticosteroids, or other medications that affect the immune system, for 2 weeks or longer Cancer
PCV13		
Swelling, redness and tenderness at site of injection Fever Irritability Drowsiness Anorexia	Anaphylactic reaction to any vaccine containing diphtheria toxoid	
HepA		
Tenderness at the injection site Headache Anorexia Malaise	Severe allergy to latex	Pregnancy
HepB		
Tenderness at the injection site Temperature of 37.7° C (99.9° F) or higher	Anaphylactic allergy to yeast	Infant weight less than 2 kg (4.4 lb)

ADVERSE EFFECTS	CONTRAINDICATIONS	PRECAUTIONS
IIV		
Swelling, redness and tenderness at the injection site Hoarseness Fever Malaise Headache Cough Aches Increased risk for Guillain-Barré syndrome Increased risk of seizures in young children receiving PCV13 and/or DTaP simultaneously		Guillain-Barré syndrome within 6 weeks of prior influenza vaccine Allergic reaction (other than hives) to eggs
MenACWY		
Redness and tenderness at the injection site Fever		
HPV4 and HPV9		
Redness, swelling, and tenderness at the injection site Mild to moderate fever Headache Fainting (shortly after receiving the vaccine)	Pregnancy Severe allergy to yeast	
HPV2		
Redness, swelling and tenderness at the injection site Temperature of 37.7° C (99.9° F) or higher Headache Fatigue Nausea, vomiting, abdominal pain Myalgia Fainting (shortly after receiving the vaccine)	Pregnancy Severe allergy to latex	

Application Exercises

1. A nurse is preparing to administer immunizations to a 4-month-old infant. Which of the following actions should the nurse take to provide atraumatic care?

   A. Administer 81 mg of aspirin.

   B. Use the deltoid muscle when injecting.

   C. Ask the parents to leave the room during the injection.

   D. Provide sucrose solution on the pacifier.

2. A nurse is planning to administer recommended immunizations to a 2-month-old infant. Which of the following vaccines should the nurse plan to give? (Select all that apply.)

   A. Rotavirus (RV)

   B. Diphtheria, tetanus, and acellular pertussis (DTaP)

   C. *Haemophilus influenzae* type b (Hib)

   D. Hepatitis A (HepA)

   E. Pneumococcal conjugate (PCV13)

   F. Inactivated poliovirus (IPV)

3. A nurse is planning to administer recommended immunizations to a 4-year-old child. Which of the following vaccines should the nurse plan to give? (Select all that apply.)

   A. Inactivated poliovirus (IPV)

   B. *Haemophilus influenzae* type b (Hib)

   C. Measles, mumps, rubella (MMR)

   D. Varicella (VAR)

   E. Hepatitis B (HepB)

   F. Diphtheria, tetanus, and acellular pertussis (DTaP)

4. A nurse is reviewing the allergy history of a child prior to administration of the varicella vaccine. A prior anaphylactic reaction to which of the following is a contraindication to this immunization? (Select all that apply)

   A. Eggs

   B. Gelatin

   C. Neomycin

   D. Latex

   E. Yeast

5. A nurse in a clinic is reviewing the immunization record for a toddler. Which of the following vaccines should the nurse administer? (See the chart for additional client information.)

   DEMOGRAPHICS

   15 months old
   Female

   IMMUNIZATION RECORD

   HepB: 1 month, 2 months, 12 months
   Rotavirus: 2 months, 4 months, 6 months
   DTaP: 2 months, 4 months, 6 months
   Hib: 2 months, 4 months, 12 months
   IPV: 2 months, 4 months, 6 months
   MMR: 12 months
   Varicella: 12 months
   HepA: 12 months

   A. DTaP

   B. RV

   C. MMR

   D. HepA

PRACTICE Active Learning Scenario

A nurse is preparing to administer IIV, HPV2, and MenACWY to a 12-year-old female client. Use the ATI Active Learning Template: Medication to complete this item.

COMPLICATIONS: Include adverse effects for each vaccine.

Application Exercises Key

1. A. The nurse should avoid administering aspirin to an infant due to the risk of Reye syndrome.

    B. The nurse should give IM immunizations in the vastus lateralis or ventrogluteal muscle in infants and young children, and into the deltoid muscle for older children and adolescents.

    C. The nurse should allow the parent to remain with the infant during immunization to reduce the infant's level of anxiety.

    D. **CORRECT:** The nurse should encourage breastfeeding during immunization or allow an infant to suck on a pacifier with sucrose solution to decrease the infant's level of pain during immunization.

    Ⓝ *NCLEX® Connection: Health Promotion and Maintenance, Aging Process*

2. A. **CORRECT:** RV is given as a two-or three-dose series starting at 2 months of age.

    B. **CORRECT:** DTaP is given as a five-dose series starting at 2 months of age.

    C. **CORRECT:** Hib is given as a three-or four-dose series starting at 2 months of age.

    D. HepA is given as a two-dose series starting at 12 months of age.

    E. **CORRECT:** PCV13 is given as a four-dose series starting at 2 months of age.

    F. **CORRECT:** IPV is given as a four-dose series starting at 2 months of age.

    Ⓝ *NCLEX® Connection: Health Promotion and Maintenance, Health Promotion/Disease Prevention*

3. A. **CORRECT:** Four doses of IPV are given during childhood with the final dose given at 4 to 6 years of age.

    B. The series of Hib vaccines is complete by the age of 15 months.

    C. **CORRECT:** Two doses of MMR are given during childhood with the final dose given at 4 to 6 years of age.

    D. **CORRECT:** Two doses of VAR are given during childhood with the final dose given at 4 to 6 years of age.

    E. The series of HepB vaccines is complete by the age of 18 months.

    F. **CORRECT:** Five doses of DTaP are given during childhood with the final dose given at 4 to 6 years of age.

    Ⓝ *NCLEX® Connection: Health Promotion and Maintenance, Health Promotion/Disease Prevention*

4. A. An allergic reaction, other than hives, is a precaution for the administration of the IIV.

    B. **CORRECT:** A history of an anaphylactic reaction to gelatin is a contraindication to the varicella vaccine.

    C. **CORRECT:** A history of an anaphylactic reaction to neomycin is a contraindication to the varicella vaccine.

    D. A history of a severe allergy to latex is a contraindication to the HepA and HPV2 vaccines.

    E. A history of an anaphylactic reaction or severe allergy to yeast are contraindications to the HepB, HPV4, and HPV9 vaccines.

    Ⓝ *NCLEX® Connection: Health Promotion and Maintenance, Health Promotion/Disease Prevention*

5. A. **CORRECT:** Five DTaP immunizations are given during childhood, with the fourth dose at 15 to 18 months of age. This toddler is due for the fourth dose and should receive the fifth and final dose at 4 to 6 years.

    B. This toddler completed the three-dose rotavirus vaccine series at age 6 months.

    C. This toddler is due for the second and final dose of the MMR vaccine at 4 to 6 years.

    D. The second and final dose of the HepA vaccine is administered 6 to 18 months following the initial dose. This toddler will need to wait at least 3 more months to receive the second dose of the HepA vaccine.

    Ⓝ *NCLEX® Connection: Health Promotion and Maintenance, Health Promotion/Disease Prevention*

PRACTICE Answer

Using the ATI Active Learning Template: Medication

COMPLICATIONS

IIV
- Allergic reaction
- Swelling, redness and tenderness at the injection site
- Hoarseness
- Fever
- Malaise
- Headache
- Cough
- Aches

HPV2
- Redness, swelling and tenderness at the injection site
- Temperature of 37.7° C (99.9° F) or higher
- Headache
- Fatigue
- Nausea, vomiting, abdominal pain
- Myalgia
- Fainting (shortly after receiving the vaccine)

MenACWY
- Allergic reaction
- Redness and tenderness at the injection site
- Fever

Ⓝ *NCLEX® Connection: Health Promotion and Maintenance, Health Promotion/Disease Prevention*

UNIT 2 NURSING CARE OF CHILDREN WHO HAVE SYSTEM DISORDERS
SECTION: IMMUNE AND INFECTIOUS DISORDERS

CHAPTER 35 # Communicable Diseases

Communicable diseases are easily spread through airborne, droplet, or direct contact transmission. Most communicable diseases can be prevented with immunizations.

Antibiotics and antitoxins reduce serious complications. Immunizations are a form of primary prevention. Secondary prevention includes the control of the spread of the disease to others.

Check the CDC's website www.cdc.gov for current immunization recommendations.

HEALTH PROMOTION AND DISEASE PREVENTION

Conjunctivitis

SPREAD: Direct contact (viral and bacterial)

INCUBATION: Depends on the infection

COMMUNICABILITY
- **Viral:** Appears secondary to an upper respiratory tract infection; clears on its own in 7 to 14 days
- **Bacterial:** Starts in one eye, spreads to the other; clears with antibiotics
- **Allergic:** Occurs in people who have other allergic conditions; clears with allergy medications

Epstein-Barr virus (EBV)/mononucleosis

SPREAD: Saliva

INCUBATION: 30 to 50 days

COMMUNICABILITY
- Some individuals can carry EBV throughout their lives, transmitting it to others, without developing infection.
- People who have mononucleosis can transmit the virus for weeks.

Erythema infectiosum (fifth disease)/parvovirus B19

SPREAD
- Droplet
- Blood

INCUBATION: 4 to 21 days

COMMUNICABILITY: Onset of manifestations before rash appears

Mumps/paramyxovirus (35.1)

SPREAD
- Direct contact
- Droplet

INCUBATION: 14 to 21 days

COMMUNICABILITY: Immediately before and after swelling begins

Pertussis (whooping cough)/Bordetella pertussis

SPREAD
- Direct contact
- Droplet
- Indirect contact with freshly contaminated articles

INCUBATION: 6 to 20 days, usually 7 to 10 days

COMMUNICABILITY: Greatest during catarrhal stage before onset of paroxysmal stage

Rubella (German measles)/rubella virus

SPREAD
- Direct contact
- Droplet

INCUBATION: 14 to 21 days

COMMUNICABILITY: 7 days before to 5 days after the rash appears

Rubeola (measles)/rubeola virus

SPREAD
- Direct contact
- Droplet

INCUBATION: 10 to 20 days

COMMUNICABILITY: 4 days before to 5 days after the rash appears

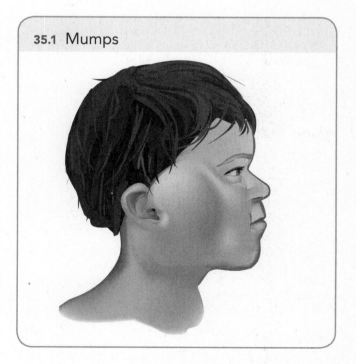

35.1 Mumps

Varicella (chickenpox)/varicella-zoster virus

SPREAD
- Direct contact
- Droplet (airborne)
- Contaminated objects

INCUBATION: 2 to 3 weeks, usually 14 to 16 days

COMMUNICABILITY: 1 day before lesions appear until all lesions have formed crusts

DATA COLLECTION

RISK FACTORS

- History of communicable disease
- Immunocompromised status
- Crowded living conditions
- Poor sanitation
- Poor nutrition
- Poor oxygenation and impaired circulation
- Chronic illness
- Recent exposure to a known case of a communicable disease
- Not immunized or up to date on immunizations

EXPECTED FINDINGS

Conjunctivitis

- Pink or red color in the sclera of the eyes
- Swelling of the conjunctiva
- Excessive tearing
- Yellow-green, purulent discharge from the eyes
- Crusting of the eyelids in the morning

Fifth disease (Erythema infectiosum)

BEFORE RASH (SEVERAL DAYS): Fever, runny nose, headache

RASH (7 DAYS TO SEVERAL WEEKS)
- Red rash on face (slapped cheek) appears from day 1 to 4.
- Maculopapular red spots symmetrically distributed on upper and lower extremities progress proximal to distal surfaces through 1 week.
- Secondary itchy rash can appear on rest of body, especially on the soles of the feet.

Measles (rubeola)

3 TO 4 DAYS PRIOR TO RASH
- Mild to moderate fever
- Conjunctivitis
- Fatigue
- Cough, runny nose, red eyes, sore throat

RASH
- Koplik spots (tiny white spots) appear in mouth 2 days before rash.
- Red or reddish-brown rash beginning on the face spreading downward.
- Spike in fever with rash.

Infectious mononucleosis

- Fever
- Lethargy
- Sore throat
- Swollen lymph glands
- Loss of appetite
- Headache
- Increased WBC
- Atypical lymphocytes
- Splenomegaly
- Hepatic involvement

Mumps

- Painful, swollen parotid glands
- Fever and muscle aches
- Headache
- Earache made worse by chewing
- Fatigue and loss of appetite

Pertussis (whooping cough)

- Common cold manifestations (runny nose, congestion, sneezing, mild fever, mild cough)
- Severe coughing starts in 1 to 2 weeks.
  - Coughing fits
  - Violent and rapid coughing
  - Loud "whooping" sound upon inspiration

Rubella (German measles)

- Low-grade fever and sore throat
- Headache
- Malaise
- Cough
- Lymphadenopathy
- Red rash that starts on the face and spreads to the rest of the body, lasting 2 to 3 days

Varicella (chickenpox)

MANIFESTATIONS 1 TO 2 DAYS PRIOR TO RASH
- Fever
- Fatigue
- Loss of appetite
- Headache

RASH
- Macules start in center of trunk, spreading to the face and proximal extremities.
- Progresses from macules, to papules, to vesicles, and crust formation follows. Lesions are present in multiple stages of progress at once.
- Scabs appear in approximately 1 week.

LABORATORY TESTS

- CBC
- Electrolyte panels
- Mono spot blood test for infectious mononucleosis

PATIENT-CENTERED CARE

NURSING CARE

SYMPTOMATIC TREATMENT
- Administer an antipyretic for fever. Do not administer aspirin, due to the risk of Reye syndrome.
- Administer an antipruritic for severe itching.
- Administer analgesics for pain.
- Provide fluids and nutritious foods of the child's preference. Qpcc
- Provide quiet diversional activities.
- Promote adequate rest with naps if necessary.
- Keep lights dim if the child develops photophobia.
- Keep the child out of the sun.
- Notify the child's school or day care of the infection. Obtain a plan from the school so that the child can continue working on schoolwork at home.
- Follow health department requirements for notification of communicable diseases. Qtc

SKIN CARE
- Provide calamine lotion for topical relief.
- Keep the skin clean and dry to prevent secondary infection.
- Keep the child cool, but prevent chilling.
- Dress the child in lightweight, loose clothing.
- Give baths in tepid water.
- Keep the child's fingernails clean and short.
- Apply mittens if the child scratches.
- Reinforce good oral hygiene. A sore throat can be managed with analgesics, lozenges, and saline rinses.
- Change linens daily.

ISOLATION PRECAUTIONS
- **Airborne/contact:** Varicella
- **Droplet**
  - Fifth disease
  - Mumps
  - Pertussis
  - Rubella
- **Standard**
  - Conjunctivitis
  - Mononucleosis

MEDICATIONS

Antihistamines

Diphenhydramine and hydroxyzine to control pruritus

NURSING ACTIONS
- Monitor the reaction to the medication because some children can become hyperalert with the administration of a medication from this group.
- Monitor for drowsiness.
- Educate the family about safety precautions. Qs

Antibiotic or antiviral therapy
- Acyclovir for high-risk clients who have varicella
- Antibiotics for pertussis
- Antibiotic eye drops for bacterial conjunctivitis

NSAIDs or acetaminophen

Decreases fever

NURSING ACTIONS: Be alert for allergies.

CLIENT EDUCATION: Use the proper dosing for acetaminophen. Qs

CLIENT EDUCATION
- Good hand hygiene prevents the spread of infection.
- Adhere with antibiotic or antiviral therapy.
- Cover nose and mouth when coughing or sneezing.
- Wash the child's bed linens daily in mild detergent.
- For children who are immunocompromised, seek prompt medical care if manifestations develop.
- Encourage adolescents to participate in decision-making.

COMPLICATIONS

Fifth disease: Self-limited arthritis and arthralgia (more common in adult females)

Mononucleosis: Ruptured spleen

Myocarditis: Fetal death if mother is infected during the second trimester of pregnancy

Mumps: Orchitis, encephalitis, meningitis, oophoritis, mastitis, deafness, myocarditis, arthritis, hepatitis, pancreatitis, sterility in adult men

Pertussis
- Infants and children: pneumonia, seizures, apnea, encephalopathy, death, ear infections, hemorrhage, weight loss, hernias, rectal prolapse
- Teens and adults: weight loss, loss of bladder control, syncope, rib fractures, pneumonia

Rubella
- Complications generally rare
- Birth defects (deafness; heart defects; mental, liver, and spleen damage) in fetus of clients infected during pregnancy

Rubeola: Ear infections, pneumonia, encephalitis, death, laryngitis

Varicella: Pneumonia, bleeding problems, bacterial infection of the skin, encephalitis

Application Exercises

1. A nurse is reinforcing teaching with a group of parents about potential complications of communicable diseases. Which of the following communicable diseases can lead to pneumonia? (Select all that apply.)

   A. Rubella (German measles)

   B. Rubeola (measles)

   C. Pertussis (whooping cough)

   D. Varicella (chickenpox)

   E. Mumps

2. A nurse is reinforcing teaching with an adolescent client who has mononucleosis. The client has a fever, fatigue, swollen lymph nodes, sore throat, and a sore upper abdomen. Which of the following instructions should the nurse include? (Select all that apply.)

   A. Take antibiotics until symptoms subside.

   B. Drink plenty of liquids.

   C. Avoid participating in strenuous activities.

   D. Allow for periods of rest.

   E. Take aspirin as needed for fever and discomfort.

   F. Gargle with saltwater every 2 to 3 hr.

3. A nurse is collecting data from a client who has pertussis. Which of the following findings should the nurse expect? (Select all that apply.)

   A. Runny nose

   B. Mild fever

   C. Cough with whooping sound

   D. Swollen salivary glands

   E. Red rash

4. A nurse is reinforcing teaching with a group of parents about communicable diseases. Which of the following actions is the best method to prevent most communicable diseases?

   A. Eating a nutritious diet

   B. Avoiding persons who have infections

   C. Covering the mouth when coughing

   D. Obtaining recommended immunizations

PRACTICE Active Learning Scenario

A nurse is assisting with the care of a group of clients who have communicable diseases. Use the ATI Active Learning Template: Basic Concept to complete this item.

RELATED CONTENT: List the communicable diseases that require more than standard isolation precautions during hospitalization.

NURSING INTERVENTIONS: Identify the type of isolation precaution to be implemented with the communicable disease identified above.

Application Exercises Key

1. A. Complications of rubella include birth defects (deafness; heart defects; mental, liver, and spleen damage) in the fetus of a client infected during pregnancy.

   B. **CORRECT:** Complications of rubeola include ear infections, pneumonia, diarrhea, encephalitis, and death.

   C. **CORRECT:** Complications of pertussis include pneumonia, convulsions, apnea, encephalopathy, and death in infants and children; and weight loss, loss of bladder control, syncope, and rib fractures in teens and adults.

   D. **CORRECT:** Complications of varicella include dehydration, pneumonia, bleeding problems, bacterial infection of the skin, sepsis, toxic shock syndrome, bone or joint infections, and death.

   E. Complications of mumps include orchitis, encephalitis, meningitis, oophoritis, mastitis, and deafness.

   Ⓝ *NCLEX® Connection: Physiological Adaptation, Alterations in Body Systems*

2. A. Clients who have streptococcal pharyngitis or pertussis often receive antibiotic therapy. However, clients who have mononucleosis—a viral infection—do not.

   B. **CORRECT:** Fluids are encouraged to prevent dehydration with illness.

   C. **CORRECT:** The spleen could rupture as a result of injury. Strenuous activities should be avoided.

   D. **CORRECT:** Fatigue is common in clients who have mononucleosis. Allowing for periods of rest facilitates healing.

   E. Acetaminophen is used to control fever and discomfort.

   F. **CORRECT:** Saltwater can soothe discomfort associated with a sore throat.

   Ⓝ *NCLEX® Connection: Physiological Adaptation, Alterations in Body Systems*

3. A. **CORRECT:** A client who has pertussis has coldlike manifestations (runny nose, congestion, mild fever).

   B. **CORRECT:** A client who has pertussis has coldlike manifestations

   C. **CORRECT:** A client who has pertussis will experience coughing fits and a whooping sound.

   D. A client who has mumps will have enlarged lymph nodes.

   E. A client who has measles will have a red rash.

   Ⓝ *NCLEX® Connection: Physiological Adaptation, Basic Pathophysiology*

4. A. Eating a nutritious diet will help decrease the spread of infection. However, this is not the best method to prevent communicable disease.

   B. Avoiding people who have infections will decrease the spread of infection. However, this is not the best method to prevent communicable disease.

   C. Covering the mouth when coughing will decrease the spread of infection. However, this is not the best method to prevent communicable disease.

   D. **CORRECT:** Obtaining recommended immunizations has decreased the rate of communicable diseases and is the best method to prevent further spread of illness.

   Ⓝ *NCLEX® Connection: Health Promotion and Maintenance, Health Promotion/Disease Prevention*

PRACTICE Answer

Using ATI Active Learning Template: Basic Concept

RELATED CONTENT
- Varicella
- Rubella
- Fifth disease
- Pertussis
- Mumps

NURSING INTERVENTIONS
- Airborne/contact: Varicella
- Droplet: Rubella, fifth disease, pertussis, mumps

Ⓝ *NCLEX® Connection: Safety and Infection Control, Standard Precautions/Transmission-Based Precautions/ Surgical Asepsis*

CHAPTER 36 *Acute Otitis Media*

Acute otitis media (AOM) is an infection of the structures of the middle ear with rapid manifestations of infection. Otitis media with effusion (OME) is a collection of fluid in the middle ear but no infection.

Repeated infections can cause impaired hearing and speech delays. Many infections clear spontaneously in a few days. The majority of incidences are related to eustachian tube malfunction.

DATA COLLECTION

RISK FACTORS

- Eustachian tubes in children are shorter and more horizontal than those of adults. Otitis media is most common in the first 24 months of life and again when children enter school (ages 5 to 6). Otitis media occurs infrequently after age 7.
- Otitis media is usually triggered by a bacterial infection (*Streptococcus pneumoniae*, *Haemophilus influenzae*, *Moraxella catarrhalis*), viral infection (respiratory syncytial virus or influenza), allergies, or enlarged adenoids.
- There is a lower incidence of otitis media in infants who are breastfed (possibly due to the presence of immunoglobulin A [IgA] in breast milk), which protects against infection. Q EBP
- Incidence is higher in the winter and spring months.
- Exposure to large numbers of children (daycare)
- Exposure to secondhand smoke
- Cleft lip and cleft palate
- Noncompliance with childhood vaccinations
- Down syndrome
- Siblings or parents who have a history of chronic otitis media

EXPECTED FINDINGS

- Recent history of upper respiratory infection
- Acute onset of changes in behavior
- Frequent crying, irritability, and fussiness
- Inconsolability
- Tugging at ear
- Reports of ear pain, loss of appetite, nausea, and vomiting

PHYSICAL FINDINGS

- **AOM**
  - Rubbing or pulling on ear
  - Crying
  - Lethargy
  - Rhinorrhea, vomiting, and diarrhea
  - Bulging yellow or red tympanic membrane
  - Purulent material in middle ear or drainage from external canal
  - Decreased or no tympanic movement with pneumatic otoscopy
  - Lymphadenopathy of the neck and head
  - Temperature as high as 40° C (104° F)
  - Hearing difficulties and speech delays if otitis media becomes chronic
- **OME**
  - Feeling of fullness in the ear
  - Low temperature, purulent discharge, no pain
  - Orange discoloration of the tympanic membrane with decreased movement
  - Transient hearing loss and balance disturbances

DIAGNOSTIC PROCEDURES

Pneumatic otoscope

A pneumatic otoscope is used to visualize the tympanic membrane and middle ear structures. The otoscope also evaluates tympanic membrane movement.

NURSING ACTIONS: Gently pull the pinna down and back to visualize the tympanic membrane of a child younger than 3 years old. For a child older than 3 years, gently pull the pinna up and back. Q PCC

PATIENT-CENTERED CARE

NURSING CARE

- Provide comfort measures.
  - Administer pain medication.
  - Administer antibiotics.
  - Provide diversional activities.
- Place the child in an upright position.
- Implement fever-reduction measures.

MEDICATIONS

Acetaminophen or ibuprofen

Used to provide analgesia and reduce fever

NURSING ACTIONS
- Obtain a liquid preparation.
- Use age-appropriate techniques to administer medication.

Antibiotics

- Amoxicillin, amoxicillin-clavulanate, or azithromycin PO (10 to 14 days)
- Ceftriaxone IM (once)

NURSING ACTIONS
- Wait 72 hr for spontaneous resolution of otitis media before starting antibiotics.
- Antibiotic administration depends on the age of the child, and the presence and severity of manifestations.
- Administer in high doses orally, usually 80 to 90 mg/kg/day in two divided doses.
- The usual course of oral treatment is 10 days in children younger than 6 years of age. The course can be shorter for older children.
- The IM route is used for resistant organisms or for client-specific reasons (difficulty taking oral medications, inability to complete the oral course). Qᴘᴄᴄ

CLIENT EDUCATION
- Complete the total course of treatment.
- Observe for manifestations of allergy to the antibiotic (rash, difficulty breathing).
- Decongestants and antihistamines are not recommended for the treatment of otitis media.

Benzocaine or lidocaine

Ear drops for topical pain relief

CLIENT EDUCATION: Properly administer ear drops.

THERAPEUTIC PROCEDURES

A child who has multiple episodes of otitis media can require myringotomy with tympanostomy tube placement. Laser-assisted myringotomy is a less invasive form of this treatment.
- This procedure is performed in an outpatient setting with the administration of general anesthesia. It is usually completed in 15 min.
- A small incision is made in the tympanic membrane, and tiny plastic or metal tubes are placed into the eardrum to equalize pressure and minimize effusion.
- Recovery takes place in a PACU, and discharge usually occurs within 1 hr.
- Postoperative pain is not common and is expected to be mild if present.
- The tubes come out spontaneously (usually in 6 to 12 months).

CLIENT EDUCATION
- Limit the child's activities for a few days following surgery.
- Notify the provider when tubes come out. This usually does not require replacement of tubes.
- Avoid getting water into the child's ears while the tubes are in place. The effectiveness of earplugs is not conclusive. Follow the provider's instructions.

CLIENT EDUCATION

- Use comfort measures.
- Feed the child in an upright position when bottle- or breastfeeding.
- If drainage is present, clean the external ear with sterile cotton swabs. Apply antibiotic ointment.
- Avoid exposure to risk factors if possible (secondhand smoke, individuals who have viral/bacterial respiratory infections).
- Seek medical care at initial indication of infections (change in behavior, tugging on ear).
- Keep the child's immunizations up to date.

COMPLICATIONS

Hearing loss or speech delays

NURSING ACTIONS
- Monitor for deficits.
- Recommend referral for audiology testing if needed.

CLIENT EDUCATION: Speech therapy can be necessary.

Application Exercises

1. A nurse is caring for a toddler who has acute otitis media. Which of the following is the priority action for the nurse to take?

   A. Provide emotional support to the family.

   B. Instruct the family on care of the child.

   C. Encourage the child to socialize with other toddlers.

   D. Administer analgesics.

2. A nurse in an outpatient facility is caring for an infant who has manifestations of acute otitis media (AOM). The nurse should identify which of the following as risk factors for otitis media? (Select all that apply.)

   A. Breastfeeding without formula supplementation

   B. Attending daycare 4 days/week

   C. Immunizations up to date

   D. History of a cleft palate repair

   E. Parents who smoke cigarettes outside

3. A nurse is caring for a toddler who has had rhinitis, cough, and diarrhea for 2 days. The toddler's tympanic membrane has an orange discoloration and decreased movement. Which of the following statements should the nurse make?

   A. "Your child has an ear infection that requires antibiotics."

   B. "Your child could experience transient hearing loss."

   C. "Your child will need to be on a decongestant until this clears."

   D. "Your child will need to have a myringotomy."

4. A nurse is caring for a 2-year-old child who has had three ear infections in the past 5 months. Which of the following complications is the child at risk for developing long-term?

   A. Balance difficulties

   B. Rash

   C. Speech delays

   D. Mastoiditis

5. A nurse is collecting data from an infant. The nurse should identify which of the following findings as manifestations of acute otitis media? (Select all that apply.)

   A. Decreased pain in the supine position

   B. Rolling head side to side

   C. Loss of appetite

   D. Increased sensitivity to sound

   E. Crying

PRACTICE Active Learning Scenario

A nurse is preparing to care for an infant who has acute otitis media for the first time. What information about AOM should the nurse be aware of prior to providing care?

Use the ATI Active Learning Template: System Disorder to complete this item.

ALTERATION IN HEALTH (DIAGNOSIS)

NURSING CARE: Describe two interventions.

MEDICATIONS: List two.

CLIENT EDUCATION: Describe two education points to reinforce.

COMPLICATIONS: Identify one.

Application Exercises Key

1. A. Providing emotional support to the family is important because it promotes psychological esteem. However, another action is the priority.

   B. Instructing the family on the care of the child is important to promote recovery from illness and security of the child's health. However, another action is the priority.

   C. Encouraging the child to socialize with other toddlers is important to meet the child's need for love and belonging. However, another action is the priority.

   D. **CORRECT:** The priority action when using Maslow's hierarchy of needs is to meet the toddler's physiological need first. Administering analgesics to alleviate or decrease physical pain is the priority action for the nurse to take.

   Ⓝ *NCLEX® Connection: Physiological Adaptation, Alterations in Body Systems*

2. A. Breastfeeding helps to protect against AOM because breast milk contains secretory immunoglobulin A.

   B. **CORRECT:** Infants who attend daycare have an increased risk of OM due to the increased potential of exposure to infants and children who have viral/bacterial respiratory infections.

   C. The pneumococcal conjugate vaccine decreases the incidence of OM.

   D. **CORRECT:** Infants born with cleft palate are more prone to AOM because micro-organisms can easily enter the eustachian tubes.

   E. **CORRECT:** Exposure to secondhand smoke increases an infant's risk for AOM.

   Ⓝ *NCLEX® Connection: Health Promotion and Maintenance, Health Promotion/Disease Prevention*

3. A. Rhinitis, cough, diarrhea, and orange discoloration of the tympanic membrane are findings of otitis media with effusion (OME). The child does not require antibiotics at this time

   B. **CORRECT:** Rhinitis, cough, diarrhea, and an orange discoloration of the tympanic membrane are findings of OME. Transient hearing loss is a complication of OME.

   C. Rhinitis, cough, diarrhea, and an orange discoloration of the tympanic membrane are findings of OME. Decongestants are not recommended for the treatment of OME.

   D. Clients who have chronic OME require a myringotomy to facilitate drainage of fluid from behind the tympanic membrane.

   Ⓝ *NCLEX® Connection: Physiological Adaptation, Alterations in Body Systems*

4. A. Balance difficulties can be present with otitis media. However, it is not a long-term complication.

   B. Rash is not a complication of otitis media. However, the nurse should monitor a client prescribed antibiotic therapy for acute otitis media for a rash, which can indicate antibiotic sensitivity.

   C. **CORRECT:** Speech delay is a potential complication of otitis media.

   D. Mastoiditis can be a result of otitis media. However, it is not a long-term complication.

   Ⓝ *NCLEX® Connection: Physiological Adaptation, Basic Pathophysiology*

5. A. Infants who have acute otitis media have an increase in pain in the supine position from the fluid and pressure in the ear.

   B. **CORRECT:** Infants who have acute otitis media roll their head side to side because of the pain and pressure in the ear.

   C. **CORRECT:** Infants who have acute otitis media exhibit a loss of appetite due to the pain and pressure in the ear.

   D. Infants who have acute otitis media have a decreased sensitivity to sound from the fluid and pressure in the ear.

   E. **CORRECT:** Infants who have acute otitis media exhibit crying and irritability from the pain.

   Ⓝ *NCLEX® Connection: Physiological Adaptation, Basic Pathophysiology*

PRACTICE Answer

Using the ATI Active Learning Template: System Disorder

ALTERATION IN HEALTH (DIAGNOSIS): Acute otitis media is an infection of the structures of the middle ear with rapid manifestations of infection.

NURSING CARE
- Provide comfort care with pain medications and distraction.
- Provide management of fever.
- Place child in an upright position.

MEDICATIONS
- Amoxicillin, amoxicillin-clavulanate, or azithromycin PO; or ceftriaxone IM for antibiotic therapy
- Acetaminophen or ibuprofen for pain and fever
- Benzocaine or lidocaine ear drops for topical pain relief

Ⓝ *NCLEX® Connection: Physiological Adaptation, Pathophysiology*

CLIENT EDUCATION
- Use comfort measures.
- Feed the child in an upright position when bottle- or breastfeeding.
- If drainage is present, clean the external ear with sterile cotton swabs. Apply antibiotic ointment.
- Avoid risk factors (secondhand smoke, individuals who have viral/bacterial respiratory infections).
- Seek medical care at the onset of findings of infections (change in child's behavior, tugging on ear).
- Keep the child's immunizations up to date.

COMPLICATIONS: Hearing loss and speech delays

CHAPTER 37 *HIV/AIDS*

HIV is a viral infection that primarily affects a specific subset of T-lymphocytes, the CD4 T-cells, resulting in decreased function of the immune system. This leads to impaired organ function and a variety of opportunistic illnesses in a weakened host.

DATA COLLECTION

RISK FACTORS

- Clients who are infected with HIV/AIDS can transmit the virus to the fetus or infant perinatally or through breast milk.
- Exposure to blood products or body fluids that contain the HIV virus
- Sexual abuse
- Risky behaviors (unprotected sexual activity, IV substance use)
- Sexually transmitted infections
- Lack of awareness

EXPECTED FINDINGS

37.1 HIV infection stages

	LESS THAN 12 MONTHS (CELLS/µL*)	1 TO 5 YEARS (CELLS/µL)	6 YEARS AND OLDER (CELLS/µL)
STAGE 1	1,500 or more	1,000 or more	500 or more
STAGE 2	750 to 1,499	500 to 999	200 to 499
STAGE 3	Less than 750	Less than 500	Less than 200

*CD4+ T-lymphocyte count

HIV categories of infection

To read more about HIV, go to the website of the Centers for Disease Control and Prevention (www.cdc.gov).

Category N: Not symptomatic
No manifestations considered to be the result of HIV infection are present, or the child has only one of the conditions listed in the mildly symptomatic category.

Category A: Mildly symptomatic
Children have two or more of the following mildly symptomatic manifestations, but none of the conditions listed in the moderately or severely symptomatic categories.
- Lymphadenopathy (greater than 0.5 cm at more than 2 sites)
- Hepatomegaly
- Splenomegaly
- Recurrent upper respiratory infections, sinusitis, or otitis media
- Dermatitis
- Parotitis

Category B: Moderately symptomatic
Children have more serious manifestations.
- Anemia
- Bacterial meningitis, pneumonia, or sepsis (single episode)
- Oropharyngeal candidiasis (thrush)
- Cardiomyopathy
- Cytomegalovirus infection onset before 1 month
- Hepatitis
- Herpes simplex virus (HSV), bronchitis, pneumonitis, or esophagitis
- Diarrhea (recurrent/chronic)
- Herpes zoster
- Leiomyosarcoma
- Lymphoid interstitial pneumonia (LIP) or pulmonary lymphoid hyperplasia complex
- Persistent fever (lasting more than 1 month)
- Toxoplasmosis before 1 month of age
- Disseminated varicella
- Nocardiosis

Category C: Severely symptomatic
- Multiple serious bacterial infections (meningitis, bone or joint, abscesses of internal organ or body cavity, septicemia, pneumonia)
- Esophageal or pulmonary candidiasis, (bronchi, trachea, lungs)
- Cytomegalovirus disease (greater than 1 month of age with site other than liver, spleen, or lymph nodes)
- HSV stomatitis, bronchitis, pneumonitis, or esophagitis lasting longer than 1 month
- Kaposi's sarcoma
- Disseminated or extrapulmonary mycobacterium tuberculosis
- Encephalopathy with developmental delays
- Disseminated coccidioidomycosis
- Extrapulmonary cryptococcosis
- Cryptosporidiosis or isosporiasis with diarrhea
- Disseminated histoplasmosis
- *Pneumocystis carinii* pneumonia
- Multifocal leukoencephalopathy
- Salmonella septicemia
- Toxoplasmosis of the brain (onset before 1 month of age)
- Wasting syndrome
- Lymphoma

HIV infection: 13 to 20 years

Refer to **ADULT MEDICAL SURGICAL REVIEW MODULE, CHAPTER 76: HIV/AIDS.**

DIAGNOSTIC PROCEDURES

LABORATORY CRITERIA FOR DIAGNOSIS

- 18 months or older: Positive result from HIV enzyme-linked immunosorbent assay (ELISA) and Western blot immunoassay. Two positive results from separate blood specimens diagnose HIV positive status.
- Infants less than 18 months of age who were born to infected mothers: Positive result from polymerase chain reaction and virus culture.
- CD4 counts and viral load help track disease status and progression.

CLASSIFICATION: Children are classified by the following criteria.
- **N**: No signs or symptoms
  - N1 = no evidence of suppression
  - N2 = evidence of moderate suppression
  - N3 = severe suppression
- **A**: Mild signs or symptoms
  - A1 = no evidence of suppression
  - A2 = evidence of moderate suppression
  - A3 = severe suppression
- **B**: Moderate signs or symptoms
  - B1 = no evidence of suppression
  - B2 = evidence of moderate suppression
  - B3 = severe suppression
- **C**: Severe signs or symptoms
  - C1 = no evidence of suppression
  - C2 = evidence of moderate suppression
  - C3 = severe suppression

PATIENT-CENTERED CARE

NURSING CARE

- Encourage a balanced diet that is high in calories and protein. Provide the child's preferred food and beverages. Give nutritional supplements.
- Administer total parental nutrition if indicated by the child's nutritional status.
- Provide oral care, and report abnormalities for treatment.
- Keep the child's skin clean and dry.
- Provide nonpharmacological methods of pain relief.
- Monitor for pain, and provide adequate pain management. Use of medications can include nonsteroidal anti-inflammatory drugs (NSAIDs), acetaminophen, opioids, muscle relaxants, and/or a eutectic mixture of local anesthetics (EMLA cream) for numerous diagnostic procedures.
- Prevent infection.
  - Use standard precautions. Qs
  - Encourage deep breathing and coughing.
  - Maintain good hand hygiene.
  - Instruct the child and parents to avoid individuals who have colds/infections/viruses.
  - Encourage immunizations (pneumococcal vaccine, yearly seasonal influenza vaccine).
  - Monitor for indications of opportunistic infections.
- Administer medications for opportunistic infections.
- Identify stressors affecting the family, and recommend appropriate referrals (school/community response to child, finances, access to health care).
- Discuss with adolescents the various routes of HIV transmission (sexual transmission, IV substance use). Ensure the adolescent understands safe sex practices. Qpcc

MEDICATIONS

Antiretroviral medications

Antiretroviral medications are given at various stages of the HIV cycle to inhibit reproduction of the virus, therefore slowing progression of the HIV disease process.
- A combination of antiretroviral medications helps decrease the child's development of medication resistance.
- Antiretroviral medication therapy is lifelong.

Nucleoside reverse transcriptase inhibitors: Zidovudine, didanosine, stavudine, lamivudine, and abacavir suppress the synthesis of viral DNA.

Nonnucleoside reverse transcriptase inhibitors: Delavirdine, efavirenz, and nevirapine bind to the viral DNA, causing direct inhibition.

Protease inhibitors: Indinavir, ritonavir, nelfinavir, saquinavir, and lopinavir inhibit an enzyme needed for the virus to replicate.

NURSING ACTIONS

- Monitor laboratory results (CBC, WBC, liver function tests). Antiretroviral medications can increase alanine aminotransferase, aspartate aminotransferase, bilirubin, mean corpuscular volume, high-density lipoproteins, total cholesterol, and triglycerides.
- Caution clients about the adverse effects of the medications and ways to decrease the severity of the adverse effects.

CLIENT EDUCATION: Take the medication on a regular schedule, and do not miss doses.

Antibiotics

Trimethoprim-sulfamethoxazole: Administer to all infants who are born to infected mothers until HIV infection is excluded. QEBP

IV gamma globulin

To prevent recurrent or serious bacterial infections

INTERPROFESSIONAL CARE

- Social services can help with access to health care and medication acquisition.
- Dietitians can assist with nutritional support and promote good nutrition.

CLIENT EDUCATION

- The illness is chronic, and lifelong medication administration is needed.
- Notify the provider if the following manifestations develop: headache, fever, lethargy, warmth, tenderness, redness at joints, and neck stiffness.
- Avoid transmission of the virus (high-risk behaviors).
- Follow safe practice when using needles/syringes and administering medications.
- Plan to receive inactivated childhood immunizations. Live, attenuated vaccines can cause disease in immunosuppressed clients.

COMPLICATIONS

Failure to thrive

NURSING ACTIONS
- Obtain a baseline height and weight, and continue to monitor.
- Promote optimal nutrition. This can require the administration of total parenteral nutrition.
- Monitor growth and development for delays.
- Provide opportunities for normal development (age-appropriate toys, playing with children of the same age). Qpcc

CLIENT EDUCATION
- Ensure adequate nutrition.
- Offer foods and fluids based on the child's preferences.

Pneumocystis carinii pneumonia

NURSING ACTIONS
- Check and monitor respiratory status (respiratory rate and effort, oxygen saturation, breath sounds).
- Administer antibiotics.
- Administer an antipyretic and/or analgesics.
- Provide adequate hydration, and maintain fluid and electrolyte balance.
- Use postural drainage and chest physiotherapy to mobilize and remove fluid from the lungs.
- Promote adequate rest.
- Instruct the child and parents about the infectious process and how to prevent infection.

CLIENT EDUCATION: Maintain the medication regimen and schedule.

PRACTICE Active Learning Scenario

A nurse is reinforcing teaching with the parent of a child who has AIDS. What information should the nurse include? Use the ATI Active Learning Template: System Disorder to complete this item.

COMPLICATIONS: List two complications of AIDS and include four nursing actions for each.

Application Exercises

1. A nurse is reviewing discharge teaching with a parent of a child who has HIV. Which of the following information should the nurse include? (Select all that apply.)
   - A. Obtain yearly influenza vaccine.
   - B. Monitor a fever for 24 hr before seeking medical care.
   - C. Avoid individuals who have colds.
   - D. Provide nutritional supplements.
   - E. Administer aspirin for pain.

2. A nurse is caring for a child who has AIDS. Which of the following isolation precautions should the nurse implement?
   - A. Contact
   - B. Airborne
   - C. Droplet
   - D. Standard

3. A nurse is helping admit a child who has HIV. The nurse should identify which of the following findings as indications that the child is in the mildly symptomatic category of HIV? (Select all that apply.)
   - A. Herpes zoster
   - B. Anemia
   - C. Dermatitis
   - D. Hepatomegaly
   - E. Lymphadenopathy

4. A nurse is reinforcing teaching with a group of adolescents about HIV/AIDS. Which of the following statements should the nurse include?
   - A. "You can contract HIV through casual kissing."
   - B. "HIV is transmitted through IV substance use."
   - C. "HIV is now curable if caught in the early stages."
   - D. "Medications inhibit transmission of the HIV virus."

5. A nurse is collecting data from a child who has severely symptomatic HIV. The nurse should recognize that which of the following conditions is part of the severely symptomatic category? (Select all that apply.)
   - A. Kaposi's sarcoma
   - B. Hepatitis
   - C. Wasting syndrome
   - D. Pulmonary candidiasis
   - E. Cardiomyopathy

Application Exercises Key

1. A. **CORRECT:** A yearly influenza vaccination is recommended to protect the child from infection.

    B. The child who has HIV should receive prompt medical care for a fever, as this indicates an infection.

    C. **CORRECT:** Avoiding individuals who have colds assists in protecting the child from opportunistic infections.

    D. **CORRECT:** Providing nutritional supplements can promote improved nutrition for a child who has HIV.

    E. The parent should administer acetaminophen, NSAIDs, or opioids for pain to a child who has HIV.

    Ⓝ *NCLEX® Connection: Physiological Adaptation, Alterations in Body Systems*

2. A. Contact isolation precautions are indicated for a client who has a disease that spreads through direct contact with clients or contaminated substances.

    B. Airborne isolation precautions are indicated for a client who has a disease that spreads through small-particle droplets.

    C. Droplet isolation precautions are indicated for a client who has a disease that is spreads through large-particle droplets.

    D. **CORRECT:** Standard isolation precautions prevent transmission of diseases that spread through blood or body fluids, such as HIV.

    Ⓝ *NCLEX® Connection: Coordinated Care, Ethical Practice*

3. A. Herpes zoster is a manifestation of the moderately symptomatic category.

    B. Anemia is a manifestation of the moderately symptomatic category.

    C. **CORRECT:** The mildly asymptomatic category includes at least two mild manifestations, such as dermatitis.

    D. **CORRECT:** The mildly asymptomatic category includes at least two mild manifestations, such as hepatomegaly.

    E. **CORRECT:** The mildly asymptomatic category includes at least two mild manifestations, such as lymphadenopathy.

    Ⓝ *NCLEX® Connection: Physiological Adaptation, Basic Pathophysiology*

4. A. Blood, semen, vaginal secretions, and breast milk can carry HIV. There is no evidence that casual contact such as kissing spreads the virus.

    B. **CORRECT:** HIV is transmitted via blood, semen, vaginal secretions, and breast milk. IV substance use is a potential mode of exposure to contaminated body fluids.

    C. Antiretroviral therapy slows the progression of HIV but does not cure the disease.

    D. Medications suppress the progression of the virus, and can reduce the risk of transmission. However, medications cannot completely prevent HIV transmission from one individual to another.

    Ⓝ *NCLEX® Connection: Health Promotion and Maintenance, High Risk Behaviors*

5. A. **CORRECT:** Kaposi's sarcoma is a manifestation in a child who is severely symptomatic.

    B. Hepatitis is a manifestation in a child who is moderately symptomatic.

    C. **CORRECT:** Wasting syndrome is a manifestation in a child who is severely symptomatic.

    D. **CORRECT:** Pulmonary candidiasis is a manifestation in a child who is severely symptomatic.

    E. Cardiomyopathy is a manifestation in a child who is moderately symptomatic.

    Ⓝ *NCLEX® Connection: Physiological Adaptation, Basic Pathophysiology*

PRACTICE Answer

Using the ATI Active Learning Template: System Disorder

COMPLICATIONS

Failure to thrive
- Obtain a baseline height and weight, and continue to monitor.
- Promote optimal nutrition. This can require the administration of total parenteral nutrition.
- Monitor growth and development patterns for delays.
- Provide opportunities for normal development (age-appropriate toys, playing with children of the same age).
- Instruct the child and parents about how to meet the child's nutritional needs and to offer the child's preferred foods and fluids.

Pneumocystis carinii pneumonia (PCP)
- Check and monitor respiratory status (respiratory rate and effort, oxygen saturation, breath sounds).
- Administer antibiotics.
- Administer an antipyretic and/or analgesics.
- Provide adequate hydration, and maintain fluid and electrolyte balance.
- Use postural drainage and chest physiotherapy to mobilize and remove fluid from the lungs.
- Promote adequate rest.
- Discuss the infectious process and how to prevent infection with the parents.
- Instruct the child and parents about the importance of medication and the need to maintain the medication regimen.

Ⓝ *NCLEX® Connection: Physiological Adaptation, Unexpected Response to Therapies*

When reviewing the following chapters, keep in mind the relevant topics and tasks of the NCLEX outline, in particular:

Physiological Adaptation

ALTERATIONS IN BODY SYSTEMS: Reinforce education to client regarding care and condition.

BASIC PATHOPHYSIOLOGY

Identify signs and symptoms related to an acute or chronic illness.

Consider general principles of client disease process when providing care (injury and repair, immunity, cellular structure).

UNEXPECTED RESPONSE TO THERAPIES: Intervene in response to client unexpected negative response to therapy (unexpected bleeding).

CHAPTER 38 *Pediatric Cancers*

Working with a child who has cancer requires caring and competency. The nurse should provide individualized care and support to the child and the child's family. Pediatric cancers have a low rate of incidence compared to cancer in adults. However, some neoplasms occur predominantly in children. Types of pediatric cancers include organ neoplasms, blood neoplasms, and bone and soft tissue cancers.

For more information, see **ADULT MEDICAL SURGICAL REVIEW MODULE, CHAPTER 79: GENERAL PRINCIPLES OF CANCER.** Refer to **ADULT MEDICAL SURGICAL REVIEW MODULE** for organ neoplasms that both adults and children can acquire, such as lymphoma and liver cancer (**CHAPTER 82**), brain tumors (**CHAPTER 12**), and testicular cancer (**CHAPTER 80**).

Organ neoplasms

- Wilms' tumor (nephroblastoma) is a malignancy that occurs in the kidneys or abdomen. The tumor is usually unilateral, with 10% of cases affecting both kidneys. Diagnosis typically occurs before age 5. Metastasis is rare.
- Neuroblastoma is a malignancy that occurs in the adrenal gland, sympathetic chain of the retroperitoneal area, head, neck, pelvis, or chest. It is usually manifested during the toddler years, with 95% of cases prior to age 10. It is more common in males than females. Half of all cases have metastasized before diagnosis.
- Treatment varies by child and can be any combination of surgery, chemotherapy, and radiation.

DATA COLLECTION

RISK FACTORS

There are no known risk factors for Wilms' tumor or neuroblastoma. Q_{EBP}

EXPECTED FINDINGS

Wilms' tumor

- Painless, firm, nontender abdominal swelling or mass
- Fatigue, malaise, weight loss
- Fever
- Hematuria
- Hypertension
- Manifestations of metastasis include dyspnea, cough, and chest pain.

Neuroblastoma

- Manifestations depend upon the location and stage of disease.
- Half of children who have neuroblastoma have few findings.
- Manifestations of metastasis include an ill appearance, periorbital ecchymoses, proptosis (bulging of the eye), bone pain, anorexia and weight loss, and irritability.

LABORATORY TESTS

Wilms' tumor

- BUN, creatinine
- CBC
- Urinalysis

Neuroblastoma

CBC and coagulation studies

DIAGNOSTIC PROCEDURES

NURSING ACTIONS

- Check the child for allergies to dye or shellfish.
- Educate the parent and child prior to procedure on expectations.
- Assist the child to remain still during the procedure.
- Instruct the child to drink oral contrast if prescribed.
- Sedation might be prescribed.
- Provide emotional support. Q_{PCC}

Wilms' tumor

- Abdominal ultrasonography
- Abdominal and chest computed tomography (CT) scan or MRI.
- Bone marrow aspiration (rule out metastasis)

Neuroblastoma

- Skeletal survey
- Skull, neck, chest, abdominal, and bone CT scans
- Bone marrow aspiration (rule out metastasis)
- Biopsy of tumor

PATIENT-CENTERED CARE

NURSING CARE

- If Wilms' tumor is suspected, do not palpate the abdomen. **Qs**
- Observe the child's and family's coping ability and available support.
- Check for developmental delays related to illness.
- Monitor physical growth (height and weight).
- Reinforce education and support to the child and family regarding diagnostic testing, treatment plan, ongoing therapy, and prognosis.
- Monitor for findings of infection, and administer antibiotics.
- Keep the child's skin clean, dry, and lubricated.
- Provide oral hygiene, and keep the child's lips lubricated.
- Provide age-appropriate diversional activities.
- Provide support to the child and family.
  - Avoid false reassurance.
  - Listen to the child's concerns.
  - Allow time for the child and family to discuss feelings regarding grief and loss.

THERAPEUTIC PROCEDURES

Treatment for Wilms' tumor

- Surgical removal of the tumor and kidney soon after diagnosis
- Preoperative chemotherapy or radiation if both kidneys are involved to decrease the size of the tumors and potentially preserve one kidney
- Postoperative radiation and/or chemotherapy for children who have large tumors, metastasis, reoccurrence, and residual disease

Treatment for neuroblastoma

- Surgical removal of the tumor
- Chemotherapy and/or radiation for metastasis and residual disease

Chemotherapy

The child can have a long-term central venous access device or peripherally inserted central catheter.

ADVERSE EFFECTS
- **Mucosal ulceration**
  - Provide frequent oral care.
  - Inspect the mouth for ulceration and hemorrhage.
  - Use a soft-bristled toothbrush or a soft, disposable toothbrush for oral care.
  - Lubricate lips with lip balm to prevent cracking.
  - Offer foods that are soft and bland.
  - Assist the child to use mouthwashes (such as 1 tsp salt mixed with 1 pint of water or 1 tsp baking soda mixed with 1 qt of water) frequently.
  - Apply local anesthetics (hydrocortisone dental paste, antiseptic mouth rinse, aluminum and magnesium hydroxide) to mucosa to minimize pain.
  - Use agents (mouthwashes, lozenges) that are effective against fungal and bacterial infections (chlorhexidine gluconate).
  - Avoid viscous lidocaine (causes risk of aspiration from depressed gag reflex), hydrogen peroxide (delays healing), milk of magnesia (dries mucous membranes), and lemon glycerin swabs (causes tooth decay and erosion of tissue).
- **Skin breakdown**
  - Inspect skin daily.
  - Check rectal mucosa for fissures.
  - Avoid rectal temperatures.
  - Provide sitz baths as needed.
  - Reposition frequently.
  - Use a pressure reduction system.
- **Neuropathy**
  - Constipation
    - Encourage a diet high in fiber.
    - Administer stool softeners and laxatives as needed.
    - Encourage fluids.
  - Foot drop, extremity numbness and weakness
    - Use a footboard in bed.
    - Assist with ambulation.
  - Jaw pain: Provide a soft or liquid diet.
- **Loss of appetite**
  - Monitor fluid intake and hydration status.
  - Weigh the child daily.
  - Monitor electrolyte values.
  - Provide small, frequent, well-balanced meals.
  - Involve the child in meal planning.
  - Administer enteral nutrition if needed.
- **Alopecia**
  - Prepare the child and parents for hair loss.
  - Encourage the use of a cotton hat or scarf, or a wig if the child is self-conscious about hair loss.
- **LATE EFFECTS:** Cardiomyopathy; cognitive and neuropsychological defects

NURSING ACTIONS
- Provide an antiemetic prior to administration.
- Allow the child several food choices, including their favorite foods.
- Observe the mouth for mucosal ulcerations.
- Offer cool fluids to prevent dehydration and soothe sore mucous membranes.
- Assist the child to manage adverse effects.
- Educate the child and family about the adverse effects of chemotherapy.
- Instruct the parents in the proper use of vascular access devices.
- Instruct the child and parents about bleeding precautions and the management of active bleeding.

CLIENT EDUCATION Qᴘᴄᴄ

- Get immunizations, and attend follow-up appointments.
- Use good infection control practices.
- The use of steroid treatment can cause moon face.
- The child can experience mood changes.
- Recognize indications of infection, skin breakdown, and nutritional deficiency.
- Maintain good hygiene.
- Avoid individuals who have infectious diseases.
- Administer medications and provide nutritional support at home.

Radiation

- Radiation is usually delivered in divided treatments over several weeks.
- Radiation affects rapidly growing cells in the body. Therefore, cells that normally have a fast turnover can be affected in addition to cancer cells.

NURSING ACTIONS

- Take care to eliminate or limit exposure when radiation is in use. Wear lead aprons.
- Educate the child and family about the procedure, and provide support.

CLIENT EDUCATION Qᴘᴄᴄ

- Do not wash off marks on skin that outline the targeted areas.
- Wash the marked areas with lukewarm water, use hands instead of a washcloth, pat dry, and take care not to remove the markings. Avoid using hot or cold water.
- Avoid soaps, creams, lotions, and powders unless prescribed.
- Wear loose cotton clothing.
- Keep the areas protected from the sun by wearing a hat and long-sleeved shirts.
- Seek medical care for blisters, weeping, and red/tender skin.

Surgical intervention: Tumor debulking

PREOPERATIVE NURSING ACTIONS

- Avoid palpation of Wilms' tumor.
- Reinforce preoperative teaching to the child and family that includes length of surgery, where the child will recover, and what equipment will be in place (nasogastric tube, IV line, indwelling urinary catheter).

POSTOPERATIVE NURSING ACTIONS

- Monitor gastrointestinal activity (bowel sounds, bowel movements, distention, nausea, vomiting).
- Provide pain relief.
- Monitor vital signs and for indications of infection.
- Encourage pulmonary hygiene.

INTERPROFESSIONAL CARE

- Social services can assist with access to medications and durable medical equipment if needed.
- A dietitian may be consulted for development of a diet plan.

COMPLICATIONS

Metastasis, kidney failure, and pancytopenia are possible.

Bone marrow depression

Resulting in anemia, neutropenia, and/or thrombocytopenia

NURSING ACTIONS

- Monitor vital signs and report them to the charge nurse and provider. Report a temperature greater than 37.8° C (100° F).
- Monitor for indications of infection (lung congestion; redness, swelling, and pain around IV sites) and lesions in the mouth. Monitor the wound site.
- Instruct the family to keep the child's immunizations up-to-date.
- Administer antimicrobial, antiviral, and antifungal medications.
- Protect the child from sources of possible infection.
  - Use good hand hygiene.
  - Encourage the child and family to use good hand hygiene.
- Screen visitors and staff for indications of infection.
- Avoid invasive procedures (injections, rectal temperatures, catheters). Apply pressure to puncture sites for 5 min.
- Monitor for indications of bleeding.
- Avoid aspirin and NSAIDs.
- Administer filgrastim, a granulocyte colony-stimulating factor that stimulates WBC production, subcutaneously daily.
- Monitor for headache, fever, and mild to moderate bone pain.
- Administer epoetin alfa subcutaneously two to three times per week to stimulate RBC formation.
- Monitor blood pressure.
- Administer oprelvekin subcutaneously daily to stimulate platelet formation.
- Encourage the use of a soft toothbrush.
- Use gentle handling and positioning to protect from injury.
- Organize care to provide for rest. Schedule rest periods.
- Provide support.

CLIENT EDUCATION

- Practice infection control procedures at home. Qᴘᴄᴄ
- Avoid crowds while undergoing chemotherapy.

Online Image: Petechiae

Anorexia, nausea, vomiting

Adverse effects of chemotherapy and radiation therapy

NURSING ACTIONS
- Avoid strong odors. Provide a pleasant atmosphere for meals.
- Avoid offering the child's favorite foods during chemotherapy because they can develop an aversion to these foods.
- Suggest and assist in selecting foods/fluids.
- Provide small, frequent meals.
- Administer antiemetics, usually before meals.

Alteration in bowel elimination

Diarrhea is a result of radiation to the abdominal area. Some chemotherapeutic agents can cause constipation. If mobility and nutrition decrease, the child is more likely to develop constipation.

NURSING ACTIONS
- Provide meticulous skin care.
- Provide a nutritious diet.
- Determine if specific foods or drinks (high-fiber, lactose-rich) worsen the child's condition.
- Monitor I&O and daily weight.

Mucositis and dry mouth

NURSING ACTIONS
- Provide a soft toothbrush or swabs.
- Lubricate the child's lips.
- Give soft, nonacidic foods. A pureed or liquid diet can be required.
- Provide analgesics.
- Avoid hydrogen peroxide and lemon glycerin swabs due to mucosal drying and irritation on eroded tissue.

CLIENT EDUCATION Qpcc
- Visit a dentist before therapy.
- Use chlorhexidine mouth wash or salt rinses using ½ tsp table salt mixed with 1 tsp baking soda and 1 quart water.

Alopecia

Occurs with chemotherapy and radiation of the head and neck

NURSING ACTIONS
- Discuss the child's feelings and monitor for indications of altered body-image.
- Discuss cutting long hair short.
- Suggest wearing a disposable surgical cap for hair collection during heavy loss periods.
- Use gentle shampoos. Gently brush the child's hair.
- Suggest wearing a cotton hat or scarf.
- Discuss the use of a wig, turbans, or hats.

CLIENT EDUCATION Qpcc
- Avoid blow dryers and curling irons.
- Practice proper scalp hygiene.
- Hair grows back in 3 to 6 months.

Blood neoplasms

- Leukemia is a group of malignancies that affect the bone marrow and lymphatic system. Leukemia is classified by the type of WBCs that becomes neoplastic and is commonly divided into two groups.
  - Acute lymphoid leukemia
  - Acute myelogenous or nonlymphoid leukemia
- Leukemia causes an increase in the production of immature WBCs, which leads to infiltration of organs and tissues.
- Bone marrow infiltration causes crowding of cells that would normally produce RBCs, platelets, and mature WBCs. Deficient RBCs cause anemia. Deficient mature WBCs (neutropenia) increase the risk for infection. Deficient platelets (thrombocytopenia) cause bleeding and bruising.
- Infiltration of spleen, liver, and lymph nodes leads to tissue fibrosis. Infiltration of the central nervous system (CNS) causes increased intracranial pressure. Other tissues can also be infiltrated (testes, prostate, ovaries, gastrointestinal tract, kidneys, and lungs).

DATA COLLECTION

RISK FACTORS
- Leukemia is the most common cancer of childhood.
- Male sex
- Peak onset between 2 and 5 years of age.
- Family history of leukemia
- Trisomy 21 (Down syndrome)

EXPECTED FINDINGS

History and data collection findings can reveal vague reports (anorexia, headache, fatigue).

PHYSICAL FINDINGS
- EARLY MANIFESTATIONS
  - Low-grade fever
  - Pallor
  - Increased bruising and petechiae
  - Listlessness
  - Enlarged liver, lymph nodes, and joints
  - Abdominal, leg, and joint pain
  - Headache
  - Vomiting and anorexia
  - Unsteady gait
- LATE MANIFESTATIONS
  - Pain
  - Hematuria
  - Ulcerations in the mouth
  - Enlarged kidneys and testicles
  - Manifestations of increased intracranial pressure

LABORATORY TESTS

Complete blood count
- Anemia (low Hgb and Hct)
- Thrombocytopenia (low platelets)
- Neutropenia (low neutrophils)
- Leukemic blasts (immature WBCs)

DIAGNOSTIC PROCEDURES

Bone marrow aspiration or biopsy analysis

The most definitive diagnostic procedure. If leukemia is present, the specimen will show prolific quantities of immature leukemic blast cells and protein markers indicating a specific type of leukemia.

NURSING ACTIONS
- Assist the provider with the procedure.
- Topical anesthetic, such as a eutectic mixture of local anesthetic cream, may be applied over the biopsy area 45 min to 1 hr prior to the procedure.
- Unconscious sedation is induced using a general anesthetic, such as propofol.
- Positioning depends on the access site to be used (posterior or anterior iliac crest is most common; tibia can be used in infants because it is easier to access and hold the infant).
- The provider obtains a specimen.
- Educate the child and parents about the procedure and postprocedure care.

POSTPROCEDURE
- Apply pressure to the site for 5 to 10 min, then apply a pressure dressing.
- Check vital signs frequently.
- Monitor for manifestations of bleeding and infection for 24 hr. Monitor dressing for bleeding every 15 minutes for the first hour after procedure and then every 1 to 2 hours for the first 24 hours.

Cerebrospinal fluid (CSF) analysis

CSF, obtained by lumbar puncture, is analyzed to determine CNS involvement.

NURSING ACTIONS
- Have the child empty his bladder.
- Assist the provider with the procedure.
- A topical anesthetic cream may be applied over the biopsy area 45 min to 1 hr prior to the procedure.
- Place the child in the side-lying position with the head flexed and knees drawn up toward the chest, and assist in maintaining the position. Distraction might need to be used.
- The child may be sedated with fentanyl and midazolam.
- The provider will clean the skin and inject a local anesthetic.
- The provider will take pressure readings and collect three to five test tubes of CSF.
- Pressure and an elastic bandage will be applied to the puncture site after the needle is removed.
- Label specimens appropriately, and deliver them to the laboratory.
- Monitor the site for bleeding, hematoma, or infection.

CLIENT EDUCATION: Remain in bed for 4 to 8 hr in a flat position to prevent leakage and a resulting spinal headache. This might not be possible for an infant, toddler, or preschooler.

Liver and kidney function studies

Used for baseline functioning before chemotherapy

NURSING ACTIONS
- Draw the appropriate amount of serum.
- Educate the child and parents about the length of time to receive results.

PATIENT-CENTERED CARE

NURSING CARE
- Provide emotional support to the child and parents.
- Encourage peer contact if appropriate.
- Evaluate pain using an age-appropriate pain scale.
- Use pharmacological and nonpharmacological interventions to provide around-the-clock pain management.

THERAPEUTIC PROCEDURES

Hematopoietic stem cell transplant

NURSING ACTIONS
- Implement protective isolation. Qs
  - Private, positive-pressure room
  - At least 12 air exchanges/hr
  - HEPA filtration for incoming air
  - Respirator mask, gloves, and gowns
  - No dried or fresh flowers, and no potted plants

CLIENT EDUCATION: The child is at an increased risk for infection and bleeding until transfused stem cells grow.

Radiation therapy to the brain

NURSING ACTIONS
- Assist with positioning.
- Provide support to the child and family.
- Manage adverse effects.
- Educate the child and parents regarding adverse effects (fatigue, infection).
- Encourage adequate rest and a healthy diet.

LATE EFFECTS
- Second malignancy
- Cognitive and neuropsychological defects

INTERPROFESSIONAL CARE

Reinforce information regarding support services for the child and family.

COMPLICATIONS

Infection

Infection can be a complication of myelosuppression.

NURSING ACTIONS
- Provide the child with a private room designed to allow for adequate air flow to reduce airborne pathogens.
- Restrict visitors and health personnel who have active illnesses.
- Adhere to strict hand hygiene.
- Monitor potential sites of infections (oral ulcer, open cut), and monitor temperature.
- Administer antibiotics after source of infection identified through chest radiographs and blood, stool, urine, and nasopharyngeal cultures.
- Encourage adequate protein and caloric intake.
- Educate the child and parents about infection control practices.

CLIENT EDUCATION
- Monitor for manifestations of infection and notify the provider.
- Avoid live vaccines while the immune system is depressed.

Hemorrhage

Bleeding (thrombocytopenia) can be a complication of myelosuppression.

NURSING ACTIONS
- Monitor for findings of bleeding (petechiae, ecchymoses, hematuria, bleeding gums, hematemesis, tarry stools).
- Avoid unnecessary skin punctures, and use surgical aseptic technique when performed. Apply pressure for 5 min to stop bleeding.
- Treat a nosebleed with cold and pressure.
- Avoid obtaining temperatures rectally.
- Inform the parents on measures for controlling epistaxis.

CLIENT EDUCATION Qpcc
- Perform meticulous oral care to prevent gingival bleeding. Use a soft toothbrush, and avoid astringent mouthwashes.
- Avoid activities that can lead to injury or bleeding.

Anemia

Can be a complication of myelosuppression

NURSING ACTIONS
- Monitor the child who is receiving blood transfusions.
- Allow for frequent rest periods.
- Administer oxygen therapy.
- Assist with IV fluid replacement.

CLIENT EDUCATION: Consume foods high in iron. Qpcc

Bone and soft tissue cancers

- Malignant tumors in bone can originate from tissues involved in bone growth (osteoid matrix, blood vessels, cartilage).
  - Osteosarcoma usually occurs in the metaphysis of long bones, most often in the femur. Treatment frequently includes amputation or limb salvage procedure of the affected extremity as well as chemotherapy.
  - Ewing's sarcoma (a primitive neuroectodermal tumor) occurs in the shafts of long bones and of trunk bones. Treatment includes surgical biopsy, intensive radiation therapy to tumor site, and chemotherapy, but not amputation. Prognosis depends on how quickly the disease is diagnosed and whether metastasis has occurred.
- Soft tissue malignancies arise from undifferentiated cells in the soft tissues (muscles, tendons), in connective or fibrous tissue, or in blood or lymph vessels. These malignancies can begin in any area of the body.
  - Rhabdomyosarcoma originates in skeletal muscle in any part of the body, but it most commonly occurs in the head and neck, with the orbit of the eye frequently affected. Treatment consists of surgical biopsy, local radiation therapy, and chemotherapy, rather than radical surgical procedures.
- Children who undergo irradiation for malignancies in or near the pelvic area can experience sterilization and secondary cancers.

Bone tumors

DATA COLLECTION

RISK FACTORS

- Osteosarcoma peaks at age 15 during growth spurts and is more common in males than females.
- Ewing's sarcoma occurs prior to 30 years of age and is more common in Caucasian children.

EXPECTED FINDINGS

- Nonspecific bone pain that is often mistaken for an injury or growing pains
- Temporary relief of pain when extremity is flexed
- Weakness, swelling, or decreased movement of the extremity
- Palpable lymph nodes near the tumor
- Anemia, generalized infection
- Unexplained weight loss
- Limpness or inability to hold a heavy object

LABORATORY TESTS

CBC and other common tests can help rule out infection, iron deficiency anemia, and other possible causes of findings.

DIAGNOSTIC PROCEDURES

- X-rays, computed tomography (CT) scans, or magnetic resonance imaging (MRI) of the primary site
- Bone marrow biopsy
- CT of the chest and bone scans to evaluate metastasis

PATIENT-CENTERED CARE

NURSING CARE

- Be honest when answering questions and discussing information about the disease and treatment.
- Allow the child time, usually several days, to prepare emotionally for surgery and chemotherapy.
- Avoid overwhelming the child with information.
- Provide emotional support for the child and family.

THERAPEUTIC PROCEDURES

Surgical biopsy

Tumor is biopsied under anesthesia to determine presence and tissue type of cancer.

NURSING ACTIONS
- Provide routine preoperative and postoperative care.
- Provide for adequate pain relief.
- Monitor wound for manifestations of infection.
- Educate the child and family regarding postprocedure care.

Limb salvage procedure for bone cancers

Includes a course of chemotherapy to shrink the tumor and then total bone and joint replacement after the tumor and affected bone are removed.

NURSING ACTIONS
- Check site distal to surgery for pulses, warmth, and capillary refill.
- Assist with managing adverse effects.
- Provide routine postoperative care.
- Provide for adequate pain relief.

CLIENT EDUCATION: Hair loss is an expected effect of preoperative chemotherapy.

Limb amputation for bone cancer

The child can receive chemotherapy both preoperatively and postoperatively.

NURSING ACTIONS
- Provide routine preoperative and postoperative care.
- Provide emotional support.
- Monitor for adequate circulation
- Care for the stump.
- Monitor for the presence of phantom limb pain, and medicate appropriately.

- Prepare the child for fitting of a temporary prosthesis, which can occur immediately after surgery. Qpcc
- Work with the child and family to plan for issues such as appropriate clothing to wear with prosthesis.
- Role-play issues that the child will need to deal with after discharge, such as talking to strangers who ask about the prosthesis.

CLIENT EDUCATION
- Cooperate with postoperative physical therapy.
- The child's emotions, such as anger, are normal grief reactions after amputation, chemotherapy, and other treatments.

INTERPROFESSIONAL CARE

- Older children and adolescents can benefit from attending a support group for children who have cancer and/or have had amputations.
- Assist with a referral for mental health counseling to assist the child to resume normal activities.
- Assist in coordinating physical and occupational therapy referrals to start while in the hospital and to continue after discharge.

Rhabdomyosarcoma

DATA COLLECTION

RISK FACTORS

Rhabdomyosarcoma occurs in children of all ages (but more commonly in children 6-years-old and younger) and is more common in males.

EXPECTED FINDINGS

- Pain in local areas related to compression by the tumor (sore throat can occur with tumor of the nasopharynx)
- Possible absence of pain in some parts of the body, such as in the retroperitoneal area, until the tumor begins to obstruct organs

BASED ON AFFECTED AREA
- **CNS:** headaches, diplopia, vomiting
- **Orbit:** unilateral proptosis, ecchymosis of conjunctiva, strabismus
- **Nasopharynx:** stuffy nose, pain, nasal obstruction, epistaxis, palpable neck nodes, visible mass (late)
- **Neck:** hoarseness, dysphagia, visible palpable neck mass
- **Paranasal sinuses:** nasal obstruction, pain, discharge, sinusitis, swelling
- **Middle ear:** chronic otitis media, pain, sanguinopurulent discharge, facial paralysis
- **Retroperitoneal area:** usually no manifestations; abdominal mass, pain, intestinal or genitourinary obstruction
- **Perineum:** visible superficial mass, bowel or bladder obstruction
- **Extremity:** pain, palpable fixed mass, lymph node enlargement

DIAGNOSTIC PROCEDURES

- CT scan or MRI of the primary site
- Biopsy of tumor
- CT of the chest, bone scan, bone marrow biopsy, and lumbar puncture to evaluate metastasis

PATIENT-CENTERED CARE

NURSING CARE

- Be honest when answering questions and discussing information about the disease and treatment.
- Allow the child time, usually several days, to prepare emotionally for surgery and chemotherapy.
- Avoid overwhelming the child with information.
- Provide emotional support for the parents and child.

THERAPEUTIC PROCEDURES

Localized radiation therapy

Radiation therapy can be used in combination with chemotherapy and surgery.

NURSING ACTIONS
- Assist the child with positioning.
- Monitor for adverse effects.
- Educate the child and family regarding the course of therapy.

Surgical biopsy

Tumor is biopsied under anesthesia to determine presence and tissue type of cancer.

NURSING ACTIONS
- Provide routine preoperative and postoperative care.
- Provide for adequate pain relief.
- Monitor wound for manifestations of infection.
- Actions vary with extent and area of surgery, but should include preprocedure and postprocedure data collection, including vital signs, medication for pain, and wound care as necessary.
- Educate the child and family regarding postprocedure care.

INTERPROFESSIONAL CARE

- Older children and adolescents can benefit from attending a support group for children who have cancer.
- Assist with a referral for mental health counseling to assist the child to resume normal activities.
- Assist in coordinating physical and occupational therapy referrals to start while in the hospital and to continue after discharge.

Application Exercises

1. A nurse is caring for a toddler who has a Wilms' tumor. Which of the following actions should the nurse take?

   A. Palpate the child's abdomen to identify the size of the tumor.

   B. Prepare the child for surgery.

   C. Reinforce teaching with the parents about dialysis.

   D. Administer an antiemetic 1 hr after chemotherapy begins.

2. A nurse is collecting data from a child who has neuroblastoma of the adrenal gland. Which of the following findings are indications of metastasis from the primary site? (Select all that apply.)

   A. Weight gain

   B. Bone pain

   C. Periorbital ecchymoses

   D. Proptosis

   E. Ill appearance

3. A nurse is collecting data from a child who has leukemia. Which of the following are early manifestations of leukemia? (Select all that apply.)

   A. Hematuria

   B. Anorexia

   C. Petechiae

   D. Ulcerations in the mouth

   E. Pallor

4. A nurse is caring for a child who has mucosal ulceration. Which of the following actions should the nurse take? (Select all that apply.)

   A. Swab the mucosa with lemon glycerin swabs.

   B. Apply viscous lidocaine.

   C. Offer soft foods.

   D. Use a soft, disposable toothbrush for oral care.

   E. Encourage gargling with a warm saline mouthwash.

5. A nurse is collecting data for a child who has rhabdomyosarcoma of the upper arm. Which of the following findings should the nurse expect? (Select all that apply.)

   A. Pain

   B. Discoloration of the skin

   C. Lymph node enlargement

   D. Easy bruising

   E. Palpable mass

PRACTICE Active Learning Scenario

A nurse is reinforcing teaching about myelosuppression with the parent of a child who has bone cancer and is receiving chemotherapy. Use the ATI Active Learning Template: System Disorder to complete this item.

NURSING CARE: Describe two actions related to each of the following areas.
- Evaluating laboratory data to monitor for complications
- Preventing infection
- Preventing hemorrhage or injury from bleeding
- Preventing anemia or injury from anemia

Application Exercises Key

1. A. The nurse should avoid palpating the child's abdomen. Pressure applied to the abdomen could rupture the encapsulated tumor.

   B. **CORRECT:** The nurse should prepare a child who has Wilms' tumor for surgical removal of the tumor and kidney. Surgery is performed soon after diagnosis.

   C. The nurse should inform the parents that Wilms' tumor is usually unilateral, therefore dialysis is not indicated if the remaining kidney is unaffected.

   D. The nurse should administer an antiemetic prior to the administration of chemotherapy.

   Ⓝ *NCLEX® Connection: Physiological Adaptation, Alterations in Body Systems*

2. A. A child who has metastatic neuroblastoma is expected to have weight loss rather than weight gain.

   B. **CORRECT:** A child who has metastatic neuroblastoma is expected to have bone pain.

   C. **CORRECT:** A child who has metastatic neuroblastoma is expected to have periorbital ecchymoses.

   D. **CORRECT:** A child who has metastatic neuroblastoma is expected to have proptosis.

   E. **CORRECT:** A child who has metastatic neuroblastoma is expected to have an ill appearance.

   Ⓝ *NCLEX® Connection: Reduction of Risk Potential, Potential for Complications from Surgical Procedures and Health Alterations*

3. A. Hematuria is a late manifestation of leukemia.

   B. **CORRECT:** Anorexia is an early manifestation of leukemia.

   C. **CORRECT:** Petechiae is an early manifestation of leukemia.

   D. Ulcerations in the mouth are a late manifestation of leukemia.

   E. **CORRECT:** Pallor is an early manifestation of leukemia.

   Ⓝ *NCLEX® Connection: Physiological Adaptation, Basic Pathophysiology*

4. A. Lemon glycerin swabs can cause tooth decay and erosion of the tissues.

   B. Viscous lidocaine can depress the gag reflex and cause aspiration.

   C. **CORRECT:** Offering soft foods decreases the amount of chewing needed and possible irritation.

   D. **CORRECT:** A soft toothbrush allows for adequate cleaning of the mouth and decreases irritation.

   E. **CORRECT:** A warm saline mouthwash is effective in soothing mucosal ulcerations.

   Ⓝ *NCLEX® Connection: Basic Care and Comfort, Nonpharmacological Comfort Interventions*

5. A. **CORRECT:** Pain is an expected finding in a child who has rhabdomyosarcoma of an extremity.

   B. Rhabdomyosarcoma is a soft tissue cancer. Discoloration of the skin is not an expected finding.

   C. **CORRECT:** Lymph node enlargement is an expected finding in a child who has rhabdomyosarcoma of an extremity.

   D. Easy bruising is not an expected finding in a child who has rhabdomyosarcoma.

   E. **CORRECT:** Palpable mass is an expected finding in a child who has rhabdomyosarcoma of an extremity.

   Ⓝ *NCLEX® Connection: Physiological Adaptation, Basic Pathophysiology*

PRACTICE Answer

Using the ATI Active Learning Template: System Disorder

NURSING CARE

Evaluating laboratory data to monitor for complications
- Infection: elevated WBC and fever
- Hemorrhage: blood in urine or stool, bruising, and petechiae
- Anemia: fatigue and decreased hemoglobin/hematocrit

Preventing infection
- Provide the child with a private room. The room should be designed to allow for adequate air flow to reduce airborne pathogens.
- Restrict visitors and health personnel who have active illnesses.
- Adhere to strict hand hygiene.
- Monitor potential sites of infections (oral ulcer, open cut) and temperature.
- Administer antibiotics after source of infection is identified through chest radiographs and blood, stool, urine, and nasopharyngeal cultures.
- Encourage adequate protein and caloric intake.

Preventing hemorrhage or injury from bleeding
- Monitor for findings of bleeding (petechiae, ecchymoses, hematuria, bleeding gums, hematemesis, tarry stools).
- Avoid unnecessary skin punctures, and use surgical aseptic technique when performed. Apply pressure for 5 min to stop bleeding.
- Treat a nosebleed with cold and pressure.
- Avoid obtaining temperatures rectally.

Preventing anemia or injury from anemia
- Provide rest periods as needed. Administer oxygen therapy
- Assist with IV fluid replacement.

Ⓝ *NCLEX® Connection: Physiological Adaptation, Pathophysiology*

NCLEX® Connections

When reviewing the following chapters, keep in mind the relevant topics and tasks of the NCLEX outline, in particular:

Psychosocial Integrity

ABUSE OR NEGLECT
Identify signs and symptoms of physical, psychological, or financial abuse in the client (family involvement, inadequate weight gain, poor hygiene).

Provide safe environment for abused/neglected client.

Physiological Adaptation

ALTERATIONS IN BODY SYSTEMS: Reinforce education to client regarding care and condition.

BASIC PATHOPHYSIOLOGY: Identify signs and symptoms related to an acute or chronic illness.

MEDICAL EMERGENCIES: Respond/intervene to a client life-threatening situation (cardiopulmonary resuscitation).

UNIT 3   NURSING CARE OF CHILDREN WHO
          HAVE OTHER SPECIFIC NEEDS

CHAPTER 39 # Complications of Infants

It is essential to immediately identify complications of newborns and infants, notify the charge nurse and provider, and assist to implement appropriate interventions. Ongoing emotional support to an infant's parents is also imperative to contribute to the plan of care.

Complications include phenylketonuria (PKU), meningocele, necrotizing enterocolitis (NEC), respiratory distress syndrome (RDS), congenital hypothyroidism, substance-exposed infants, hyperbilirubinemia, chromosomal abnormalities, neonatal seizures, newborn sepsis, failure to thrive (FTT), and plagiocephaly.

Phenylketonuria

- PKU is an inherited metabolic disorder in which the newborn lacks the enzyme phenylalanine hydroxylase. This enzyme converts phenylalanine, an essential amino acid, into tyrosine. The lack of this enzyme leads to the accumulation of phenylalanine in the newborn's bloodstream and tissues, which causes cognitive impairment.
- Pregnant clients must adhere to strict dietary guidelines from 3 months before conception throughout pregnancy. Failure to follow strict dietary guidelines during pregnancy can result in fetal microcephaly and cognitive impairment. Clients who have PKU have phenylalanine levels monitored one to two times per week throughout pregnancy.
- All newborns are screened for PKU by blood spot analysis after the newborn has ingested a source of protein as close as possible to discharge. Immediate identification and implementing a diet with low phenylalanine significantly decreases the occurrence of cognitive impairment.

DATA COLLECTION

EXPECTED FINDINGS

NEWBORN PHYSICAL FINDINGS
- Growth failure
- Frequent vomiting
- Irritability
- Musty odor to urine
- Microcephaly
- Blue eyes, very fair skin, light blonde hair

PATIENT-CENTERED CARE

NURSING CARE

Nursing care focuses on dietary intake.
- Initiate dietary restrictions as soon as PKU is diagnosed, or within 7 to 10 days of birth.
- Place newborn on a formula low in phenylalanine.
  - Intake should be 20 to 30 mg phenylalanine per kilogram of body weight per day.
  - Monitor phenylalanine level.
  - Goal is a phenylalanine level between 2 and 8 mg/dL.
- Monitor phenylalanine levels in newborns who are breastfeeding. Breast milk contains phenylalanine, so exclusively breastfeeding might not be recommended.
- Monitor the newborn for findings of PKU.
- Provide parents with emotional support and reinforce teaching.

COMPLICATIONS

EXPECTED FINDINGS
- Cognitive impairment (can be severe)
- Hyperactivity with erratic behavior
- Bizarre behavior such as fright reactions
- Head banging
- Arm biting
- Disorientation
- Spasticity or catatonic-like positions
- Seizures

Meningocele/ Myelomeningocele

Meningocele and myelomeningocele are neural tube defects (NTDs) that are present at birth and affect the CNS and spine. These defects occur when the neural tube fails to close during the third to fourth week of embryonic development.

Meningocele is the protrusion of a sac-like cyst that contains meninges and spinal fluid.

Myelomeningocele is the protrusion of a sac-like cyst that contains meninges, spinal fluid, and a portion of the spinal cord and nerves.

DATA COLLECTION

EXPECTED FINDINGS

PHYSICAL FINDINGS
- Protrusion of a sac-like cyst midline of the spine: Cysts are most commonly found in the lumbar or lumbosacral area.
- Sensory and neuromotor dysfunction
  - Type and severity of dysfunction dependent on location of defect
  - Observe lower extremities for movement and response to stimuli
- Possible constant dribbling of urine and loss of feces
- Possible limb deformities

PATIENT-CENTERED CARE

NURSING CARE

- Observe for infant-parent attachment.
- Check the cyst.
- Perform routine newborn examinations.
- Obtain accurate measurements of output.
- Check fontanels and monitor head circumference.

THERAPEUTIC PROCEDURES

Closure of the meningocele/myelomeningocele sac

Done as soon as possible to prevent complications due to injury or infection

PREOPERATIVE NURSING ACTIONS

- Assist with preparing the family for the newborn's surgery (within 24 to 72 hr after birth).
- Protect the sac from injury.
- Place the infant in a radiant warmer, without clothing.
- Apply a sterile, moist nonadhering dressing with 0.9% sodium chloride on the cyst, re-wetting to prevent drying.
- Inspect the cyst closely for leakage of fluid or manifestations of irritation.
- Monitor for manifestations of infection (fever, irritability, lethargy).
- Avoid measuring temperature rectally.
- Avoid putting pressure on the sac.

POSTOPERATIVE NURSING ACTIONS

- Monitor vital signs.
- Monitor I&O.
- Monitor weight.
- Inspect for manifestations of infection.
- Monitor for leakage of cerebrospinal fluid (CSF).
- Maintain prone position until other positions are prescribed.
- Resume oral feedings.
- Assist with range of motion (ROM) exercises to extremities.
- Monitor fontanels for bulging.
- Measure head circumference.
- Reinforce education to the parents on postoperative home care.

ONGOING CARE

- Monitor head circumference.
- Monitor skin integrity.
- Check for allergies, such as latex.
- Monitor for infections.
- Offer support to family.

Necrotizing enterocolitis

NEC is an inflammatory disease of the gastrointestinal mucosa caused by ischemia or hypoxia. Ischemia results in death of mucosal cells, leading to necrotic patches that interfere with digestion.

DATA COLLECTION

RISK FACTORS

- Preterm birth
- Respiratory distress syndrome
- Polycythemia
- Asphyxia
- Receiving enteral feedings
- Pre-existing infection

EXPECTED FINDINGS

PHYSICAL FINDINGS

- Abdominal distention
- Gastric residuals
- Bloody stools
- Periods of apnea
- Hypotension
- Lethargy
- Poor feeding
- Decreased urinary output

LABORATORY TESTS

- CBC with differential
- ABGs
- Coagulation studies
- Blood cultures
- Electrolytes

DIAGNOSTIC PROCEDURES

Abdominal x-rays
- Sausage-shaped dilation of intestine
- Marked distention of intestine
- Characteristic "soapsuds" appearance of the intestinal wall due to air infiltration
- Free air in abdominal cavity if perforation has occurred

PATIENT-CENTERED CARE

NURSING CARE

- Treatment begins with prevention. Withhold feedings for 24 to 48 hr from newborns who suffered birth asphyxia.
- Initiate feeding with breast milk, which has a protective effect against the development of NEC.
- Discontinue all feedings at first sign of NEC.
- Handle the abdomen carefully to prevent intestinal perforation.
- Measure abdominal girth just above the umbilicus every 4 to 8 hr.
- Assist with serial abdominal x-rays every 4 to 6 hr.
- Monitor vital signs.
- Perform all routine newborn examinations.
- Assist with preparing the newborn and family for surgical intervention.
  - Removal of necrotized portion of bowel
  - Temporary colostomy is a possibility.

Respiratory distress syndrome

RDS occurs as a result of surfactant deficiency in the lungs and is characterized by lung immaturity.
- Surfactant is a phospholipid that assists in alveoli expansion. Surfactant keeps alveoli from collapsing and allows gas exchange to occur.
- Atelectasis (collapsing of a portion of lung) increases the work of breathing. As a result, respiratory acidosis and hypoxemia can develop.
- Complications from RDS are related to oxygen therapy and mechanical ventilation.

DATA COLLECTION

RISK FACTORS

- Preterm birth
- Perinatal asphyxia (meconium staining, cord prolapse, nuchal cord)
- Maternal diabetes mellitus
- Premature rupture of membranes
- Cesarean section birth
- Multifetal pregnancy
- Cold stress
- Sepsis
- Airway obstruction
- Hypoglycemia
- Cardiac defects

EXPECTED FINDINGS

PHYSICAL FINDINGS

- Tachypnea (respiratory rate greater than 60/min)
- Nasal flaring
- Expiratory grunting
- Retractions
- Labored breathing with prolonged expiration
- Fine crackles on auscultation
- Cyanosis
- Unresponsiveness, flaccidity, and apnea with decreased breath sounds (manifestations of worsened RDS)

LABORATORY TESTS

- Culture and sensitivity of blood, urine, and cerebrospinal fluid
- Blood glucose

DIAGNOSTIC PROCEDURES

- ABGs reveal hypercapnia (excess of carbon dioxide in the blood) and respiratory or mixed acidosis.
- Chest x-ray

PATIENT-CENTERED CARE

NURSING CARE

- Suction the mouth, trachea, and nose as needed.
- Maintain thermoregulation.
- Provide mouth and skin care.
- Maintain adequate oxygenation.
- Decrease stimuli.

MEDICATIONS

Beractant

CLASSIFICATION: Lung surfactant

INTENDED EFFECT: Restore surfactant and improve respiratory compliance in premature newborns who have RDS

NURSING ACTIONS
- Assist with performing a respiratory assessment (ABGs; respiratory rhythm, rate, and color) before and after administration of agent.
- Provide suction prior to medication administration.
- Monitor endotracheal tube placement.

Congenital hypothyroidism

Congenital hypothyroidism occurs due to an absent or nonfunctioning thyroid gland in a newborn. Thyroid hypofunction can be caused by maternal iodine deficiency or maternal antithyroid medications during pregnancy.

- Findings might not appear until 3 months of age in a formula-fed infant and 6 months of age in a breastfed infant.
- Early diagnosis is crucial due to severe progressive physical and cognitive dysfunction that occurs if left untreated.

DATA COLLECTION

EXPECTED FINDINGS

PHYSICAL FINDINGS
- Sleeping excessively
- Enlarged tongue
- Respiratory difficulty
- Poor sucking
- Cool, dry skin on extremities
- Jaundice
- Subnormal temperature, respiratory rate, and heart rate
- Short, thick neck
- Hypotonia with decreased deep tendon reflexes
- Abdominal distention and constipation

PATIENT-CENTERED CARE

NURSING CARE

- Monitor vital signs, respiratory status, and weight.
- Check for feeding difficulties.
- Administer synthetic thyroid hormone (sodium levothyroxine).
- Administer supplemental vitamin D to support rapid bone growth.
- Monitor thyroid levels (T3, T4, TSH).
- Reinforce teaching with parents on the importance of proper medication administration.

Substance-exposed infants

Maternal substance use during pregnancy consists of any use of alcohol or drugs. Intrauterine drug exposure can cause anomalies, neurobehavioral changes, and evidence of withdrawal in the neonate. These changes depend on the specific drug or combination of drugs used, dosage, route of administration, metabolism and excretion by the mother and her fetus, timing of exposure, and length of exposure.

- Substance withdrawal in the newborn occurs when the mother uses drugs that have addictive properties during pregnancy. This includes illicit substances, heroin, opiates, alcohol, tobacco, methadone, and prescription medications.
- Fetal alcohol spectrum disorder (FASD) and fetal alcohol syndrome (FAS) result from exposure of the fetus to the chronic or periodic intake of alcohol during pregnancy. FASD is an umbrella term used to describe the range of effects. FAS is a form of FASD that refers specifically to children who exhibit a triad of characteristic facial features, growth restriction, and neurodevelopmental deficits, as well as a confirmed history of maternal alcohol consumption.
- Newborns who have FAS are at risk for specific congenital physical defects, along with long-term complications.
  - Feeding problems
  - Central nervous system dysfunction (learning disabilities, low IQ, seizures)
  - Behavioral difficulties, such as hyperactivity (ADHD)
  - Language abnormalities
  - Delayed growth and development
  - Poor maternal-newborn bonding

DATA COLLECTION

RISK FACTORS

- Maternal use of substances prior to knowing she is pregnant
- Maternal substance use and addiction

EXPECTED FINDINGS

PHYSICAL FINDINGS
Monitor the neonate for abstinence syndrome (withdrawal) and increased wakefulness using the neonatal abstinence scoring system that checks for and scores the following.

- **CNS:** increased wakefulness; high-pitched, shrill cry; incessant crying; irritability; tremors; hyperactivity with increased Moro reflex; increased muscle tone; abrasions and excoriations on face and knees; convulsions
- **Metabolic, vasomotor, and respiratory:** nasal congestion with flaring, frequent yawning, sneezing, skin mottling, tachypnea greater than 60/min, sweating, or temperature greater than 38.3° C (101° F)
- **Gastrointestinal:** poor feeding; regurgitation (projectile vomiting); diarrhea; excessive, uncoordinated, constant sucking

Heroin withdrawal

Neonatal abstinence syndrome
- Low birth weight and small for gestational age (SGA)
- Decreased Moro reflexes (rather than increased)
- Jitteriness, hyperactivity
- Hypothermia or hyperthermia
- Shrill, persistent cry

Methadone withdrawal

Neonatal abstinence syndrome
- Tremors, irritability, fever, sleep pattern disturbances
- Higher birth weight
- Increased risk of sudden infant death syndrome (SIDS)

Cocaine exposure

- Newborn can appear normal or exhibit neurologic problems at birth
- Neurobehavioral depression or excitability
- High-pitched cry, abnormal sleep patterns, excessive sucking, hypertonicity, tremors, irritability, inability to console, and poor tolerance to changes in routine

Marijuana exposure

Associated with a decrease in newborn birth weight and length, and fetal growth

Methamphetamine withdrawal

Small head circumference, SGA, agitation, vomiting, rapid respiratory rate, bradycardia or tachycardia, lethargy, frequent infections, emotional disturbances, and delayed growth and development

Fetal alcohol syndrome

- Craniofacial features (microcephaly, short palpebral fissures, thin upper lip, flat midface, indistinct philtrum)
- Hearing disorders
- Many vital organ anomalies (limb and heart defects, including ventricular septal defects)
- Prenatal and postnatal growth restriction
- Developmental delays and neurologic abnormalities
- Cognitive impairment
- Attention deficit disorder

Tobacco exposure

- Prematurity, low birth weight, developmental delays
- Increased risk for SIDS and respiratory tract illnesses

PATIENT-CENTERED CARE

NURSING CARE

Nursing care for maternal substance use and neonatal effects or withdrawal include the following in addition to normal newborn care.
- Assist with neonatal abstinence scoring system assessment.
- Elicit and check reflexes.
- Monitor the ability to feed and digest intake.
- Monitor fluids and electrolytes with skin turgor, mucous membranes, fontanels, and I&O.
- Observe the newborn's behavior.

MEDICATIONS

Phenobarbital

CLASSIFICATION: Anticonvulsant

INTENDED EFFECT: Decrease CNS irritability and control seizures for newborns who are susceptible to seizures

NURSING ACTIONS
- Decrease environmental stimuli.
- Cluster care for newborns to minimize stimulation.
- Swaddle the newborn to reduce self-stimulation and protect the skin from abrasions.
- Monitor and maintain fluids and electrolytes.
- Administer frequent, small feedings of high-calorie formula. The newborn can require gavage feedings.
- Elevate the newborn's head during and following feedings, and burp the newborn to reduce vomiting and aspiration. Qs
- Try various nipples to compensate for a poor suck reflex.
- For newborns addicted to cocaine, avoid eye contact. Use vertical rocking and a pacifier.
- Prevent infection.

Hyperbilirubinemia

Hyperbilirubinemia is an elevation of serum bilirubin levels resulting in jaundice. Jaundice normally appears in the sclera, nails, or skin.

Jaundice can be either physiologic or pathologic

- **Physiologic jaundice** is considered benign (resulting from normal newborn physiology of increased bilirubin production due to the shortened lifespan and breakdown of fetal RBCs and liver immaturity). The newborn who has physiological jaundice has no other manifestations and shows evidence of jaundice after 24 hr of age.
- **Hemolytic disease of the newborn (HDN)**, or pathologic jaundice, is a result of an underlying disease. HDN appears before 24 hr of age. In the term newborn, normal unconjugated bilirubin levels are 0.2 to 1.4 mg/dL. Levels must exceed 5 mg/dL before jaundice is observed.

Kernicterus (bilirubin encephalopathy): When some pathologic conditions exist in addition to increased bilirubin levels, the newborn has an increased permeability of the blood-brain barrier to unconjugated bilirubin. The newborn has the potential for irreversible brain damage. It is a neurological syndrome caused by bilirubin depositing in brain cells. Survivors can experience neurological damage, cerebral palsy, and seizures, and display cognitive impairment, ADHD, delayed or abnormal motor movement, behavioral disorders, perceptual problems, and hearing loss.

DATA COLLECTION

RISK FACTORS

Pathologic hyperbilirubinemia
- Increased serum bilirubin levels
- Rh or ABO incompatibility
- Significant bruising
- Jaundice within 24 hr of birth
- Ineffective, difficult breastfeeding
- Gestational age 35 to 36 weeks
- Sibling who had jaundice

EXPECTED FINDINGS

Hypoxia, hypothermia, hypoglycemia, and metabolic acidosis can increase the risk of brain damage despite lower serum levels of bilirubin.

PHYSICAL FINDINGS
- Yellowish tint to skin, sclera, mucous membranes, and nails
- Yellowish skin
- Lethargy
- Hypotonic
- Poor feeding
- Decreased activity
- High-pitched cry
- Temperature instability

PATIENT-CENTERED CARE

NURSING CARE

- To verify jaundice, press the tip of the newborn's nose or sternum (bony prominences) lightly with one finger. Then release pressure, and observe the skin color for yellowish tint as the skin is blanched.
- Note the time of jaundice onset to distinguish between physiologic and pathologic jaundice.
- Observe the skin and mucous membranes for jaundice.
- Monitor vital signs.
- Assist with phototherapy.
  - Maintain an eye mask over the newborn's eyes for protection of corneas and retinas.
  - Keep the newborn undressed except for a diaper.
  - Avoid applying lotions or ointments to the skin because they absorb heat and can cause burns.
  - Remove the newborn from phototherapy every 4 hr, and unmask the newborn's eyes, checking for inflammation or injury.
  - Reposition the newborn every 2 hr to expose all body surfaces to the phototherapy lights and prevent pressure sores.
- Observe for effects of phototherapy.
  - Bronze discoloration: not a serious complication
  - Maculopapular skin rash: not a serious complication
  - Development of pressure areas
  - Dehydration (poor skin turgor, dry mucous membranes, decreased urinary output)
  - Elevated temperature
- Reinforce with the parents to hold and interact with the newborn when phototherapy lights are off.
- Monitor elimination and daily weights for evidence of dehydration.
- Check the newborn's axillary temperature every 4 hr during phototherapy because temperature can become elevated.
- Feed the newborn early and frequently, every 3 to 4 hr. This promotes bilirubin excretion in the stools.
- Encourage breastfeeding of the newborn. Supplementation with donor breast milk or formula can be prescribed.

Newborn sepsis

Infection can be contracted by the newborn before, during, or after delivery. Newborns are highly susceptible to micro-organisms due to their limited immunity and inability to localize infection. The infection can spread rapidly into the bloodstream.

Newborn sepsis is the presence of micro-organisms or their toxins in the blood or tissues of the newborn during the first month after birth. Manifestations of sepsis are subtle and can resemble other diseases. The nurse often notices them during routine care of the newborn.

Organisms frequently responsible for newborn infections include *Staphylococcus aureus*, *Staphylococcus epidermidis*, *Escherichia coli*, *Haemophilus influenzae*, group A beta-hemolytic streptococcus, *Klebsiella pneumoniae*, and *Pseudomonas aeruginosa*.

Prevention of infection and newborn sepsis starts with maternal screening for infections, prophylactic interventions, and the use of sterile and aseptic techniques during delivery. Prophylactic antibiotic treatment of the eyes of all newborns and appropriate umbilical cord care also help to prevent newborn infection and sepsis.

DATA COLLECTION

EXPECTED FINDINGS

PHYSICAL FINDINGS
- Temperature instability (hypothermia common)
- Suspicious drainage (eyes, umbilical stump)
- Poor feeding pattern (weak suck, decreased intake)
- Vomiting and diarrhea
- Poor weight gain
- Abdominal distention
- Large amount of residual if feeding by gavage method
- Apnea, retractions, grunting, cyanosis, and nasal flaring
- Decreased oxygen saturation level
- Skin changes (pallor, jaundice, petechiae)
- Increased or decreased heart rate
- Rapid breaths
- Low blood pressure
- Irritability
- Possible seizure activity
- Poor muscle tone and lethargy

PATIENT-CENTERED CARE

NURSING CARE

- Monitor risk for infection. (Review maternal health record.)
- Monitor vital signs continuously.
- Monitor I&O and daily weight.
- Monitor fluid and electrolyte status.
- Monitor visitors for infection.
- Obtain specimens (blood, urine, stool) to assist in identifying the causative organism.
- Reinforce teaching with the family about the importance of infection control.
  - Instruct them to use clean bottles and nipples for each feeding.
  - Inform them to discard any unused formula.
  - Demonstrate hand hygiene and watch return demonstration.
- Reinforce the importance of adequate rest and decreased physical stimulation for the newborn.
- Provide emotional support to the family.

Failure to thrive

FTT is inadequate growth resulting from the inability to obtain or use calories required for growth. It is usually described in an infant who falls below the 5th percentile for weight (and possibly for height) or who has a pattern of consistent weight loss.
- Inadequate caloric intake
- Inadequate absorption
- Increased metabolism
- Defective utilization

DATA COLLECTION

RISK FACTORS

- Disturbed parent-child interactions
- Dysfunctional parenting behaviors
- Poverty
- Family stress
- Insufficient nutrition

EXPECTED FINDINGS

- Less than 5th percentile on growth chart
- Malnourished appearance
- No fear of strangers
- Minimal smiling
- Small stature
- Lower cognitive and academic achievement scores
- Withdrawn behavior
- Developmental delays
- Feeding disorder
- Wide-eyed gaze
- Stiff or flaccid body

PATIENT-CENTERED CARE

NURSING CARE

- Assist with obtaining a nutritional history.
- Observe parent-child interactions.
- Obtain baseline height and weight. Observe for low weight, malnourished appearance, and manifestations of dehydration.
- Weigh the newborn daily without clothing or a diaper.
- Maintain strict I&O and calorie counts.
- Instruct parents how to recognize and respond to infant's hunger cues.
- Establish an eating routine that includes usual times, duration, and setting.
- Reinforce proper positioning, latching on, and timing for breastfeeding.
- Provide 24 kcal/oz formula. Instruct parents how to mix formula properly.
- Administer multivitamin supplements.
- Provide developmental stimulation.

CLIENT EDUCATION

- Maintain eye contact and face-to-face posture during feedings.
- Talk to the infant while feeding.
- Burp the infant frequently.
- Keep the environment quiet and avoid distractions.
- Be persistent and remain calm during 10 to 15 min of refusal to eat.
- Never force the infant to eat.

Plagiocephaly

Plagiocephaly is an acquired condition that occurs from cranial molding in infancy. The infant's head becomes asymmetric or oblique in shape due to flattening of the occiput. Plagiocephaly is attributed to the supine sleep position, as its occurrence has increased significantly since the initiation of the Safe to Sleep campaign. The campaign was initiated to assist in the prevention of sudden infant death syndrome (SIDS) and recommends that infants sleep on their backs.

- The key to prevention of plagiocephaly is reinforcing education to parents on the importance of allowing the infant to lie in the prone position (tummy time) for 30 to 60 min/day while awake. Parents should also alternate the infant's head position each night to avoid persistent pressure on the occiput.
- Treatment for plagiocephaly includes physical therapy and the wearing of a customized helmet to reshape the skull.

DATA COLLECTION

RISK FACTORS

- Placing the infant in the supine position for sleeping
- Torticollis

EXPECTED FINDINGS

PHYSICAL FINDINGS

- Oblique shape of head
- Asymmetrical skull and facial features
- Flattened occiput
- Frontal and parietal projection
- Prominent cheekbone
- Anterior displacement of an ear
- Possible decreased range of motion in neck if torticollis is present

PATIENT-CENTERED CARE

NURSING CARE

- Reinforce the need for physical therapy for neck exercises.
- Assist parents in the proper use of the skull-molding helmet.

CLIENT EDUCATION

- Perform daily tummy time when the infant is awake.
- Limit the time the infant is in a car seat, bouncer, or swing.
- Alternate the infant's head position during sleep.
- Place infant in the supine position for sleep,
- There is no evidence that plagiocephaly leads to permanent cognitive delays or neurological damage.
- Torticollis, or tightening of the sternocleidomastoid muscle on one side of the neck, can develop.
- Physical therapy can successfully treat torticollis within 4 to 8 weeks.

Newborn seizures

Newborn seizures are usually a manifestation of a serious underlying disease. The most common causes for newborn seizures are hypoxic-ischemic encephalopathy (HIE) or cellular damage due to a hypoxic perinatal episode.

- Newborn seizures are divided into four subtypes: clonic, tonic, myoclonic, and subtle.
- Newborn seizures can be difficult to identify due to subtle manifestations. Seizures must be differentiated from normal newborn jitteriness and tremors. Newborns typically exhibit oral movements, oculomotor deviations, and apnea during seizure activity.

DATA COLLECTION

EXPECTED FINDINGS

Findings vary based on type of seizure.

Clonic: Slow rhythmic jerking movements; one to three movements per second

- **Focal:** Involves face, or upper or lower extremities on one side of the body; can involve neck or trunk; newborn is conscious during seizure
- **Multifocal:** Can migrate randomly from one part of the body to another; movements can start at different times

Tonic: Extension, stiffening movements
- **Generalized:** Extension of all limbs; upper limbs maintain a stiffly flexed position
- **Focal:** Sustained posturing of one limb; asymmetric posturing of trunk or neck

Subtle: Most common in premature newborns, often overlooked
- Horizontal eye deviation, repetitive blinking, fluttering of eyelids, staring
- Sucking or other oral/buccal/tongue movements
- Arm movements resembling swimming or rowing
- Leg movements resembling pedaling
- Apnea is common.

Myoclonic: Rapid jerks that involve flexor muscle groups
- **Focal:** Involves upper extremity flexor muscles; no changes in EEG
- **Multifocal:** Asynchronous twitching of several parts of the body; no changes in EEG
- **Generalized:** Bilateral jerks of upper and lower limbs; associated with EEG discharges

PATIENT-CENTERED CARE

NURSING CARE

Early recognition and reporting of seizure activity
- Monitor vital signs.
- Continue routine newborn examinations.
- Administer antiseizure medications.
- Administer medications for the underlying cause.
- Assist with respiratory support if hypoxia is present
- Encourage infant-parent bonding.
- Instruct parents about the newborn's status and reinforce teaching about the current treatment plan.
- Reinforce teaching to parents about home medications and safe administration.

PRACTICE Active Learning Scenario

A nurse is contributing to the plan of care for a newborn who has a myelomeningocele. What interventions should the nurse include? Use the ATI Active Learning Template: System Disorder to complete this item.

NURSING CARE: Include nursing actions before and after surgery for a newborn who has a myelomeningocele.

Application Exercises

1. A nurse is reviewing the medical record of a newborn who has necrotizing enterocolitis (NEC). Which of the following findings is a risk factor for NEC?

   A. Macrosomia

   B. Transient tachypnea of the newborn (TTN)

   C. Maternal gestational hypertension

   D. Preterm birth

2. A nurse is collecting data from a newborn who has congenital hypothyroidism. Which of the following manifestations should the nurse expect? (Select all that apply.)

   A. Hypertonicity

   B. Cool extremities

   C. Short neck

   D. Tachycardia

   E. Hyperreflexia

3. A nurse is reinforcing teaching with the parent of a newborn who has plagiocephaly. Which of the following statements by the parent indicates understanding?

   A. "I should put my baby to sleep on her belly during her afternoon nap."

   B. "I should alternate my baby's head position each time she sleeps."

   C. "I should expect my baby to require therapy for cognitive delays."

   D. "I should allow my baby to sleep in her infant swing."

4. A nurse is contributing to the plan of care for a newborn who is receiving phototherapy for hyperbilirubinemia. Which of the following interventions should the nurse include?

   A. Reposition the newborn every 4 hr.

   B. Lotion the newborn's skin twice per day.

   C. Check the newborn's temperature every 8 hr.

   D. Remove the newborn's eye mask during feedings.

5. A nurse is reinforcing preconception teaching with a client who has phenylketonuria (PKU). Which of the following information should the nurse include?

   A. "You should follow a low-phenylalanine diet once pregnancy is confirmed."

   B. "You will have your phenylalanine levels checked one to two times per week throughout pregnancy."

   C. "You should plan to increase intake of dietary proteins toward the end of pregnancy."

   D. "You will require a cesarean section birth due to the likelihood of the fetus having macrosomia."

Application Exercises Key

1. A. Macrosomia does not place a newborn at risk for NEC.

   B. TTN does not place a newborn at risk for NEC.

   C. Maternal gestational hypertension does not place a newborn at risk for NEC.

   D. **CORRECT:** A gestational age of 36 weeks, or a preterm birth, places a newborn at risk for NEC.

   (N) *NCLEX® Connection: Health Promotion and Maintenance, Health Promotion/Disease Prevention*

2. A. Hypertonicity is not an expected finding in a newborn who has congenital hypothyroidism.

   B. **CORRECT:** Cool extremities are an expected finding in a newborn who has congenital hypothyroidism.

   C. **CORRECT:** A short neck is an expected finding in a newborn who has congenital hypothyroidism.

   D. Tachycardia is not an expected finding in a newborn who has congenital hypothyroidism.

   E. Hyperreflexia is not an expected finding in a newborn who has congenital hypothyroidism.

   (N) *NCLEX® Connection: Physiological Adaptation, Basic Pathophysiology*

3. A. A newborn who has plagiocephaly should not be placed in the prone position to sleep.

   B. **CORRECT:** A newborn's head should not be placed in the same position each time she sleeps. The nurse should reinforce to the parent that the positioning of the head for sleeping should be alternated.

   C. There is no evidence that plagiocephaly leads to neurological damage or cognitive delays.

   D. A newborn who has plagiocephaly should not be allowed to sleep in an infant swing.

   (N) *NCLEX® Connection: Physiological Adaptation, Alterations in Body Systems*

4. A. A newborn undergoing phototherapy should be repositioned every 2 hr.

   B. A newborn undergoing phototherapy should not have lotion applied to the skin because it can cause burns.

   C. A newborn undergoing phototherapy should have their temperature monitored every 4 hr.

   D. **CORRECT:** A newborn undergoing phototherapy should have the eye mask removed for each feeding to allow for bonding and assessment of the eyes.

   (N) *NCLEX® Connection: Reduction of Risk Potential, Potential for Complications of Diagnostic Tests/Treatments/Procedures*

5. A. A client who has PKU should follow a low-phenylalanine diet for at least 3 months prior to conception and throughout the pregnancy.

   B. **CORRECT:** A client who has PKU will have phenylalanine levels monitored one to two times per week throughout pregnancy.

   C. A client who has PKU should decrease dietary intake of protein prior to conception.

   D. A client who has PKU is at no higher risk of fetal macrosomia and will not require a cesarean birth.

   (N) *NCLEX® Connection: Physiological Adaptation, Basic Pathophysiology*

PRACTICE Answer

Using the ATI Active Learning Template: System Disorder

NURSING CARE

Preoperative
- Protect the sac from injury.
- Place the infant in a radiant warmer, without clothing.
- Apply sterile, moist nonadhering dressing saturated with 0.9% sodium chloride, re-wetting as needed.
- Monitor cysts for findings of fluid leak or infection.
- Avoid measuring temperature rectally.

Postoperative
- Monitor vital signs.
- Monitor I&O.
- Monitor the surgical site for redness, edema, and drainage.
- Monitor for leakage of cerebrospinal fluid.
- Maintain prone position until other positions are prescribed.

(N) *NCLEX® Connection: Safety and Infection Control, Complications of Infants*

CHAPTER 40 *Pediatric
Emergencies*

In caring for children, nurses deal with emergent care situations that require rapid data collection and intervention. These situations offer opportunities for parent and community education.

Respiratory emergencies

Respiratory insufficiency: Increased work of breathing with mostly adequate gas exchange or hypoxia with acidosis

Respiratory failure: Inability to maintain adequate oxygenation of the blood

Apnea
- Cessation of respirations for more than 20 seconds
- Can be associated with hypoxemia or bradycardia
- Can be central or obstructive

Respiratory arrest: Complete cessation of respirations

Airway obstruction: Can be due to aspiration of a foreign body

DATA COLLECTION

RISK FACTORS

- Toddlers
- Primary inefficient gas exchange due to cerebral trauma, brain tumor, overdose, asphyxia, or CNS infection
- Obstructive lung disease caused by aspiration, infection, tumor, anaphylaxis, laryngospasm, or asthma
- Restrictive lung disease resulting from cystic fibrosis, pneumonia, or respiratory distress syndrome

EXPECTED FINDINGS

- History of illnesses (chronic or acute)
- History of events leading to respiratory emergency
- Allergies

EARLY INDICATIONS OF RESPIRATORY DISTRESS
- Restlessness
- Tachypnea
- Tachycardia
- Diaphoresis
- Nasal flaring
- Retractions
- Grunting
- Dyspnea
- Wheezing

ADVANCED HYPOXIA
- Bradypnea
- Bradycardia
- Peripheral or central cyanosis
- Stupor
- Coma

INDICATIONS OF CHOKING
- Universal choking sign (clutching neck with hands)
- Inability to speak
- Weak, ineffective cough
- High-pitched sounds or no sound
- Dyspnea
- Cyanosis

LABORATORY TESTS

Arterial blood gases (ABGs)

DIAGNOSTIC PROCEDURES

Chest x-rays

PATIENT-CENTERED CARE

NURSING CARE

- Follow American Heart Association (AHA) guidelines for CPR for respiratory and cardiac arrest.
- Follow the facility's protocol for activating the rapid response team. Q**EBP**
- Use current basic life support guidelines for neonates and pediatric clients.
- Position the client to maintain patent airway. Monitor respiratory status. Monitor vital signs.
- Administer oxygen.
- Suction as needed.
- Assist with preparations for intubation.
- Use a calm approach with the child and family.
- Administer medications.
- Keep the family informed of the child's status.
- Reinforce teaching with the family about manifestations of respiratory distress
- Encourage the family to learn CPR.

Obstructed airway
- Follow AHA guidelines for a choking child.
- For infants, use a combination of back blows and chest thrusts.
- For children and adolescents, use abdominal thrusts.
- Remove any visual obstruction or large debris from the mouth, but do not perform a blind finger sweep.
- Place the recovered child (one who resumes breathing) into the recovery position (side-lying position with legs bent at knees for stability).

CLIENT EDUCATION: Use strategies to prevent respiratory emergencies, such as recognizing choking hazards for toddlers.

Drowning

Asphyxiation while child is submerged in fluid can occur in any standing body of water that is at least 1 inch deep (bathtub, toilet, bucket, pool, pond, lake).
- Submersion injury (near-drowning) incidents are those in which children survive for 24 hr after being submerged in fluid.
- Inform families about preventive measures.

DATA COLLECTION

RISK FACTORS

- Age older than 12 months
- Swimming (can be overconfident or lack ability)
- Inadequate supervision or unattended in bathtub, pools
- Not wearing life jackets when in water
- Diving
- Child maltreatment

EXPECTED FINDINGS

Assist in collecting the following data.
- History of event including location and time of submersion
- Type and temperature of the fluid
- Respiratory system data collection
  (SEE RESPIRATORY EMERGENCIES)
- Body temperature (hypothermia)
- Bruising, spinal cord injury, or other physical injuries

LABORATORY TESTS

- ABGs
- Blood glucose (monitor for both hyper- and hypoglycemia)

DIAGNOSTIC PROCEDURES

Chest x-rays

PATIENT-CENTERED CARE

NURSING CARE

Based on degree of cerebral insult
- Administer oxygen (might need mechanical ventilation).
- Monitor vital signs.
- Administer medications.
- Provide chest physiotherapy.
- Monitor for complications that can occur 24 hr after incident (cerebral edema, respiratory distress).
- Use a calm approach with the child and family.
- Keep the family informed of the child's status.

CLIENT EDUCATION

- Lock toilet seats when child is at home.
- Do not leave the child unattended in the bathtub.
- Even a small amount of water can lead to accidental drowning.
- Do not leave the child unattended in a swimming pool, even if the child can swim.
- Make sure private pools are fenced with locked gates to prevent children from wandering into the pool area.
- Provide life jackets when boating.

Apparent life-threatening event

Sudden event where the infant exhibits apnea, change in color, change in muscle tone, and choking

DATA COLLECTION

RISK FACTORS

- Gastroesophageal reflux
- Respiratory infections
- Seizure
- Metabolic problems
- Child maltreatment
- Urinary tract infection (UTI)

EXPECTED FINDINGS

EVENT: Apnea can be present during event.
- Change in color: pallor, redness, cyanosis
- Change in muscle tone: hypotonia
- Choking, gagging, coughing

LABORATORY TESTS

- Blood cultures: bacterial or viral infection
- Urine culture: UTI
- CBC
- Serum glucose
- Electrolytes

DIAGNOSTIC PROCEDURES

Electrocardiogram: long QT syndrome or dysrhythmias

Electroencephalogram: epilepsy

pH study: reflux

Magnetic resonance imaging: hemorrhage or cerebral abnormalities/injuries

Sleep study: sleep apnea

PATIENT-CENTERED CARE

NURSING CARE

- Assist in collecting the following data.
  - Description of the event by the observer
  - CPR efforts provided
  - Maternal history
  - Family history of seizures
- Prepare the infant and family for testing.
- Monitor the infant for recurrent events.
- Encourage the family to learn CPR.

CLIENT EDUCATION: Use an apnea monitor.

Sudden infant death syndrome

- Sudden infant death syndrome (SIDS) is the sudden, unpredictable death of an infant without an identified cause, even after investigation and autopsy.
- Inform the family about preventive measures.

DATA COLLECTION

RISK FACTORS
- Maternal smoking during pregnancy
- Secondhand smoke
- Co-sleeping with parent or adult
- Nonstandard bed (sofa, soft bedding, water bed, pillows)
- Prone or side-lying sleeping
- Low birth weight
- Prematurity
- Multiple birth
- Low Apgar score
- Viral illness
- Family history of SIDS

EXPECTED FINDINGS
- History of events prior to discovery of infant
- History of illnesses
- Pregnancy and birth history
- Presence of risk factors

PATIENT-CENTERED CARE

NURSING CARE

- Provide support.
- Allow the infant's family an opportunity to express feelings.
- Assist with scheduling a home health visit to follow a death.
- Assist with referrals to support groups, counseling, or community groups.

CLIENT EDUCATION: Take precautions to reduce the risks of SIDS.
- Place the infant on the back for sleep. Qs
- Avoid exposure to tobacco smoke.
- Prevent overheating.
- Use a firm, tight-fitting mattress in the infant's crib.
- Remove pillows, quilts, and stuffed animals from the crib during sleep.
- Ensure that the infant's head is kept uncovered during sleep.
- Offer pacifier when infant is sleeping.
- Encourage breastfeeding.
- Avoid co-sleeping.
- Maintain immunizations up to date.

Poisoning

- Ingestion of or exposure to toxic substances
- Inform families about preventive measures.

DATA COLLECTION

RISK FACTORS
- Children younger than 6 years of age
- Improperly stored medications, household chemicals, and hazardous substances
- Exposure to plants, cosmetics, and heavy metals, which are potential sources of toxic substances
- Lead ingestion from lead-based paint or soil contamination

EXPECTED FINDINGS

INFORMATION REGARDING POISONOUS AGENT
- Name and location
- Amount ingested
- Time of ingestion

Specific poisons

Physical response depends on specific poison. QEBP

Acetaminophen
- **2 to 4 hr after ingestion:** Nausea, vomiting, sweating, pallor
- **24 to 36 hr after ingestion:** Improvement in condition
- **36 hr to 7 days or longer (hepatic stage):** Pain in upper right quadrant, confusion, stupor, jaundice, coagulation disturbances
- **Final stage:** Death or gradual recovery

Acetylsalicylic acid (aspirin)
- **Acute poisoning:** Nausea, vomiting, disorientation, diaphoresis, tachypnea, tinnitus, oliguria, lightheadedness, seizures
- **Chronic poisoning:** Subtle version of acute manifestations, bleeding tendencies, dehydration, seizures more severe than acute poisoning

Supplemental iron
- **Initial period (30 min to 6 hr after ingestion):** Vomiting, hematemesis, diarrhea, gastric pain, bloody stools
- **Latency period (up to 24 hr after ingestion):** Improvement of condition
- **Systemic toxicity period (12 to 24 hr after ingestion):** Metabolic acidosis, hyperglycemia, bleeding, fever, shock, possible death
- **Hepatic injury period (48 hr to 5 days after ingestion):** Impaired liver function, jaundice, hypoglycemia, coma
- Scarring causing pyloric stenosis or duodenal obstruction (2 to 5 weeks after ingestion)

Hydrocarbons: Gasoline, kerosene, lighter fluid, paint thinner, turpentine
- Gagging, choking, coughing, nausea, vomiting
- Lethargy, weakness, tachypnea, cyanosis, grunting, retractions

Corrosives: Household cleaners, batteries, bleach, denture cleaners
- Pain and burning in mouth, throat, and stomach
- Edematous lips, tongue, and pharynx with white mucous membranes
- Violent vomiting with hemoptysis
- Drooling
- Anxiety
- Shock

Lead
- **Low-dose exposure:** Distractibility, impulsiveness, hyperactivity, hearing impairment, mild intellectual difficulty
- **High-dose exposure:** Cognitive delays varying in severity, blindness, paralysis, coma, seizures, death
- **Other manifestations:** Kidney impairment, impaired calcium function, anemia

LABORATORY TESTS

- Serum lead
- CBC with differential
- ABGs
- Serum iron
- Serum acetaminophen
- Liver function tests
- Blood alcohol and toxicology screening

PATIENT-CENTERED CARE

NURSING CARE

Depends on the poison ingested
- Monitor for ongoing changes.
- Terminate exposure.
- Provide cardiorespiratory support as needed.
- Notify local or regional poison control center.
- Assist with administration of IV fluids.
- Assist with cardiac monitoring.
- Monitor vital signs and oxygen saturation.
- Monitor I&O.
- Administer antidote.
- Assist with gastric decontamination.
  - Activated charcoal
  - Gastric lavage
  - Increasing bowel motility
  - Syrup of ipecac is contraindicated for routine poison control treatment.
- Keep the family informed of the child's condition.

Interventions for specific substances

Acetaminophen: N–acetylcysteine given orally

Acetylsalicylic acid
- Activated charcoal
- Gastric lavage
- Sodium bicarbonate
- Oxygen and ventilation
- Vitamin K
- Hemodialysis for severe cases

Supplemental iron
- Emesis or lavage
- Chelation therapy

Hydrocarbons (gasoline, kerosene, lighter fluid, paint thinner, turpentine)
- Do not induce vomiting.
- Intubation with cuffed endotracheal tube prior to any gastric decontamination
- Treatment of chemical pneumonia

Corrosives (household cleaners, batteries, denture cleaners, bleach)
- Airway maintenance
- NPO
- Analgesics for pain
- Do not induce vomiting.

Lead: Chelation therapy

CLIENT EDUCATION

POISON PREVENTION
- Keep toxic agents out of reach of children. Qs
- Lock cabinets containing potentially harmful substances.
- Do not take medication in front of children.
- Discard unused medications.
- When giving a child medication, do not say it is candy.
- Use nonmercury thermometers.
- Eliminate lead-based paint in the environment.
- Encourage hand hygiene prior to eating.
- Do not store food in lead-based containers.

COMPLICATIONS

Cognitive impairments

Varies with degree of anoxic insult or lead levels in blood

NURSING ACTIONS
- Provide prevention measures to families.
- Recommend routine screening for lead levels at 1, 2, and 3 years of age.
- Collaborate with the interprofessional team to assist with care for children who have elevated lead levels.
- Assist with appropriate referrals (community nurse, teacher, early intervention).

Application Exercises

1. A nurse is assisting with the care of a child who is experiencing respiratory distress. Which of the following findings are manifestations of respiratory distress? (Select all that apply.)

   A. Bradypnea

   B. Peripheral cyanosis

   C. Tachycardia

   D. Diaphoresis

   E. Restlessness

2. A nurse in an urgent care clinic is assisting with the care of a child whose parent reports that the child has swallowed paint thinner. The child is lethargic, gagging, and cyanotic. Which of the following actions should the nurse take?

   A. Induce vomiting with syrup of ipecac.

   B. Insert a nasogastric tube, and administer activated charcoal.

   C. Obtain a cuffed endotracheal tube for the provider.

   D. Assist with chelation therapy

3. A nurse is assisting with admission of an infant who experienced a life-threatening event. Which of the following prescriptions should the nurse anticipate? (Select all that apply.)

   A. Electroencephalogram

   B. Electrocardiogram

   C. Serum glucose

   D. Lipid panel

   E. Blood culture

4. A nurse is reinforcing teaching with a parent about acetaminophen poisoning. Which of the following information should the nurse include?

   A. Nausea begins 24 hr after ingestion.

   B. Treatment is most effective if administered within 8 hr of ingestion.

   C. Jaundice will appear 12 hr after ingestion.

   D. Children show indications of improvement 4 hr after ingestion.

5. A nurse in a community center is assisting with an informational presentation for a group of parents on management of airway obstructions in toddlers. Which of the following responses by the parents indicates understanding? (Select all that apply.)

   A. "I will push on my child's abdomen."

   B. "I will apply back blows until the obstruction clears."

   C. "I will turn my child on his side when he starts breathing again."

   D. "I will use my finger to check my child's mouth for objects that I'm not able to see."

   E. "I will immediately place my child in my car and take him to the closest emergency facility."

PRACTICE Active Learning Scenario

A nurse is discussing prevention of sudden infant death syndrome (SIDS) with a group of parents. What information should the nurse include? Use the ATI Active Learning Template: System Disorder to complete this item.

NURSING CARE: Identify at least seven preventive measures to reduce the risk of SIDS.

Application Exercises Key

1. A. Bradypnea is a manifestation of advanced respiratory distress and hypoxia.

   B. Peripheral cyanosis is a manifestation of advanced respiratory distress and hypoxia.

   C. **CORRECT:** Tachycardia is an early manifestation of respiratory distress.

   D. **CORRECT:** Diaphoresis is an early manifestation of respiratory distress.

   E. **CORRECT:** Restlessness is an early manifestation of respiratory distress.

   Ⓝ *NCLEX® Connection: Physiological Adaptation, Basic Pathophysiology*

2. A. Inducing vomiting with syrup of ipecac is contraindicated as a poison control treatment for hydrocarbons.

   B. Activated charcoal is indicated for acetylsalicylic acid poisoning.

   C. **CORRECT:** The nurse should obtain a cuffed endotracheal tube for the provider to use for intubation. Treatment for poisoning with hydrocarbons includes intubation to protect the airway before proceeding with gastric decontamination.

   D. Chelation therapy is indicated for lead poisoning.

   Ⓝ *NCLEX® Connection: Physiological Adaptation, Medical Emergencies*

3. A. **CORRECT:** EEG is performed to check for epilepsy.

   B. **CORRECT:** ECG is performed to check for long QT syndrome or dysrhythmias.

   C. **CORRECT:** Serum glucose is performed to check for metabolic problems related to hyper- or hypoglycemia.

   D. A lipid panel is not routinely performed for an infant who experienced an apparent life-threatening event.

   E. **CORRECT:** A blood culture is obtained to check for bacterial or viral infections.

   Ⓝ *NCLEX® Connection: Reduction of Risk Potential, Diagnostic Tests*

4. A. Nausea is a manifestation that begins 2 to 4 hr after ingestion.

   B. **CORRECT:** Treatment is most effective if administered within 8 hr of ingestion, but it is still beneficial if administered within 24 hr.

   C. Jaundice will appear in 36 hr to 7 days following ingestion.

   D. Children show an improvement in condition 24 to 36 hr after ingestion. This improvement in condition precedes the hepatic stage.

   Ⓝ *NCLEX® Connection: Physiological Adaptation, Medical Emergencies*

5. A. **CORRECT:** The nurse should instruct the parents to use abdominal thrusts to clear an obstructed airway in a toddler as part of AHA guidelines.

   B. The nurse should inform the parents that back blows alternating with chest thrusts are recommended by AHA guidelines for clearing the obstructed airway of an infant.

   C. **CORRECT:** The nurse should instruct the parents to place the recovered toddler (one who resumes breathing) into a side-lying recovery position with legs bent at the knees for stability.

   D. The nurse should inform the parents that blind finger sweeps to check for an obstructed airway are not recommended by AHA guidelines because this action can cause an object to be pushed further down into the toddler's throat, causing injury and further obstruction.

   E. The nurse should instruct the parents to attempt to clear the toddler's obstructed airway according to AHA guidelines and to call 911. Attempting to personally transport the child to an emergency facility delays treatment.

   Ⓝ *NCLEX® Connection: Physiological Adaptation, Medical Emergencies*

PRACTICE Answer

Using the ATI Active Learning Template: System Disorder

NURSING CARE

- Place the infant on the back for sleep.
- Avoid exposure to tobacco smoke.
- Prevent overheating.
- Use a firm, tight-fitting mattress in the infant's crib.
- Remove pillows, quilts, and stuffed animals from the crib during sleep.
- Ensure that the infant's head is kept uncovered during sleep.
- Offer a pacifier at naps and night.
- Encourage breastfeeding.
- Avoid co-sleeping.
- Maintain immunizations up to date.

Ⓝ *NCLEX® Connection: Psychosocial Integrity, Abuse/Neglect*

CHAPTER 41 Psychosocial Issues of Infants, Children, and Adolescents

Nurses care for pediatric clients who have psychosocial issues as well as physical illnesses. Psychosocial issues (such as depression) can occur as a result of a physical illness, be independent from physical illness, or be the cause for somatic manifestations (such as pain). It is important that the nurse be familiar with various psychosocial issues to assist the interprofessional team in providing the child with appropriate screenings, referrals, and treatment.

Depression

- Difficult to detect and often overlooked in school-aged children because children have limitations in expressing their feelings.
- At least five manifestations of depression (insomnia, feelings of worthlessness, irritable mood, persistent thoughts of death, weight loss) must be present for a minimum of 2 weeks to diagnose major depressive disorder in children and adolescents.

DATA COLLECTION

RISK FACTORS

- Family history
- Traumatic event
- Inadequate support system (family or social)

EXPECTED FINDINGS

- Sad facial expressions
- Withdrawal from family, friends, and activities
- Fatigue
- Tearfulness/crying
- Ill feeling
- Feelings of worthlessness
- Weight loss or gain
- Alterations in sleep
- Lack of interest in school, drop in school performance
- Statements regarding low self-esteem
- Hopelessness
- Suicidal ideation or persistent thoughts of death
- Irritability

PATIENT-CENTERED CARE

NURSING CARE

- Assist with planning care that is individualized.
- Assist with obtaining health history and growth and development information.
- Screen for substance use.
- Determine if there is an actual or potential risk to self (suicide plan, lethality of the plan, means to carry out the plan).
- Reinforce coping strategies.
- Encourage individual or family counseling (peer group discussions, mentoring, counseling).
- Interview the child.

MEDICATIONS

Tricyclic antidepressants or selective serotonin reuptake inhibitors (SSRIs)

Trazodone, sertraline, paroxetine, bupropion, venlafaxine

NURSING ACTIONS
- Monitor for adverse effects.
- Monitor for suicidal ideation.

CLIENT EDUCATION
- Identify adverse effects.
- Therapeutic effectiveness can take up to 2 weeks.
- Do not abruptly discontinue the medication.

COMPLICATIONS

Suicide attempt

Posttraumatic stress disorder (PTSD)

Develops following a traumatic or catastrophic event

DATA COLLECTION

RISK FACTORS

- Potential genetic predisposition
- Traumatic incident
- Repeated trauma
- Psychiatric disorder
- Natural disaster
- Sexual abuse
- Witnessing homicide, suicide, or other violent act

EXPECTED FINDINGS

INITIAL RESPONSE
- Lasts a few minutes to 2 hr
- Increased stress hormones (fight or flight)
- Psychosis

SECOND PHASE
- Lasts approximately 2 weeks
- Period of calm (numbness, denial)
- Decreased defense mechanisms

THIRD PHASE (COPING)
- Extends 2 to 3 months
- Getting worse instead of better
- Depression, phobias, anxiety, conversion reactions, repetitive movements, flashbacks, or obsessions

PATIENT-CENTERED CARE

NURSING CARE

- Assist with referral to psychotherapy services.
- Monitor for behavior changes/problems.
- Monitor school work.
- Assist the client and family with coping strategies.
- Allow the client and family to express their feelings.
- Prevent or reduce long-term effects.

MEDICATIONS

Selective norepinephrine reuptake inhibitors may be used on an individual basis.

Attention-deficit/ hyperactivity disorder

- Inattentiveness, hyperactivity, and impulsiveness usually revealed prior to age 7
- Common in childhood and can persist into adulthood
- A child must meet diagnostic criteria for diagnosis of attention-deficit hyperactivity disorder (ADHD).
  - Manifestations between 4 and 18 years of age
  - Manifestations in more than one setting
  - Evidence of social or academic impairment
  - Six or more findings from a category (inattention or hyperactivity-impulsivity)

DATA COLLECTION

RISK FACTORS

- Family history of ADHD
- Exposure to toxins or medicines
- Chronic otitis media, meningitis, or head trauma
- Higher incidence in males

EXPECTED FINDINGS

INATTENTION
- Failing to pay close attention to detail or making careless mistakes
- Blocking incoming stimuli
- Difficulty sustaining attention
- Does not seem to listen
- Failing to follow through on instructions

- Difficulty organizing activities
- Avoiding or disliking activities that require mental effort for a period of time, such as reading
- Losing things
- Easy distractibility
- Forgetfulness

HYPERACTIVITY
- Fidgeting
- Failing to remain seated
- Inappropriate running
- Difficulty engaging in quiet play
- Seeming to be busy all the time
- Talking excessively

IMPULSIVITY
- Blurting out responses before questions are asked
- Difficulty waiting turns
- Interrupting often
- Striking out, biting, shouting

PATIENT-CENTERED CARE

NURSING CARE

- Obtain medical, developmental, or behavioral history.
- Use behavioral checklists with adaptive scales.
- Use a calm, firm, respectful approach with the child.
- Use modeling to demonstrate acceptable behavior.
- Obtain the child's attention before giving directions. Provide short and clear explanations.
- Set clear limits on unacceptable behaviors, and be consistent.
- Suggest physical activities through which the child can use energy and obtain success.
- Focus on the child's and family's strengths, not just the problems.
- Support the parents' efforts to remain hopeful.
- Provide a safe environment for the child and others.
- Provide the child with specific positive feedback when expectations are met.
- Identify issues that result in power struggles.
- Assist the child in developing effective coping mechanisms.
- Encourage the child to participate in a form of group, individual, or family therapy.
- Assist the family with behavioral strategies.
  - Positive reinforcement
  - Rewards for good behavior
  - Age-appropriate consequences
- Assist the family with modification of the environment to help the child become successful.
  - Structured environment
  - Charts to assist with organization
  - Decreasing stimuli in the environment
  - Consistent study area
  - Modeling positive behaviors
  - Using steps when assigning chores
  - Using pastel colors

- Assist with appropriate classroom placement in the school.
  - Collaborate with the school nurse.
  - Allow more time for testing.
  - Place in classroom that has order and consistent rules.
  - Offer verbal instruction combined with visual cues.
  - Plan academic subjects in the morning.
  - Include regular breaks.
  - Provide for small classroom settings or work groups.

MEDICATIONS

Methylphenidate, dextroamphetamine

Psychostimulant, which increases dopamine and norepinephrine levels

NURSING ACTIONS
- Monitor height and weight
- Gradually increase dose to reach therapeutic results.
- Give 30 min before meal.
- Give last dose of the day prior to 1800 to prevent insomnia.
- Monitor for adverse effects (insomnia, anorexia, nervousness, hyper/hypotension, tachycardia, anemia).
- Avoid caffeine.
- Store safely. The medication has potential for misuse by others.
- Tricyclic antidepressants are used as adjunct therapy to treat insomnia.

Atomoxetine

Selective norepinephrine reuptake inhibitor

NURSING ACTIONS
- Gradually increase dose to reach therapeutic results.
- Monitor for adverse effects (suicidal ideation).

Autism spectrum disorder

Complex neurodevelopmental disorders with spectrum of behaviors affecting an individual's ability to communicate and interact with others in a social setting.

DATA COLLECTION

RISK FACTORS
- Possible genetic component
- Exact cause unknown
- Current research does not indicate a link between autism spectrum disorder (ASD) and vaccines containing thimerosal.

EXPECTED FINDINGS
- Delays in at least one of the following
  - Social interaction
  - Social communication
  - Imaginative play prior to age 3 years
- Distress when routines are changed
- Unusual attachments to objects
- Inability to start or continue conversation

- Delayed or absent language development uses gestures instead of words
- Grunting or humming
- Inability to adjust gaze to look at something else
- Not referring to self correctly
- Withdrawn, labile mood
- Decreased pain sensation
- Spending time alone rather than playing with others
- Avoiding eye contact
- Withdrawal from physical contact
- Heightened or lowered senses
- Not imitating actions of others
- Minimal pretend play
- Short attention span
- Intense temper tantrums
- Showing aggression
- Repetitive movements (rocking, hand flapping)
- Typical IQ less than 70

PATIENT-CENTERED CARE

NURSING CARE
- Assist with screening data collection tools, such as the Checklist for Autism in Toddlers (CHAT) or Pervasive Developmental Disorders Screening Test.
- Assist with referral to early intervention, physical therapy, occupational therapy, and speech and language therapy.
- Assist with behavior modification program.
  - Promote positive reinforcement.
  - Increase social awareness.
  - Encourage verbal communication.
  - Decrease unacceptable behaviors.
  - Assist in setting realistic goals.
  - Structure opportunities for small successes.
  - Set clear rules.
- Decrease environmental stimulation.
- Assist with nutritional needs.
- Introduce new situations slowly.
- Monitor for behavior changes.
- Encourage age-appropriate play.
- Communicate at an age-appropriate level (brief and concrete).
- Provide support to the family.
- Encourage support groups.
- Discuss with parents the benefits of the Autism Society for further education, support for the family including siblings, and information about treatment programs.

MEDICATIONS

Used on an individual basis to control aggression, anxiety, hyperactivity, irritability, mood swings, compulsions, and attention problems
- SSRIs can decrease aggression.
- Antipsychotics and melatonin can help with insomnia.

Cognitive impairment

- Also known as intellectual disability
- Previously called mental retardation

DATA COLLECTION

RISK FACTORS

- Familial, social, environmental, organic or other unknown causes
- Infections (congenital rubella, syphilis)
- Fetal alcohol syndrome
- Chronic lead ingestion
- Chromosomal disorders
- Trauma to the brain
- Gestational disorders
- Pre-existing disease (Down syndrome, microcephaly, hydrocephaly, psychiatric disorders, metabolic disorders, cerebral palsy)

EXPECTED FINDINGS

- Can range from mild to severe
- Delayed developmental milestones
- Inability to reason or problem solve

EARLY MANIFESTATIONS
- Abnormal eye contact
- Feeding difficulties
- Language difficulties
- Fine and gross motor delays
- Decreased alertness
- Irritability
- Decreased responsiveness to contact

PATIENT-CENTERED CARE

NURSING CARE

- Determine the child's deficiency.
- Contribute to a plan of care individualized to the client's needs.
- Assist with appropriate referrals (early intervention program, social work, speech therapy, physical therapy, occupational therapy).
- Add visual cues with verbal instruction.
- Give one-step instructions.
- Assist the family in teaching the child self-cares.
- Assist the family in promoting development.
- Encourage play and exercise.
- Assist the family with appropriate activities and toys.
- Assist with communication skills.
- Encourage social activities.

Failure to thrive

Inadequate growth resulting from the inability to obtain or use calories required for growth. It is usually described in an infant or child who falls below the fifth percentile for weight (and possibly for height) or who has persistent weight loss.

DATA COLLECTION

RISK FACTORS

- Preterm birth with low birth weight or intrauterine growth restriction
- Parental neglect, lack of parental knowledge, or disturbed maternal-child attachment
- Poverty
- Health or childrearing beliefs
- Family stress
- Feeding resistance
- Inadequate caloric intake such as incorrect formula prep or juice consumption
- Insufficient breast milk
- Improper latching or uncoordinated sucking and swallowing

ORGANIC CAUSES: Cerebral palsy, chronic kidney failure, congenital heart disease, increased metabolism (hyperthyroidism), inadequate absorption (cystic fibrosis, celiac disease, Crohn's disease), hepatic disease, impaired utilization (Down syndrome), prematurity, and gastroesophageal reflux

EXPECTED FINDINGS

- Less than the fifth percentile on the growth chart for weight
- Malnourished appearance
- Poor muscle tone, lack of subcutaneous fat
- No fear of strangers
- Minimal smiling
- Decreased activity level
- Lethargy
- Withdrawn behavior
- Developmental delays
- Feeding disorder
- Wide-eyed gaze, absent eye contact
- Stiff or flaccid body

PATIENT-CENTERED CARE

NURSING CARE

- The nurse might have to remove child from parental care to evaluate carefully and administer therapy.
- Obtain a nutritional history.
- Observe parent-child interactions.
- Obtain accurate baseline height and weight. Observe for low weight, malnourished appearance, and indications of dehydration.
- Weigh the child daily without clothing or a diaper.
- Maintain strict I&O and calorie counts.

- Reinforce with parents how to recognize and respond to the infant's cues of hunger.
- Establish a routine for eating that encourages usual times, duration, and setting.
- Reinforce proper positioning, latching on, and timing for breastfeeding.
- Provide high-calorie milk supplements for children.
- Administer multivitamin supplements (zinc, iron).
- Instruct parents how to mix formula and provide step-by-step written instructions.
- Limit juice to 4 oz/day.
- Provide developmental stimulation.
- Nurture the child (rocking, talking to the child).
- Reinforce behavior modification techniques during mealtimes.

COMPLICATIONS

Extreme malnourishment

NURSING ACTIONS: Prepare the child and parents for tube feedings or IV therapy.

Maltreatment of infants and children

Maltreatment of infants and children is attributed to a variety of predisposing factors, which include parental, child, and environmental characteristics. Child maltreatment can occur across all economic and educational backgrounds and racial/ethnic/religious groups.

Maltreatment of children is made of several specific types of behaviors.
- **Physical:** causing pain or harm to a child (shaken baby syndrome, fractures, factitious disorder imposed on another)
- **Sexual:** occurring when sexual contact takes place without consent, whether or not the victim is able to give consent (includes any sexual behavior toward a minor and dating violence among adolescents)
- **Emotional:** humiliating, threatening, or intimidating a child (includes behavior that minimizes an individual's feelings of self-worth)
- **Neglect:** includes failure to provide the following
  - **Physical care:** food, clothing, shelter, medical or dental care, safety, education
  - **Emotional care** and/or stimulation to foster normal development: nurturing, affection, attention

DATA COLLECTION

RISK FACTORS

WARNING SIGNS OF MALTREATMENT
- Physical evidence of maltreatment
- History of injury incompatible with findings
- Vague explanation of injury
- Other injuries that are not related to the original client concern
- Delay in seeking care
- Multiple fractures at different stages of healing
- Bruising in a nonmobile client or in areas not prone to injury
- Caregivers/client report conflicting histories
- Statement of possible maltreatment from a caregiver or client

PARENTAL CHARACTERISTICS
- Younger parents
- Single parents who have a partner unrelated to the child
- Social isolation
- Low-income situation
- Lack of education
- Low self-esteem
- Lack of parenting knowledge
- Substance use disorder
- History of having been maltreated
- Lack of support systems

CHARACTERISTICS OF THE CHILD
- Child 1 year old or younger is at greater risk due to the need for constant attention and increased demands of caregiving.
- Infants and children who are unwanted, hyperactive, or who have physical or mental disabilities are at risk due to their increased demands and need for constant attention.
- Premature infants are at risk due to the possible failure of parent-child bonding at birth.

ENVIRONMENTAL CHARACTERISTICS
- Chronic stress
- Divorce, alcohol use disorder, substance use disorder, poverty
- Unemployment, inadequate housing, crowded living conditions
- Substitute caregivers

EXPECTED FINDINGS
- Inconsistencies between the parent/caregiver's report and the child's injuries
- Inconsistency between nature of injury and developmental level of the child
- Repeated injuries requiring emergency treatment
- Inappropriate responses from the parents or child

Physical neglect
- Failure to thrive, malnutrition
- Lack of hygiene
- Frequent injuries
- Being dressed inappropriately for weather
- Delay in seeking health care
- Dull affect
- School absences
- Self-stimulating behaviors

Physical maltreatment
- Bruises, welts in various stages of healing
- Burns
- Fractures
- Lacerations
- Fear of parents
- Lack of emotional response/reaction

- Superficial relationships
- Withdrawal
- Aggression
- Bruising in an infant before 6 months of age should be deemed suspicious by the nurse.

Emotional neglect and maltreatment
- Failure to thrive
- Eating disorder
- Enuresis
- Sleep disturbances
- Self-stimulating behaviors
- Withdrawal
- Lack of social smile (infant)
- Extreme behaviors
- Delayed development
- Attempted suicide
- Parent/caregiver rejects, isolates, terrorizes, ignores, verbally assaults, or overpressures the child

Sexual maltreatment is defined as the employment, use, persuasion, or inducement of a child to engage in any sexually explicit conduct. Examples include pedophilia, prostitution, incest, molestation, and pornography.
- Bruises, lacerations on genitals
- Bleeding of genitalia, anus, or mouth
- Sexually transmitted infection
- Difficulty walking or standing
- UTI
- Regressive behavior
- Withdrawal
- Personality changes
- Bloody, torn, or stained underwear
- Unusual body odor

Shaken baby syndrome or abusive head trauma (AHT):
Shaking can cause intracranial hemorrhage. Caregiver's frustrations with persistent crying can lead to this.
- Can have no external indications of injury
- Vomiting, poor feeding, and listlessness
- Respiratory distress
- Bulging fontanels
- Retinal hemorrhages
- Seizures
- Posturing
- Alterations in level of consciousness
- Apnea
- Bradycardia
- Blindness
- Unresponsiveness

LABORATORY TESTS

CBC, urinalysis, and other tests that check for sexually transmitted infections or bleeding

DIAGNOSTIC PROCEDURES

Depend upon the data collection findings and injuries
- Radiograph
- Computed tomography or magnetic resonance imaging scan

PATIENT-CENTERED CARE

NURSING CARE

- Identify maltreatment as soon as possible. Conduct detailed history and physical examination.
- Inspect for unusual bruising on the abdomen, back, and buttocks. Document thoroughly with size, shape, and color. Use diagrams to represent location.
- Identify the mechanism of injury, which might not be congruent with the physical appearance of the injury. Many bruises at different stages of healing can indicate ongoing beatings.
- Observe for bruises or welts in the shape of a belt buckle or other objects.
- Observe for burns that appear glove- or stocking-like on hands or feet, which can indicate forced immersion into boiling water. Small, round burns can be caused by lit cigarettes. Document detailed descriptions of all findings.
- Note fractures that have unusual features, such as forearm spiral fractures, which could be caused by twisting the extremity forcefully. The presence of multiple fractures is suspicious.
- Check the child for head injuries. Identify the child's level of consciousness, making sure to note equal and reactive pupils. Monitor for nausea and vomiting.
- The nursing priority is the child's safety and ensuring the child is in a safe environment.
- Mandatory reporting is required of all health care providers, including suspected cases of child maltreatment. There are civil and criminal penalties for not reporting.
- Clearly and objectively document information obtained in the interview and during data collection.
- Photograph and detail all visible injuries.
- Conduct the interview with the child and parents individually.
- Be direct, honest, and professional.
- Use language the child understands.
- Be understanding and attentive.
- Client circumstances are case-sensitive, and referrals are made to always keep the client safe. Explain the process if a referral is made to child protective services.
- Use open-ended questions that require a descriptive response. These questions are less threatening and elicit more relevant information.
- Provide support for the child and parents.
- Demonstrate behaviors for child-rearing with the parents and child.
- Provide consistent care to the child.
- Avoid asking the child probing questions.
- Promote self-esteem.
- Assist with alleviating feelings of shame and guilt.
- Assist the child with grieving the loss of parents, if indicated.
- Discharge can begin once legal determination of placement has been decided.

INTERPROFESSIONAL CARE

Assist with appropriate referrals.

Bullying

- Physical, verbal, or emotional maltreatment that is repetitive by a person to another person with intent to establish power and dominance with intimidation
- Can be with or without face–to–face contact

SETTINGS: School, playground, bus, text messages, Internet

DATA COLLECTION

RISK FACTORS

PERPETRATORS OF BULLYING BEHAVIOR
- Male gender
- Depression
- Decreased academic performance
- Decreased social involvement with peers
- Exposure to domestic violence
- Conduct problems
- Criminal acts
- Peer pressure
- Ineffective communication with parents
- Dropping out of school

RECIPIENTS OF BULLYING BEHAVIOR
- Low self–esteem
- Loneliness
- Somatic reports
- Anxiety
- Depression

PATIENT-CENTERED CARE

NURSING CARE

- Obtain support from the family.
- Assist with referral for counseling and bullying prevention programs.
- Follow procedures for investigating and reporting

CLIENT EDUCATION

- Observe for indications of bullying and be inquisitive.
- Assist teens with making decisions.

PRACTICE Active Learning Scenario

A nurse is discussing shaken baby syndrome with a group of parents. What manifestations should the nurse include? Use the ATI Active Learning Template: Basic Concept to complete this item.

UNDERLYING PRINCIPLES: Include seven manifestations.

Application Exercises

1. A nurse is reinforcing teaching with a group of parents about characteristics of infants who have failure to thrive. Which of the following characteristics should the nurse include?

   A. Intense fear of strangers

   B. Increased risk for childhood obesity

   C. Inability to form close relationships with siblings

   D. Developmental delays

2. A nurse is reinforcing instruction to the teacher of a child who has attention-deficit/hyperactivity disorder (ADHD). Which of the following classroom strategies should the nurse recommend? (Select all that apply.)

   A. Eliminate testing.

   B. Allow for regular breaks.

   C. Combine verbal instruction with visual cues.

   D. Establish consistent classroom rules.

   E. Increase stimuli in the environment.

3. A nurse is reinforcing teaching with a parent about posttraumatic stress disorder (PTSD). Which of the following information should the nurse include? (Select all that apply.)

   A. Children who have PTSD can benefit from psychotherapy.

   B. A manifestation of PTSD is phobias.

   C. Personality disorders are a complication of PTSD.

   D. PTSD develops following a traumatic event.

   E. There are six stages of PTSD.

4. A nurse is discussing with the parent of a child risk factors for attention-deficit/hyperactivity disorder (ADHD). Which of the following should the nurse include?

   A. Formula-feeding as an infant

   B. History of head trauma

   C. History of postterm birth

   D. Child of a single parent

5. A nurse is caring for a child who has depression. Which of the following findings should the nurse expect? (Select all that apply.)

   A. Preferring being with peers

   B. Weight loss or gain

   C. Report of low self-esteem

   D. Sleeping more than usual

   E. Hyperactivity

Application Exercises Key

1. A. These infants do not exhibit the expected fear of strangers.

   B. These infants are not at an increased risk for childhood obesity.

   C. These infants can form close relationships with siblings.

   D. **CORRECT:** These infants can exhibit developmental delays due to decreased nutritional intake needed for brain development.

   Ⓝ *NCLEX® Connection: Health Promotion and Maintenance, Developmental Stages and Transitions*

2. A. Allowing for added time when testing can assist the client who has ADHD to be successful.

   B. **CORRECT:** Allowing for regular breaks will assist the client who has ADHD to focus on the required tasks.

   C. **CORRECT:** Combining verbal instruction with visual cues will assist the client who has ADHD with learning information.

   D. **CORRECT:** Providing consistent classroom rules will assist the client who has ADHD to be successful.

   E. Stimuli in the environment distract the client who has ADHD, so it should be decreased.

   Ⓝ *NCLEX® Connection: Psychosocial Integrity, Behavioral Management*

3. A. **CORRECT:** Children who have PTSD should be referred to psychotherapy to assist with resolution of the traumatic event.

   B. **CORRECT:** The child who is experiencing PTSD often has new phobias that can be related to the traumatic event.

   C. Depression and anxiety, rather than personality disorders, are possible complications of PTSD.

   D. **CORRECT:** PTSD develops following a traumatic event such as assault, serious injury, or a life-threatening episode.

   E. PTSD has three phases: the initial response, second phase, and third phase (coping).

   Ⓝ *NCLEX® Connection: Psychosocial Integrity, Mental Health Concepts*

4. A. Receiving formula as an infant is not a risk factor for ADHD.

   B. **CORRECT:** History of head trauma is a risk factor for ADHD.

   C. History of a post-term birth is not a risk factor for ADHD.

   D. Being the child of a single parent does not increase the risk of ADHD.

   Ⓝ *NCLEX® Connection: Health Promotion and Maintenance, Health Promotion/Disease Prevention*

5. A. A preference for being alone is associated with depression.

   B. **CORRECT:** Weight loss or gain are associated with depression.

   C. **CORRECT:** Low self-esteem and feelings of worthlessness are associated with depression.

   D. **CORRECT:** Alterations in sleep, such as sleeping more than usual, is a finding associated with depression.

   E. Fatigue is associated with depression.

   Ⓝ *NCLEX® Connection: Psychosocial Integrity, Mental Health Concepts*

PRACTICE Answer

Using the ATI Active Learning Template: Basic Concept

UNDERLYING PRINCIPLES

- Vomiting, poor feeding, and listlessness
- Respiratory distress
- Bulging fontanels
- Retinal hemorrhages
- Seizures
- Posturing
- Alterations in level of consciousness
- Apnea
- Bradycardia
- Blindness
- Unresponsiveness

Ⓝ *NCLEX® Connection: Physiological Adaptation, Illness Management*

References

Berman, A., Snyder, S., & Frandsen, G. (2016). *Kozier & Erb's fundamentals of nursing: Concepts, process, and practice* (10th ed.). Upper Saddle River, NJ: Prentice-Hall.

Burchum, J. R., & Rosenthal, L. D. (2016). *Lehne's pharmacology for nursing care* (9th ed.). St. Louis, MO: Elsevier.

Centers for Disease Control and Prevention (2017). *Diseases and conditions.* Retrieved from https://www.cdc.gov/diseasesconditions/index.html

Centers for Disease Control and Prevention. (2017). *Vaccines and immunizations.* Retrieved from https://www.cdc.gov/vaccines/index.html

Dudek, S. G. (2014). *Nutrition essentials for nursing practice* (7th ed.). Philadelphia: Lippincott Williams & Wilkins.

Grodner, M., Escott-Stump, S., & Dorner, S. (2016). *Nutritional foundations and clinical applications of nutrition: A nursing approach* (6th ed.). St. Louis, MO: Mosby.

Halter, M. J. (2014). *Varcarolis' foundations of psychiatric mental health nursing: A clinical approach* (7th ed.). St. Louis, MO: Saunders.

Hockenberry, M. J., & Wilson, D. (2015) *Wong's nursing care of infants and children* (10th ed.). St. Louis, MO: Mosby.

Immunization Action Coalition. (2017). *Advisory Committee on Immunization Practice.* Retrieved from http://www.immunize.org/acip/

Lowdermilk, D. L., Perry, S. E., Cashion, M. C., & Aldean, K. R. (2016). *Maternity & women's health care* (11th ed.). St. Louis, MO: Elsevier.

Pagana, K. D., & Pagana, T. J. (2014). *Mosby's manual of diagnostic and laboratory tests* (5th ed.). St. Louis, MO: Elsevier.

Pillitteri, A. (2014). *Maternal and child health nursing: Care of the childbearing and childrearing family* (7th ed.). Philadelphia: Lippincott Williams & Wilkins

Potter, P. A., Perry, A. G., Stockert, P., & Hall, A. (2017). *Fundamentals of nursing* (9th ed.). St. Louis, MO: Elsevier

Taketomo, C. K., Hodding, J. H., & Kraus, D. M. (2016). *Lexi-Comp's Pediatric & Neonatal Dosage Handbook: A universal resource for clinicians treating pediatric and neonatal patients* (23rd ed.). Hudson, OH: Lexi-Comp.

Vallerand, A. H., & Sanoski, C. A. (2017). *Davis's drug guide for nurses* (15th Ed.). Philadelphia: Elsevier.

STUDENT NAME _____

CONCEPT_____   REVIEW MODULE CHAPTER_____

Related Content

(E.G., DELEGATION, LEVELS OF PREVENTION, ADVANCE DIRECTIVES)

Underlying Principles

Nursing Interventions

WHO? WHEN? WHY? HOW?

STUDENT NAME _____

PROCEDURE NAME _____ REVIEW MODULE CHAPTER_____

Description of Procedure

Indications

CONSIDERATIONS

Nursing Interventions (pre, intra, post)

Interpretation of Findings

Client Education

Potential Complications

Nursing Interventions

STUDENT NAME _____

DEVELOPMENTAL STAGE _____ REVIEW MODULE CHAPTER_____

EXPECTED GROWTH AND DEVELOPMENT

Physical Development	Cognitive Development	Psychosocial Development	Age-Appropriate Activities

Health Promotion

Immunizations	Health Screening	Nutrition	Injury Prevention

ACTIVE LEARNING TEMPLATE: *Medication*

STUDENT NAME _____

MEDICATION _____

REVIEW MODULE CHAPTER_____

CATEGORY CLASS_____

PURPOSE OF MEDICATION

Expected Pharmacological Action

Therapeutic Use

Complications

Medication Administration

Contraindications/Precautions

Nursing Interventions

Interactions

Client Education

Evaluation of Medication Effectiveness

ACTIVE LEARNING TEMPLATE: *Nursing Skill*

STUDENT NAME _____

SKILL NAME_____ REVIEW MODULE CHAPTER_____

Description of Skill

Indications

CONSIDERATIONS

Nursing Interventions (pre, intra, post)

Outcomes/Evaluation

Client Education

Potential Complications

Nursing Interventions

STUDENT NAME _____

DISORDER/DISEASE PROCESS _____ REVIEW MODULE CHAPTER_____

Alterations in Health (Diagnosis)

Pathophysiology Related to Client Problem

Health Promotion and Disease Prevention

ASSESSMENT

Risk Factors

Expected Findings

Laboratory Tests

Diagnostic Procedures

SAFETY CONSIDERATIONS

PATIENT-CENTERED CARE

Nursing Care

Medications

Client Education

Therapeutic Procedures

Interprofessional Care

Complications

ACTIVE LEARNING TEMPLATE: *Therapeutic Procedure*

STUDENT NAME _____

PROCEDURE NAME _____ REVIEW MODULE CHAPTER_____

Description of Procedure

Indications

CONSIDERATIONS

Nursing Interventions (pre, intra, post)

Outcomes/Evaluation

Client Education

Potential Complications

Nursing Interventions